ISBN 978-0-484-89018-2
PIBN 10149573




FB &c Ltd, Dalton House, 60 Windsor Avenue, London, SW19 2RR.
Company number 08720141. Registered in England and Wales.

For support please visit www.forgottenbooks.com

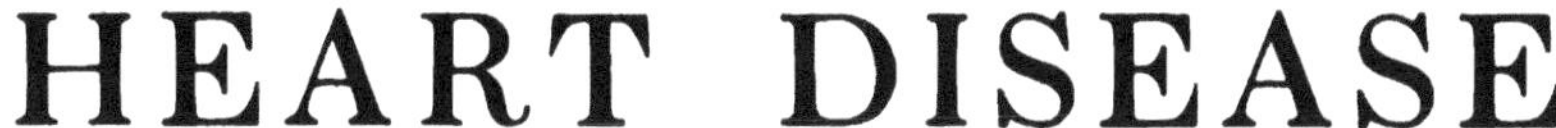

# HEART DISEASE

AND

## ANEURYSM OF THE AORTA

WITH SPECIAL REFERENCE TO

## PROGNOSIS AND TREATMENT.

BY


SIR WILLIAM H. BROADBENT, BART., K.C.V.O.

M.D. LOND., F.R.S., D.SC. LEEDS, LL.D. EDIN. AND ST. ANDREWS, F.R.C.P.

PHYSICIAN IN ORDINARY TO H.M. THE KING, AND TO H.R.H. THE PRINCE OF WALES; COMMANDEUR DE LA LÉGION D'HONNEUR; HON. MEMBER OF VEREIN FÜR INNERE MEDICIN, BERLIN AND OF GESELLSCHAFT FÜR INNERE MEDICIN UND KINDERHEILKUNDE IN WIEN, AND OF SOCIÉTÉ IMPÉRIALE, CONSTANTINOPLE; VICE-PRESIDENT IMPERIAL CANCER RESEARCH; CHAIRMAN OF COUNCIL OF NATIONAL ASSOCIATION FOR PREVENTION OF TUBERCULOSIS; CONSULTING PHYSICIAN TO ST. MARY'S HOSPITAL AND TO THE LONDON FEVER HOSPITAL;

AND

JOHN F. H. BROADBENT

M.A., M.D. (OXON.), F.R.C.P.,

PHYSICIAN TO OUT-PATIENTS, ST. MARY'S HOSPITAL; ASSISTANT PHYSICIAN TO THE LONDON FEVER HOSPITAL; HON. PHYSICIAN TO THE METROPOLITAN CONVALESCENT INSTITUTION; FORMERLY ASSISTANT PATHOLOGIST AND MEDICAL REGISTRAR TO ST. MARY'S HOSPITAL.


FOURTH EDITION.

# PREFACE TO FOURTH EDITION.

My father, Sir William Broadbent, has entrusted to me the preparation of the new edition of this work, and with his approval I have rearranged the subject-matter, and have added chapters on the pulse, disease of the coronary arteries, bradycardia, and atheroma of the aorta. I have also revised and rewritten the chapters on acute and malignant (or pernicious) endocarditis, and that on affections of the myocardium, a subject at which I have been working recently. I am indebted to Messrs. Green for permission to make use of the article I wrote for the *Encyclopædia Medica* on affections of the pericardium. My father has made several important additions to the chapters on angina pectoris and functional affections of the heart, and has carefully revised the whole of the proofs.

JOHN F. H. BROADBENT.

*April*, 1906.

# PREFACE TO THIRD EDITION.

ADVANTAGE is taken of the demand for a new edition of the work on the Heart to make the book more complete, and with this view chapters on acute affections of the heart, Endocarditis, Pericarditis, Myocarditis, and on Aneurysm of the Arch of the Aorta, have been added. In these, as in the original work, no attempt is made to give a systematic and complete treatise on each subject, or to enter into a discussion of conflicting views which have been entertained on various points of pathology and etiology. The object has been rather to endeavour to place before the reader a clinical picture of each disease and to emphasize the points which are of chief importance in diagnosis and prognosis.

The task of revision and of making the considerable additions which have been specified has fallen almost entirely on my son, Dr. John Broadbent, as I myself have not had the requisite leisure. The chapters on the inflammatory affections of the heart are entirely his work, and the chapter on Aneurysm has been arranged and compiled by him from notes and papers of my own which have been published elsewhere. While making this acknowledgment, however, I accept the responsibility, as I have carefully perused all the new matter and made some additions. Several illustrations have been added, for which, with the exception of Fig. 23, I am indebted to Dr. A. W. Sanders, whose coloured drawing of acute aortitis from a recent specimen is worthy of special notice.

W. H. BROADBENT.

NOVEMBER, 1899.

# PREFACE TO FIRST EDITION.

This book is, for the most part, a reproduction of lectures on "Prognosis in Valvular Disease of the Heart," delivered before the Harveian Society in 1884, and of the Lumleian Lectures at the Royal College of Physicians on "Prognosis in Structural Diseases of the Heart," delivered in 1891.

The prognosis of heart disease already engaged my attention when I was house-physician under Sibson at St. Mary's Hospital, and my first paper on this subject was read before the Harveian Society in 1866. Up to that time there had not, so far as I am aware, been any systematic study and exposition of the indications by which the probable course of disease of the heart in different cases might be foreseen, and ideas which tended to obscure the interpretation of the symptoms and physical signs were held by physicians of great experience and authority. Traces of the controversies of those days will still be found in the present work. They have lost much of their interest, but references to them could not well be entirely omitted.

The prognosis of heart disease is worthy of special study, not only on account of its inherent importance, but also because the knowledge which enables the medical man to forecast clearly the course of the disease constitutes the best preparation for its treatment. The subject of treatment did not, however, enter into the scheme of the lectures, but it is engrafted upon them in the present work, and for this, and for the rearrangement rendered necessary by it, I am indebted to my son, Dr. John Broadbent, without whose efficient assistance and co-operation the task of preparing this book could not have been accomplished.

The lectures on which the book is based having been addressed to the College of Physicians and to the Harveian Society, presupposed a knowledge of heart disease on the part of my audience, and a minute exposition and analysis of the symptoms and physical signs, by means of which the diagnosis of the different valvular and structural affections of the heart is arrived at, were therefore unnecessary. This is still taken for granted, but a brief chapter on the examination of the cardiac region, and on the significance of the various departures from normal conditions, has been added.

The principal motive for reproducing the lectures has been the frequently expressed wish on the part of old pupils to see my teachings on heart disease in a collected form. They have had to wait long, and to them I now dedicate the book.

W. H. BROADBENT.

SEPT. 15TH, 1897.

# CONTENTS.

CHAPTER I.



CHAPTER II.

THE PULSE.



CHAPTER III.

DISEASES OF THE PERICARDIUM.



CHAPTER IV.



CHAPTER V.

"MALIGNANT" OR "PERNICIOUS" ENDOCARDITIS.

## CHAPTER VI.



## CHAPTER VII.

### VALVULAR LESIONS.



## CHAPTER VIII.



## CHAPTER IX.

### AORTIC STENOSIS.



## CHAPTER X.

### AORTIC INCOMPETENCE.

## CHAPTER XI.

### Mitral Incompetence or Regurgitation.



## CHAPTER XII.

### Mitral Stenosis.



## CHAPTER XIII.

### Valvular Disease of the Right Side of the Heart.



## CHAPTER XIV.

### Congenital Malformations.



## CHAPTER XV.

### Prognosis in Valvular Disease (General).

## CHAPTER XVI.



## CHAPTER XVII.

### TREATMENT (GENERAL).



## CHAPTER XVIII.

### TREATMENT BY DRUGS.



## CHAPTER XIX.

### STRUCTURAL CHANGE IN THE HEART.



## CHAPTER XX.

### DILATATION.

## CHAPTER XXI.

### Structural Change in the Right Ventricle.



## CHAPTER XXII.

### Disease of the Coronary Arteries.



## CHAPTER XXIII.

### Affections of the Myocardium.



## CHAPTER XXIV.

### Affections of the Myocardium (*Continued*).



## CHAPTER XXV.

### Angina Pectoris.



## CHAPTER XXVI.

### Functional Affections (so-called) of the Heart.

## CHAPTER XXVIII.

### ACUTE AORTITIS OR ACUTE DEGENERATIVE LESIONS OF THE AORTA.



## CHAPTER XXIX.

### ATHEROMA OR CHRONIC DEGENERATIVE LESIONS OF THE AORTA.



## CHAPTER XXX.

### ANEURYSM OF THE ARCH OF THE AORTA.

# HEART DISEASE.

## CHAPTER I.

THE RELATIONS OF THE HEART TO THE CHEST WALLS—MOVEMENTS OF THE HEART—ON THE METHODS OF EXAMINATION BY INSPECTION: PALPATION, PERCUSSION, AND AUSCULTATION.

A SYSTEMATIC description of the anatomy and relations of the heart, and a text-book exposition of the physical signs by means of which departures from the normal condition of the heart are recognized, would be out of place in a work of this character. A brief reminder, however, of the relations of the heart to the chest wall, together with a short description of the method in which a clinical examination of the heart should be conducted, and an indication of the significance of the various points observed, will form a useful preliminary to the study of heart disease. This will therefore form the subject of the introductory chapter.

The first portion of this chapter, dealing with the position and relations of the heart, is mainly taken from the works of Sibson,* who devoted much time and labour to the study of this subject, and under whom I worked while he was engaged upon it.

* Sibson's Works, edited by Orel. Vol. iii.

## The Position of the Heart and the Relation of its Cavities to the Chest Walls.

The heart and great vessels, with their pericardial covering, occupy the central portion of the thoracic cavity. The right auricle and ventricle compose the whole of the front of the heart, with the exception of a narrow strip to

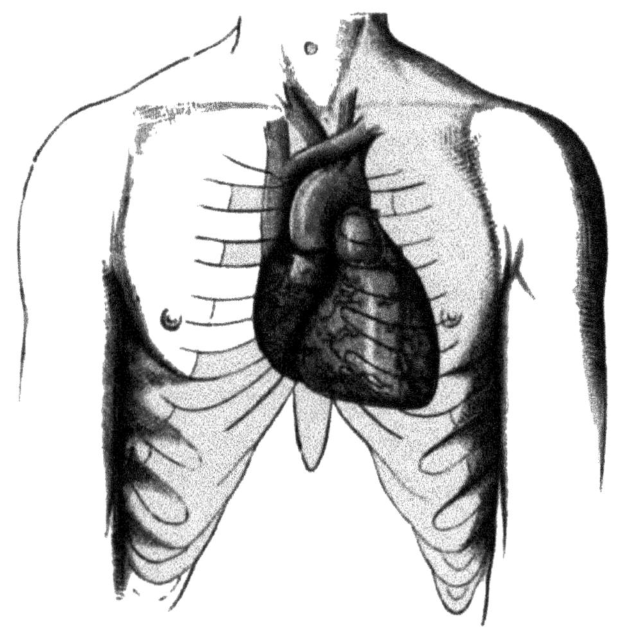

FIG. 1.—RELATION OF HEART TO CHEST WALLS (*Sibson*).

the left, where the left ventricle comes into view from behind.

The **right auricle** lies behind the sternum, its upper border being on a level with the third costal cartilages, and extending from a point about one inch to the right of the sternum nearly to its left border. It is broadest above, and narrows down almost to a point at the lower end of the auriculo-ventricular furrow, which forms its left border and runs obliquely downwards from the sternal end of the third left to the sternal end of the seventh right costal cartilage. Its right border is convex, and lies behind the right costal cartilages, just beyond the right margin of the sternum.

The right auricle undergoes more change in form during

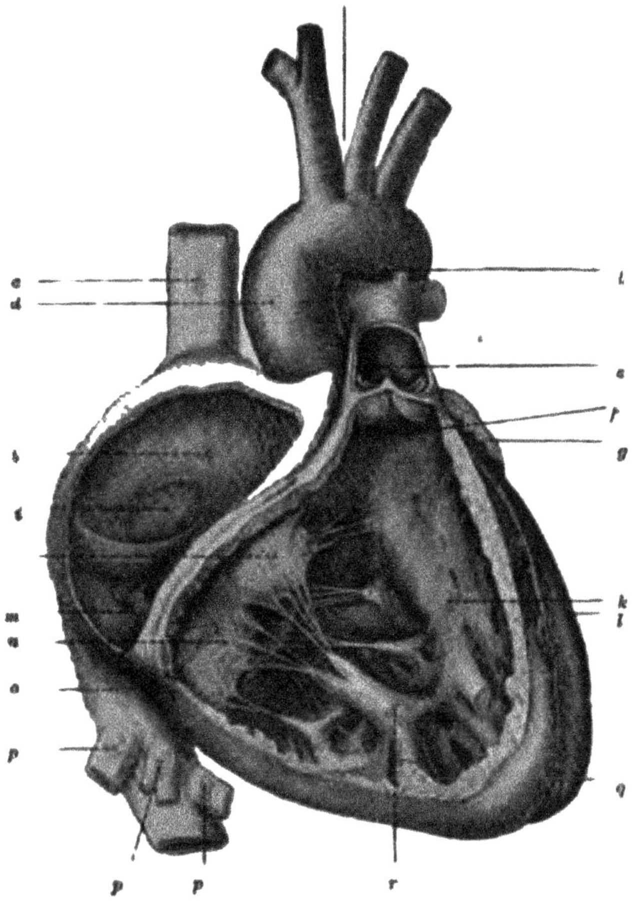


FIG. 2.—THE HEART AND GREAT VESSELS, WITH THE ANTERIOR WALLS OF THE RIGHT AURICLE AND RIGHT VENTRICLE DISSECTED OFF TO SHOW POSITION OF THE VALVES AND SEPTA (QUAIN'S *Anatomy*).

*a*, Innominate and left carotid arteries; *b*, Transverse part of arch; *c*, Vena cava superior; *d*, Ascending part of arch of aorta; *e*, Pulmonary artery; *f*, Pulmonic valves; *g*, Appendix of left auricle; *h*, Inter-auricular septum; *i*, Fossa ovalis, with Eustachian valve below; *j*, Left segment of tricuspid valve; *k*, Inter-ventricular septum; *l*, Left ventricle; *m*, Coronary vein; *n*, Right segment of tricuspid valve; *o*, Inferior vena cava; *p*, Hepatic veins; *q*, Left ventricle; *r*, Anterior papillary muscle.

the action of the heart than any other portion of the organ, becoming nearly twice as wide in systole of the ventricles as in diastole. The auriculo-ventricular furrow also sweeps backwards and forwards to so great an extent, to the left during systole and to the right during diastole of the ventricles, that it presents no fixed position during life.

The right ventricle, when exposed to view, presents a pyramidal shape. The base of the pyramid is formed by the lower boundary of the ventricle, which rests on the central tendon of the diaphragm; the apex of the pyramid is crowned and completed by the pulmonary artery; the left side is formed by the furrow which divides the left from the right ventricle; the right side, by the furrow separating the right auricle and ventricle.

The furrow separating the two ventricles runs from the third to the fifth left costal cartilages, just behind their junction with the ribs.

The left ventricle forms the convex left border of the heart as seen from the front, and forms a long, narrow strip extending from the third left intercostal space down to the fifth, where it terminates in the apex of the heart. This occupies the fifth space, being usually situated just internal to a line drawn vertically downwards from the nipple.

The appendix of the left auricle lies just behind the third left costal cartilage, close to its junction with the third rib, and fills up the space between the upper end of the left and right ventricles at the top of the longitudinal or interventricular furrow.

The area which would be marked out on the chest wall by percussion, indicating the position of the heart beneath and its relation to the chest wall, is termed "the area of deep cardiac dulness."

The lungs cover the great vessels and the whole of the heart except a portion of the right ventricle.

The inner margins of the right and left lungs in front meet behind the sternum for its upper two-thirds. The inner margin of the left lung diverges from that of the right at the level of the fourth left costal cartilage. It passes thence to the left along the lower edge of the fourth cartilage in front of the body of the right ventricle, curving downwards just before it reaches the junction of the cartilage with the rib; it then crosses the fourth space and fifth cartilage, and curving, so as to form a hollow space

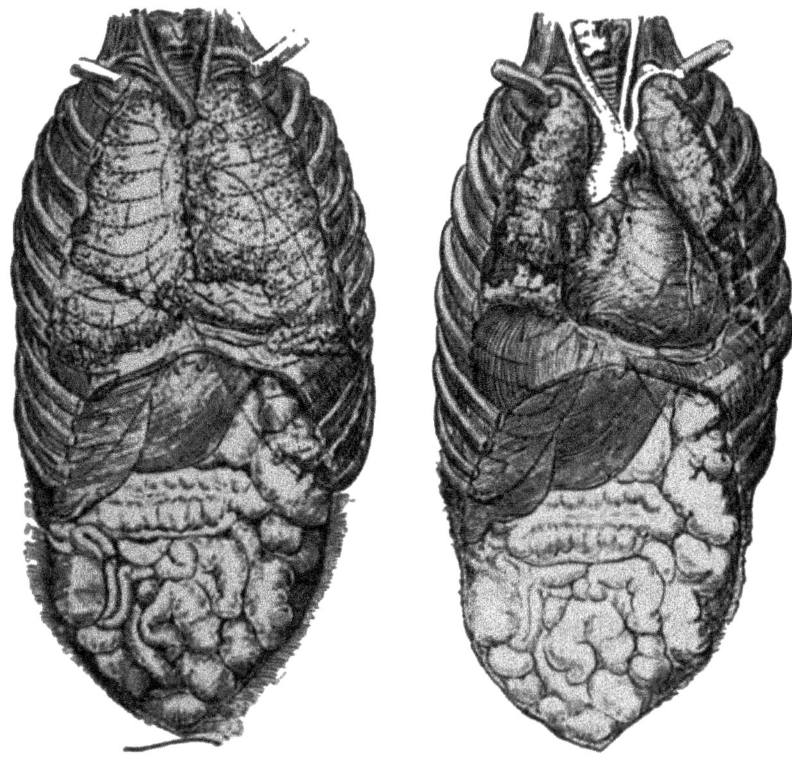

FIG. 3.—THE HEART WITH LUNGS IN SITU TO ILLUSTRATE AREA OF SUPERFICIAL CARDIAC DULNESS (*Sibson*).

FIG. 4.—THE HEART WITH OVERLYING LUNG DISSECTED OFF TO ILLUSTRATE AREA OF DEEP DULNESS (*Sibson*).

for the lodgment of the apex, ends behind the sixth cartilage.

The inner margin of the right lung continues its course nearly straight downwards behind and a little to the left of the centre of the sternum, to the level of the sixth chondrosternal articulation. It thus covers the right auricle, the auriculo-ventricular furrow, and the right border of the right ventricle.

The area on the chest wall corresponding to the part of the heart uncovered by lung can be accurately marked out by percussion, and is known as "the area of superficial cardiac dulness."

The area thus indicated would be mapped out as follows: its right margin, by a line running from above downwards slightly to the left of the middle line of the sternum from the level of the fourth costal cartilage down to that of the sixth; its highest point would be at the level of the fourth costal cartilage; its left limit would be defined by a line running outwards from the sternum at this level, along the lower edge of the fourth left costal cartilage, nearly as far as its junction with the rib, and then dipping downwards and curving slightly outwards to the point on the chest wall where the apex beat is felt. The base or lower limit corresponds to a line drawn from the sixth right costal cartilage to the apex.

## Movements of the Heart.

The heart undergoes a marked change in form and diminution in size during systole. At the end of diastole it is globular in shape. The apex is rounded, the ventricles are full, the auricles distended, the appendix of the left auricle coming forward to lie in the groove between the right ventricle and aorta. The ventricles yield on handling, and the auricles are dimpled by slight pressure of the finger. The first systolic act is the sudden swift withdrawal of the auricular appendix, due to the contraction of the auricle. Immediately afterwards the ventricles harden, and the change in form produced by the contraction begins. The septum is the centre on which the movements converge, and the most fixed point is about three-quarters of the distance from the apex to the auriculo-ventricular furrow. The pulmonary artery is drawn sharply downwards, the apex becomes more pointed, and moves spirally upwards and to the right. The left border converges slightly, and the right border more upon the axis of the heart.

The general cardiac impulse is due to the contractile hardening of the muscular walls, the apex beat to this hardening and to the rotatory movement forward and to the right. Both impulse and apex beat require a fulcrum posteriorly in order to be felt through the chest wall. This is furnished by the pericardium and spinal column, against which the shoulder of the left ventricle thrusts.

In the interior of the heart the end of diastole finds the auriculo-ventricular valves floated up into position by the action of elastic fibres on their auricular aspect, and already in contact along their free margins, so as to close the orifice. The chordæ tendineæ are slightly on the stretch. The pressure on the valves as the ventricles contract closes them more tightly, and the co-ordinate contraction of the papillary muscles neutralizes the approximation of the origin of the chordæ tendineæ to the base of the heart which results from its diminution in size during systole. The contraction of the circular muscle fibres round the orifices contributes to the complete closure of the valvular flaps.

## The Clinical Examination of the Heart.

This is conducted by inspection, palpation, percussion, and auscultation. Much is learnt by careful inspection. Bulging or other general feature of the præcordial region is to be noted. Any deformity of the chest giving rise to displacement of the heart, or fixation of one side of the thorax by pleural adhesions, or by fibroid or other disease of the lung, must be taken into account. The position and character of the apex beat should be determined as far as this is possible; the surface of the chest should be carefully scrutinized for pulsation in abnormal situations, and epigastric pulsation or any visible heave over the right ventricle should be noted.

These observations will be corroborated or checked by palpation; but there are other points which can be ascertained by the eye alone, such as retraction of intercostal spaces. This is most commonly seen in the third, fourth, and fifth left intercostal spaces and is usually systolic in time; it may either arise from a direct tug on the spaces by pericardial adhesions, or be due to atmospheric pressure: the latter condition is more common, and in such cases the heart will usually be dilated and hypertrophied, and therefore subject to great diminution in volume during systole.

Inspection also embraces the neck, where is seen the carotid throb which betrays aortic regurgitation. To be characteristic, it must be visible, not at the root of the neck only, but as high as the hollow between the ramus of the jaw and the sternomastoid. It may, exceptionally, be present where there is no aortic disease, and it may be simulated by pulsation in the deep jugular vein. This, however, is easily distinguished, being readily arrested by light pressure.

Important information may frequently be derived from careful observation of the veins of the neck. The jugulars on one or both sides may be full and distended. If the distension is present on one side only, it may be due to pressure on the innominate vein of that side by an aneurysm or some other intra-thoracic tumour. If it exists on both sides, it may be due either to pressure on the superior vena cava or both innominate veins, or to dilatation and engorgement of the right side of the heart from back pressure through the lungs. In the latter case, the veins will be temporarily more or less emptied by a forcible deep inspiration, and will become more distended during expiration: in the former, variations of the intra-thoracic pressure during inspiration and expiration will have no appreciable effect in reducing or augmenting the distension. Pulsation of the jugular veins may be present when the right side of the heart is greatly dilated and tricuspid regurgitation has set in. The pulsation is often double, both auricular and ventricular systoles transmitting backward waves. It has been studied with great care by Mackenzie, of Burnley, who has obtained graphic records of two distinct types of jugular pulsation, and established their significance.

Finally, mention may be made of enlarged and tortuous veins on the surface of the chest, constituting collateral channels between the superior and inferior venæ cavæ when one or other is compressed, and of pulsating veins occasionally seen dipping into an intercostal space near the sternum.

**Palpation.**—The information obtained by palpation is second in importance only to that afforded by auscultation. The situation, force, limits, and extent of the cardiac impulse are accurately ascertained, and the relative intensity of the apex beat and right ventricle beat must be compared. The examination, to be complete, must be conducted in various ways.

Firstly, the flat of the right hand should be placed over the cardiac area, the fingers covering the apex region. The powerful heaving impulse of the apex in hypertrophy, the diffuse shock or slap in dilatation, and the peculiar sudden tap in mitral stenosis are often at once diagnostic: a powerful heave of the lower left costal cartilages, and sometimes of the lower end of the sternum as well, will indicate stress thrown on the right ventricle by back pressure through the pulmonary circulation. Thrills or vibrations, systolic or presystolic, over the area of the apex beat or elsewhere will be recognized at the same time. Sometimes a peculiar diastolic shock or retraction may be felt over the apex or the right ventricle, caused by the presence of pericardial adhesions. Next the fingers must be pressed into the right intercostal spaces in search of pulsation, and the apex region must be explored with the tips of the fingers, and the exact position, extent, force, and deliberate or sudden character of the apex beat must be noted. This investigation must not be limited to the point at which the apex appeared to present itself, when the hand was applied to the præcordium; the real apex beat may be sometimes far out in the axilla, or high up in the fourth space, or it may be concealed behind the mamma.

Speaking generally, displacement of the apex downwards is indicative of hypertrophy of the left ventricle, dilatation giving rise to extension of the impulse outwards and downwards; displacement of the apex to the left is caused by enlargement of the right ventricle, which is usually due to combined hypertrophy and dilatation. For the most part, any considerable change in the position of the apex beat is the result of hypertrophy and dilatation of both sides of the heart. Special displacement of the apex not due to intrinsic changes in the heart may be the result of various causes, such as pericardial or pleuro-pericardial adhesions, pleural effusion, pneumo-thorax, fibroid condition or cavitation of the lung, or deformity of the chest. It is always well to ascertain whether the apex changes its position in respiration, and with change of posture of the patient from the erect to the recumbent position, and when lying first on one side, then on the other.

It is not uncommon to find that neither apex beat nor impulse of any kind is to be felt. This does not necessarily imply feeble action of the heart, but may be due to thickness of the parietes or great depth of thorax, or to overlapping emphysematous lung, or to pericardial adhesions.

Departures from the normal in the cardiac rhythm should also be noted; they are of two kinds: Irregularity and Intermission—irregularity, when the beats are of varying force and follow each other at unequal intervals; intermission, when a beat is dropped from time to time, the intervening beats being of equal force and at equal intervals.

The irregular action of the heart is usually exaggerated in the pulse, as many of the beats may fail to reach the wrist. When the pulse is intermittent, it will usually be found that there is not an entire absence of the beat of the heart, but an imperfect and hurried beat corresponding to the intermission.

The examination by palpation, to be complete, must embrace the abdomen, and the size of the liver must be carefully ascertained. As the right ventricle begins to fail, and obstruction to the return of blood to the heart from the liver through the inferior vena cava begins to be felt, the liver becomes engorged and congested, and gradually increases in size, till it may become very much enlarged, extending even below the umbilicus. The size of the liver is therefore an important index as to the degree of venous obstruction.

In examining to ascertain the size of the liver, the patient should be made to lie on his back with the legs drawn up, so that the belly is perfectly flaccid. The flat of the hand should then be placed on the abdomen, and the edge of the liver carefully felt for; at the same time the other hand should be placed beneath the back of the patient below the false ribs, and the liver lifted from behind, so that if the liver edge is not at first felt, the jogging from behind will press it up against the hand on the abdomen, and render it more obvious. Palpation with the tips of the fingers will probably provoke some rigidity of the abdominal walls, which obscures the resistance presented by the liver behind. When, however, there is fluid present in the abdominal cavity, this method of palpation will be useful, for then on dipping sharply down with the fingers, the fluid between the liver and abdominal walls will be displaced, and the firm, hard substance of the liver be felt below.

Percussion is, as a rule, a very untrustworthy method of ascertaining the size of the liver, owing to conducted resonance from distended coils of intestine ; it will, however, serve to mark out the upper margin of the liver, unless there be consolidation of lung fluid or old pleural adhesions at the base of the right pleural cavity.

Pulsation of liver is best detected by combined simultaneous palpation and inspection. The hand should be placed on a part of the liver at some distance from the epigastrium, and gentle pressure being made, it should be carefully watched. If the liver is actually pulsating, and not merely jogged by a hypertrophied right ventricle, the hand will be seen to rise and fall rhythmically even though no actual pulsation is felt on palpation.

**Percussion.**—Percussion will verify and perhaps extend the information obtained by inspection and palpation. It is specially useful when no impulse is present. There is normally, as has already been described, a small area of absolute dulness—" the superficial cardiac dulness "—where the heart is not covered by lung, which is easily defined. It may be encroached upon and obliterated when the lungs are emphysematous, or extended when they are shrunken as a result of fibroid contraction or pleural adhesion. The deep dulness indicating the true dimensions of the heart cannot be mapped out with absolute accuracy in all cases, as the overlying lung tissue varies in thickness and extent in different individuals, and in inspiration and expiration. In percussing for this purpose, the finger must be pressed firmly into the intercostal spaces, and the stroke must be delivered smartly and perpendicularly. The note changes gradually as the dull area is left with the increase in the thickness of the overlapping lung, till full lung resonance is reached. The end of expiration, when the cushion of lung is thinnest, should be chosen as the moment to attempt the definition of the comparative dulness which indicates the size and position of the heart. The so-called auscultatory percussion is, in my opinion, of no value whatever.

**Auscultation.**—The physical examination is completed by auscultation. For the most part, a diagnosis has already been arrived at before the stethoscope is applied, and in all cases the information obtained by auscultation must be checked and interpreted by evidence derived from the pulse, and from inspection, palpation, and percussion. Either a flexible or rigid stethoscope may be employed. The former is more convenient and expeditious, as it can be shifted from point to point without moving the head, and it is always under the eye, so that bulging or retraction of spaces can be timed and co-ordinated with the sounds or murmurs heard. On the other hand, it is sometimes difficult to distinguish between the first and second sound, and the rigid stethoscope, by communicating a faint jar to the ear, at once points out the sound which is produced by the systole.

The stethoscope should be applied successively to the apex region, the tricuspid, pulmonic, and aortic areas, and the character, and absolute and relative loudness of the sounds should be noted at each point; observations taken simply at the apex or base afford very imperfect information.

**The Mitral Area.**—At the apex both sounds are normally audible—the first, comparatively long and low-pitched; the second, short and sharp. The first sound may undergo various modifications. It may be prolonged, which is usually indicative of hypertrophy; or, on the other hand, it may be short and sharp. If when short it is also loud, it is among the indications of dilatation; if weak, it may be due either to degeneration or to simple asthenia of the cardiac muscle. A peculiar sharp and snapping character of the first sound at the apex is produced by mitral stenosis. Reduplication of the first sound is an important modification often met with; it is most distinct when the stethoscope is placed exactly over the septum between the apex and right ventricle, *i.e.* partly over one ventricle, partly over the other. Left of this spot the sound may be merely blurred; right of it, reduplication may still be distinct. The double sound is due to want of synchronism between the two ventricles, and may be produced whenever undue stress is put upon the left ventricle by high systemic arterial tension, or on the right by obstruction in the pulmonary circulation. The second sound heard at the apex is, for the most part, that produced at the aortic valves; occasionally it is more distinct here than at the aortic area proper. Its modifications will be described when the sounds at the base are discussed.

The interval between the first and second sounds indicating the duration of the cardiac systole, and that between the second and first sounds, or the diastolic interval, should be carefully observed, and any deviation from the normal noted. The rhythm may be disturbed in one direction by the shortening of the diastolic interval, till the sounds are equidistant and resemble the ticking of a watch, as in palpitation, or the sounds may become equidistant from prolongation of the systole, when they resemble the beat of a pendulum. In the other direction the systolic interval may be shortened till the second sound follows the first almost without an appreciable pause: this is a serious condition, indicating incomplete contraction of the ventricle, and also, in many cases, impending cardiac failure.

The murmurs heard at the apex may be systolic, presystolic, or diastolic; of these the most frequent is the systolic. It is most commonly smooth and blowing in character; sometimes a musical element may be present, or the murmur may be rumbling and indistinct; it is rarely rough and croaking, as is often the case with aortic systolic murmurs. The systolic murmur heard at the apex always signifies more or less regurgitation through the mitral orifice, and it will be necessary to note how far outside the apex the murmur is audible, and to what extent it replaces the first sound, as these will be important points in estimating its significance. An apex murmur is sometimes more distinct in the recumbent than in the sitting or erect position, or may be brought out by slight exertion.

A pulmonic or aortic systolic murmur may be conducted to the apex, but it will be of diminished intensity and will not, as a rule, be conducted towards the axilla.

The presystolic murmur, so named from the fact that it precedes and runs up to the first sound produced by the cardiac systole, is usually vibratory in character. Speaking generally, it indicates the presence of mitral stenosis, and is produced by the rush of blood from the auricle into the ventricle through the narrowed mitral orifice; but it may be present as a temporary phenomenon after acute disease. In an early stage it is brief in duration, and rises rapidly in intensity, terminating abruptly in the first sound, when it corresponds with and is produced by the auricular systole. It may, however, be greatly prolonged; that is, it may begin at a much earlier period so as to correspond with the active dilatation stage of the ventricular diastole, which precedes the auricular systole.

A diastolic murmur audible at the apex is usually that of aortic insufficiency, conducted from the base to the apex by the walls of the heart.

**The Tricuspid Area.**—The sounds heard over the tricuspid area are mainly those of the right ventricle; the first sound is rather shorter and louder than that at the apex, and the second sound is intensified when there is obstruction in the pulmonary circulation.

Systolic, presystolic, and diastolic murmurs may be heard in this region, and the former may indicate tricuspid incompetence, but the two latter varieties are most commonly murmurs conducted from the apex or base, and cannot be relied upon for diagnostic purposes.

**The Aortic Area.**—In the pulmonic and aortic areas accentuation of the second sound is the point specially to be observed, denoting increased pressure in the pulmonic or systemic circulation respectively. Reduplication of the second sound is not uncommon, and is due to a synchronous closure of the aortic and pulmonic semilunar valves.

The murmurs audible over the aortic area in the second right intercostal space may be systolic or diastolic. A systolic murmur may indicate actual obstruction, but is more frequently due to mere roughening or rigidity of the cusps of the valves, or to dilatation of the aorta beyond the valves, or other conditions not necessarily causing narrowing of the orifice. It may be loud and rough, or musical, or soft blowing. A diastolic murmur is usually blowing in character, and almost invariably indicates aortic incompetence, being produced by the regurgitant stream of blood; it can sometimes be heard lower down over the sternum, or a little to one side of it, at a point nearer the orifice of the aorta, when it is not audible in the so-called aortic area.

**The Pulmonic Area.**—Systolic and diastolic murmurs may also be heard in the pulmonic area, the third left intercostal space, and may indicate stenosis or incompetence of the pulmonic valves. These affections are, however, rare, and are usually of congenital origin. The murmurs heard in the pulmonic region are for the most part either conducted from the region of the aorta or apex, or are hæmic murmurs dependent on abnormal conditions of the blood, or they may occasionally be due to vibrations caused by the contact of the conus arteriosus with the chest wall. A diastolic aortic murmur is frequently louder in the pulmonic area than at the right second space, and may be audible here when it cannot be heard in the aortic area.

## CHAPTER II.

# THE PULSE.

METHODS OF EXAMINING THE PULSE—THE USE OF THE SPHYGMOGRAPH—ARTERIAL TENSION—HYPERTONUS OF THE VESSELS—BLOOD PRESSURE AND INSTRUMENTS FOR ESTIMATING IT—CAUSES OF HIGH ARTERIAL TENSION.

A CAREFUL and systematic examination of the pulse is of the first importance, inasmuch as the heart and arteries together constitute one system, and are in close mechanical and functional relation.

In feeling the pulse, three fingers should be placed on the vessel, and careful palpation be made with varying degrees of pressure. The following points should be carefully noted :—

1. The frequency, that is, the number of beats per minute ; the regularity or irregularity of the beats, and their equality or inequality in force.
2. The size of the vessel, whether large or small.
3. The character of the beat, whether abrupt or gradual, long-sustained or short, subsiding gradually or falling abruptly.
4. The force or strength of each beat.
5. The condition of the vessel between the beats, whether full and resistant or readily compressible.
6. The state of the arterial wall, whether smooth, regular, and supple, or irregular, tortuous, and rigid.

The determination of the frequency, the regularity or irregularity of the pulse, the size of the vessel, the character of the beat, presents little difficulty.

**To estimate the force of each beat,** three fingers should be placed on the vessel, and pressure made by the finger nearest the heart till the wave is arrested, so that it is not felt by the two lower fingers. By varying the degree of pressure with one and all three fingers, some idea is formed of the force of the pulse wave.

It must be recollected that the radial artery when compressed by the finger is more or less flattened. When distended by the increased pressure from the volume of blood injected into the arterial system at each beat of the heart it tends to resume the circular shape, and this is felt by the finger as the pulse wave. It yields gradually as the pressure within subsides, and in the normal sphygmographic tracing the cycle is represented graphically by a sudden sharp systolic rise, followed by a gradual fall, which is interrupted by a slight secondary elevation due to the dicrotic wave.

**Condition of the Artery between the Beats.**—The artery is more or less distended with blood between the beats after the wave has passed, and the degree of pressure within the vessel during that period may be termed the constant mean blood pressure. It is also known as the "diastolic pressure," but the term is misleading, as the pressure is maintained by the elastic recoil of the aorta and large vessels, and has no reference to the heart. The term "systolic pressure" is more justifiably employed to denote the increased or variable pressure due to the blood injected at each beat of the heart. If the arterial walls are relaxed and the blood pressure is low, the vessel can readily be flattened, and can scarcely be felt by the finger between the beats. The filling of the artery at each systole of the heart will then make a greater impression on the finger, and will jerk up the lever of the sphygmograph more rapidly and to a greater height, while the fall will be more abrupt and the dicrotic rebound well marked.

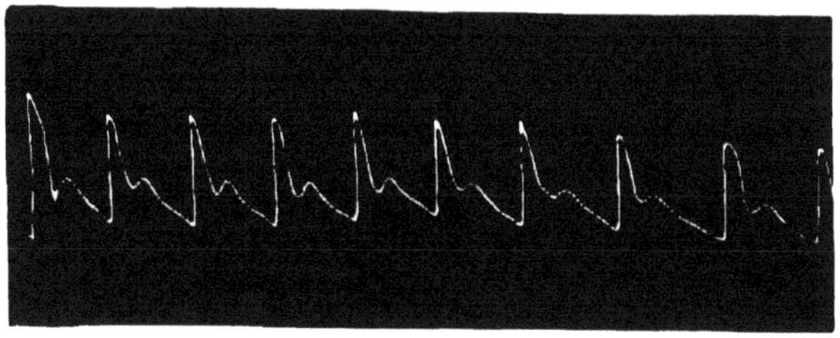

FIG. 5.—LOW-TENSION PULSE, SHOWING DICROTISM.

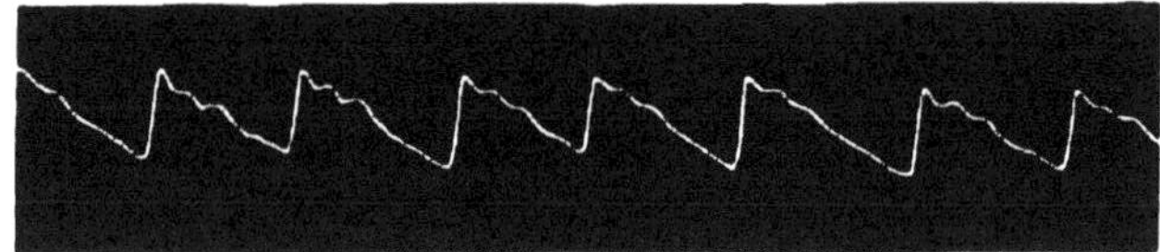

FIG. 6.—HIGH-TENSION PULSE.

When the artery is contracted and in a condition of hypertonus (to which reference will be made later), and the blood pressure is high, the vessel is not easily flattened by the finger or lever of the sphygmograph. The wave appears to be small and the excursion of the lever is limited, so that the pulse may appear to be weak, until more pressure is made, when its true character will be brought out, and the greater the pressure made the stronger the pulse will appear to be. The tracing will have a less abrupt upstroke, and will be of no great height, while the summit may be rounded, and the descent gradual, and unbroken by a dicrotic wave. By the fingers the artery will be felt as a firm rounded cord, and will not be easily compressed.

It is important, therefore, to carefully examine the artery between the beats, rolling it beneath the fingers and making varying degrees of pressure, so as to form an estimate of the mean or constant blood pressure—in other words, of the "arterial tension."

The condition of the arterial walls should also be noted, as to whether they are soft and flexible, thickened from hypertrophy, or rigid, tortuous, and deformed from degenerative changes. For this purpose the blood is pressed out of the vessel, which is then rolled under the fingers and carefully palpated by carrying them along it, so that rigidity or inequalities in its course may be detected.

Most of these points, such as the force and frequency and height of the pulse wave, the size of the vessel, its fulness or collapse between the beats, and thickening of its walls, can readily be determined by the fingers of the practised observer.

A sphygmographic tracing will form a useful supplementary graphic record of the character of the pulse wave, and will be the most trustworthy criterion as to its height and duration, as to whether its rise and subsidence are gradual or abrupt, and as to the presence or absence of dicrotism, etc. A comparison of a sphygmographic tracing from the radials of both sides will indicate whether the two pulses differ in character, and will often be of great value as an aid to the diagnosis of aneurysm. Marey's sphygmograph is the most trustworthy instrument, as the instrumental oscillations in Dudgeon's sphygmograph often vitiate results, especially when the rise of the wave is sudden and violent and its fall abrupt.

**Arterial Tension.**—There is, however, one important point as to which confusion is liable to arise. This is the question as to the meaning of the term "arterial tension." As this has an important bearing on prognosis, and reference will be frequently made to it in this volume, it may be as well to discuss the subject fully now. By "arterial tension" is here meant the strain to which the arterial wall is subjected by the contained blood between the beats of the heart—in other words, it is a measure of the constant mean blood pressure, as expressed by the strain it exerts on the arterial walls.

The factors which enter into its production are, first and foremost, the peripheral resistance in the capillaries and arterioles; secondly, the volume of blood thrown into the aorta at each systole of the heart; thirdly, the force of the heart beat.

To take a simple illustration, if we have a fire-hose with a powerful pump at one end and a narrow nozzle at the other, the hose-pipe will remain full and distended between each stroke of the pump, and the mean tension maintained will be very high. If we remove the nozzle, whatever be the force of each stroke of the pump and the quantity of water injected, the mean constant tension will be practically nil, or very low, and the hose-pipe will be flaccid between each stroke of the pump. By increasing the force of the pump and the volume of water injected, the momentary strain on the walls of the hose at each stroke will be greater, but the constant mean tension will still be very low if there is no nozzle at the distal end.

The heart corresponds to the pump, the arterial tree to the hose-pipe, and the peripheral resistance afforded by the arterioles and capillaries to that generated by the narrow nozzle at the distal end of the hose-pipe. It is true that the analogy does not hold good in all points, for in the hose-pipe we have an inelastic, more or less rigid, tube, whereas the arterial system is composed of a series of elastic contractile vessels; moreover, the aorta constitutes an elastic reservoir, which tends to make the flow of blood less jerky and more continuous, the pressure more constant, and the strain less severe, in the arteries of less size. I have thought it worth while to give this simple illustration, as the statement is made by Professor Clifford Allbutt

"That in aortic regurgitation the mean arterial tension is higher than in any other disease." * And again, "The incomprehensible statement is commonly repeated that in aortic regurgitation the tension is low." †

If we apply our illustration to aortic regurgitation (excluding that due to strain or degenerative changes), we shall see that it is impossible for the mean arterial tension to be high.

For though in aortic regurgitation we have a more powerful pump than normal from the hypertrophy of the heart, and a greater volume of blood injected into the arterial system at each beat, from the increased capacity of the dilated left ventricle, and the initial momentary strain on the vessel walls during systole is severe, yet immediately after the systole blood leaks back into the heart; the vessel walls are consequently not kept on the stretch by the contained fluid, but tend to collapse, so that the mean constant tension between each heart-beat will necessarily be low, in proportion as the regurgitation is considerable. Clifford Allbutt, in his article, obviously does not use the term "arterial tension" in the same sense as it is employed here, but rather as a synonym for the initial distensile strain at the moment of the cardiac systole.

The mean constant tension or strain on the arterial walls can be most accurately estimated by determining the blood pressure in each instance, and if in man we could, as in animals, connect the column of blood within an artery with a manometer by means of a rigid tube, this would afford a trustworthy criterion.

Obviously this method is impracticable in dealing with man, and various instruments have been devised in its place, the essential principle of which is an attempt to balance the pressure of the blood within an artery by

* "System of Medicine," vol. v. p. 937, line 32; article on "Aortic Regurgitation."

† *Ibid.*, p. 936.

graduated pressure applied externally to its walls. The degree of pressure required to arrest the flow of blood through the vessel, or the degree at which the maximum oscillations of pressure are registered by the manometer, is taken as a measure of the blood pressure within.

The instruments usually employed are of two kinds—

1. Those in which pressure is applied to the walls of a superficial artery, such as the radial, by a small rubber bag distended with air or fluid, and connected with a manometer, *e.g.* those of Hill and Barnard (small), Oliver, Vierordt, and Von Basch.

2. Those in which pressure is applied to the whole circumference of a limb, *e.g.* the arm, by a large rubber bag which completely encircles it, *e.g.* those of Riva Rocci, Hill and Barnard (large), and Gärtner.

In both groups pressure is made by the rubber bag distended with air or fluid, either till the pulse wave below is obliterated or till maximum oscillations of pressure are attained. The former indicates the systolic pressure, the latter according to Janeway the diastolic, according to Hill * the mean blood pressure. The point at which these phenomena occur is read off on a manometer.

It would be out of place to discuss these instruments so ably described by Janeway,† the merits and demerits of which have been recently reviewed in an article by C. J. Martin;‡ but it may be well to point out why the determination of the blood pressure by these methods does not give a trustworthy estimate of the arterial tension. The wall of the vessel varies greatly in elasticity and thickness in different individuals at different periods of life, and in health and disease, and the varying pressure required to overcome the resistance of the arterial wall in such diverse

* "Text-book of Physiology," edited by Schäfer, vol. ii. p. 80.

† "The Clinical Study of Blood Pressure" (Appleton).

‡ *British Medical Journal*, 1905, vol. i. pp. 865 *et seq.*

conditions must prove a source of error. Martin, as a result of a series of experiments on portions of dead arteries, claims that the range of error is small, and that an approximately accurate allowance can be made in the case of vessels the walls of which are rigid from degenerative changes. Granting that this is so, the conditions in the living vessel are essentially different, and are scarcely comparable. The element of muscular tone in the vessel wall must be taken into consideration. When the arterial tension is low and the vessel wall normal, this is perhaps a negligible quantity, but in states of high arterial tension, such as are associated with chronic Bright's disease, there is a condition of overtone or contraction of the muscular coat almost amounting to spasm, and the resistance to compression by the pneumatic rubber bag offered thereby must be very considerable. Moreover, in these circumstances there is also actual hypertrophy of the muscular coat, which will intensify this resistance, and it is scarcely possible to make accurate allowance for these sources of error, which will render the blood-pressure reading too high. Especially will this be the case in the later stages, when the heart is beginning to fail, and we have a condition of comparatively low blood pressure or arterial tension associated with hypertrophied rigid vessels, difficult to compress.

The hypertrophy of the muscular coat of the radial or other vessels can be readily demonstrated post-mortem by microscopical examination of sections of the vessel, and I have never failed to find it in some twenty or thirty cases associated with granular kidney which I have examined. The condition of overtone or hypertonus is not so readily proved, though it can be readily recognized in life by a practised observer by careful palpation of the vessel. Dr. William Russell * has, however, demonstrated clinically the existence of this hypertonus by an ingenious

* *Lancet*, 1901, vol. i. pp. 1519 *et seq.*

experiment. He argues that if this condition of hypertonus exists the diameter of the radial artery ought to vary according to the degree of tone or contraction of the muscular coat. He measured the diameter of an artery in a state of hypertonus by Oliver's arteriometer, taking at the same time a pulse tracing. He then gives erythrol tetranitrate or some vaso-dilator, and, allowing time for this to take effect, he again measures the diameter of the vessel by the arteriometer, and takes another pulse tracing. He finds that the diameter of the artery is increased and the character of the pulse altered correspondingly to the reduction of tension.

In spite of these sources of error, the determination of the blood pressure by these instruments will afford a useful comparative estimate of the blood pressure and arterial tension, and this may with advantage be supplemented by sphygmographic tracings. The scientific results obtained by Oliver, Mackenzie, and others in this way are of great value and interest. It is, however, not always practicable to employ instruments, nor is it essential for clinical purposes, as the finger can by practice be educated so that a trustworthy comparative estimate of the arterial tension can be made. For this purpose three fingers should be placed on the radial artery and varying degrees of pressure made. If the vessel remains full between the beats of the pulse, distended by the contained blood, so that it can be rolled like a cord beneath the fingers, the mean arterial tension is high. Some estimate as to the degree may be inferred from the pressure which has to be made by the finger before the flow of blood is arrested and the pulse wave obliterated. Care must be taken not to mistake a thickening of the arterial wall from degenerative changes for tension due to pressure from the contained blood. In cases of arteriosclerosis the condition can usually be diagnosed from the tortuous brachial, and the irregularity, rigidity, and loss of elasticity of the vessel wall, which is quite different to the firm, cord-like, smooth, elastic artery in a condition of hypertonus. If the vessel remains soft and flaccid between the beats, so that it can scarcely be felt, it is obvious that the tension or blood pressure is low.

I have laid some stress on the condition of hypertonus as manifested in the medium-sized and larger arteries as exemplified in the radial, but it exists throughout the arterial system, and it is the narrowing of the vast network of arterioles which entails a great increase in the peripheral resistance to the onward flow of the blood, which is of the first importance. The increased resistance necessitates greater driving power by the heart, which consequently hypertrophies sometimes to an enormous degree. The blood pressure is of necessity correspondingly raised, and the muscular coat of the large and medium-sized arteries hypertrophies, or they would give way under the strain.

It is a debatable question how far the condition of hypertonus in these vessels is due to the condition akin to spasm which affects the smaller arterioles, and how far it is a natural sequence of the increased peripheral resistance. For it is obvious that to overcome the increased resistance, increased contractile force is necessary, not only on the part of the heart, but of the whole arterial system.

This, however, is a matter of minor importance as long as we recognize that increased peripheral resistance entails increased driving power by the heart and increased contractile energy by the larger and medium-sized arteries. This gives rise to considerable increase in the blood pressure, and, consequently, to increased strain on the arterial walls, or, in other words, to high arterial tension. When the heart begins to give out under the strain, we have a decreased blood pressure and a condition of low or moderate tension, and in these circumstances we must be careful not to mistake the resistance offered to the fingers by the hypertrophied or thickened vessel walls for one of high tension due to high pressure from within.

**The Causes of Hypertonus and High Arterial Tension.**— The most typical instances of hypertonus and high arterial tension are found in association with chronic interstitial nephritis or granular kidney. A reasonable explanation of the mechanism of its production is, that poisonous products are retained in the blood as the result of imperfect elimination by the kidneys, and that these act as an irritant on the walls of the capillaries and arterioles, setting up a reflex spasm or hypertonic condition of their walls, and creating increased peripheral resistance.

Of predisposing causes heredity is the most important, and we see the tendency to high tension and vascular degeneration transmitted from generation to generation, and sometimes apparent at a very early age.

Certain constitutional diatheses, gout, diabetes, and rheumatoid arthritis, are frequently associated with high arterial tension. Over-eating, more especially excessive meat eating, in those hereditarily predisposed may be a cause, and it is probable that in this instance and in gout, perverted or defective metabolism, with resulting absorption of toxic products into the blood, and imperfect elimination, are the important etiological factors.

In the later stages of pregnancy the blood pressure is raised, and in the affection known as eclampsia the arterial tension is always extremely high. The explanation of this condition would seem to be that though the kidneys are not diseased, the extra work of eliminating the waste products of the fœtus in addition to those of the mother is too much for them, and toxic products accumulate in the blood, as in the case of granular kidney, and produce similar phenomena.

Lead poisoning is unquestionably an important and common cause. Alcohol and tobacco have been incriminated, but the part played by them is doubtful. Since the discovery of the tonic action of adrenalin on the arterial system, it has been suggested that excessive secretion of the suprarenal glands may be a cause, but there is no evidence in support of this. Whatever be the underlying cause of high arterial tension, it seems probable that it acts by generating increased peripheral resistance in the smaller arterioles and capillaries.

Confusion has arisen by mistaking the condition of hypertonus and hypertrophy of the muscular coat of the artery for arterio-sclerosis or degenerative change, because the artery feels hard and cord-like. But in the majority of cases, in the earlier stages, the radial artery will, on microscopic examination, be found to be perfectly normal except for hypertrophy of the media.

Later on degenerative changes set in in the hypertrophied vessels, and patches of atheroma or necrosis will be found in the sub-endothelial tissue, possibly as a result of the prolonged strain and impaired nutrition, or due to the action of the toxins which have given rise to the high tension. Of these, lead is especially prone to give rise to early vascular degeneration. The arteries most affected are usually the cerebral, the coronary arteries of the heart, and the aorta, so that the patient, if he escapes the perils of uræmia, is liable to succumb to cerebral hæmorrhage, or to cardiac failure from degenerative changes in the heart, or to aneurysm of the aorta.

## CHAPTER III.

# DISEASES OF THE PERICARDIUM.

PERICARDITIS — MORBID ANATOMY — ETIOLOGY — PHYSICAL SIGNS—SIGNS OF EFFUSION AND CARDIAC DILATATION—SYMPTOMS—COURSE OF THE DISEASE—DIFFERENTIAL DIAGNOSIS—PROGNOSIS: TREATMENT—ADHERENT PERICARDIUM — SUPPURATIVE PERICARDITIS — HYDROPERICARDIUM—PNEUMOPERICARDIUM, ETC.

THE pericardium is a fibro-serous sac which envelops the heart. The fibrous portion is pyramidal in shape, and at its base is firmly attached to the central tendon of the diaphragm and the adjoining muscular substance; above it is continued as a tubular prolongation on to the root of the aorta and pulmonary artery, and is gradually lost in the connective tissue of their external coats. The serous membrane lining the sac, termed the parietal layer of pericardium, passes up to the root of the great vessels, which it envelops in a common sheath for an inch to an inch and a half from their origin, and is thence reflected on to the surface of the heart, which it closely invests, constituting the visceral layer of pericardium. Laterally and anteriorly, save for a small triangular area in front termed the anterior mediastinum, the pericardium is in contact with the pleura; posteriorly it is in relation with the œsophagus, aorta, trachea, and the root of the left lung. The phrenic nerves pass down, one on either side of the sac.

**Morbid Anatomy.**—In the early stages the pericardium becomes hyperæmic and congested. Then exudation of serum and leucocytes takes place from the congested vessels, and soon both visceral and parietal layers of pericardium become coated in patches or throughout their surface with a thick layer of yellow sticky lymph. From the friction together of the two inflamed surfaces the lymph coating them acquires an irregular, ragged, or honeycomb appearance. The lymph on the surface of the pericardium may be reabsorbed, but frequently becomes vascularized and organized into fibrous tissue, gluing together the two layers of pericardium where they come into contact, and giving rise to partial or universal adhesion between the heart and pericardium.

**Effusion** may take place into the pericardial sac to a varying extent. Usually it is small in amount, but exceptionally it may be very large. In rheumatic cases a large effusion is uncommon.

The effusion consists of a yellowish serous fluid in which leucocytes, shreds of fibrin, and endothelial cells are present in varying quantity. The fluid is usually clear, but may be turbid if there is much cellular exudation, and may contain flakes of lymph. Sometimes it is blood-stained, and in scurvy may consist almost entirely of blood.

It may from the outset be purulent, constituting "suppurative pericarditis," which differs so materially in its clinical features from the simple plastic or fibrinous form that its consideration will be reserved for another section.

"Milk spots," or white opaque patches sometimes found at autopsies on the surface of the visceral pericardium, are not, as a rule, due to pericarditis, but to a localized growth of connective tissue from irritation, and they occur at some point where the heart in its movements comes into contact with the chest wall.

**The Myocardium.**—The heart muscle is almost invariably affected, and there is myocarditis to a varying degree, with resulting granular and fatty degeneration of the muscle fibres. In the more protracted cases areas of round-celled infiltration may sometimes be found in the interstitial tissue between the muscle fibres.

It is to this accompanying myocarditis that we must attribute the cardiac dilatation which is so marked a feature in pericarditis. One of the chief dangers in rheumatic inflammation of the heart, of which pericarditis is a part, lies in the damage to the cardiac muscle.

## Etiology.

Rheumatism is by far the most common and important cause of pericarditis. So close is the connection between the two that, as Dr. Frederick Roberts says,* "The pericardial inflammation is not to be looked upon as a mere complication of rheumatism, but is an integral part of the disease." Furthermore, pericarditis must not be regarded as a separate entity, but as part of a general inflammation of the heart, aptly termed "carditis" by the late Dr. Sturges,† the myocardium being almost invariably, and the endocardium frequently, affected. Pericarditis occurring in association with chorea may be regarded as of rheumatic origin.

**Rheumatism.**—In childhood and early adolescence rheumatism is especially liable to attack the heart, while the joints may be so slightly affected that attention is not drawn to them. In later life the joints are more apt to suffer severely while the heart frequently escapes.

The belief has long been held that acute rheumatism is a disease of microbic origin, and that pericarditis and endocarditis are local manifestations of the activity of a specific micro-organism. From the experimental researches

* Allbutt's "System of Medicine," vol. v. p. 752.

† Lumleian Lectures, 1894.

of Triboulet, Wasserman, Paine and Poynton, Shaw, Ainley, Walker, Beattie, and others, it would appear that acute rheumatism is due to a minute diplococcus, which may grow in chains like a streptococcus. This micro-organism they have succeeded in isolating from the pericardial fluid and blood of patients suffering from rheumatic fever, and, after growing it on suitable culture media, have inoculated it into rabbits and reproduced pericarditis, arthritis, and endocarditis, or a disease indistinguishable from acute rheumatism. Pericarditis, therefore, occurring in association with rheumatism, may be regarded as due to a micro-organism. The question as to whether this is *the* specific micro-organism of rheumatism, is further discussed in the chapter on acute endocarditis.

**Pneumonia.**—Pericarditis may occur as a complication of pneumonia or pleurisy, or even, in the absence of these affections as a primary disease, from infection by the pneumococcus, which can, as a rule, be readily isolated from the fluid in the pericardium in cases of pneumococcal origin.

**The Acute Specific Diseases.**—Acute pericarditis may ensue as a complication of scarlet fever, variola, erysipelas—rarely of measles and typhus fever.

**Bright's Disease.**—Pericarditis is met with in Bright's disease most commonly in association with the later stages of granular kidney or subacute parenchymatous nephritis.

**Traumatism.**—Injuries to the pericardium by a gunshot or punctured wound, or by a fractured rib, or by a fish-bone lodged in the œsophagus, may set up pericarditis.

**Tubercular pericarditis** may occur as part of a general miliary tuberculosis, or from the extension of the disease from a tubercular lung or bronchial gland.

## Physical Signs.

**Friction rub.**—The most trustworthy sign of pericarditis is the characteristic to-and-fro friction sound heard on auscultation. For this reason, auscultation will be considered before percussion. The friction sound is caused by the rubbing together of the two inflamed surfaces of the pericardium at each beat of the heart. It is a curious scratching rub which appears to be very superficial, and somewhat resembles the noise made by scratching a piece of rough paper with the finger-nail. It is modified by pressure with the stethoscope, and may be rendered more distinct and longer or almost extinguished. It is usually of a to-and-fro character, corresponding more or less, but not accurately, to the movements of the heart in systole and diastole. It may be only systolic in time and not present the to-and-fro character; this is usually the case when it is heard near the apex, and not over the base. On the other hand, over the base of the heart the friction sound may be triple or cantering instead of merely to and fro, the auricular systole being attended with an audible independent rub. It is said to be first heard, as a rule, over the base of the heart, but frequently it is first audible at the apex as a single scratch at each systole. As the inflammation spreads, a to-and-fro friction rub is heard over the whole or a large proportion of the præcordial area, and since the heart is usually dilated it may be heard an inch or more to the right of the sternum in children. The rub may be present for a day or two only in mild cases; in cases of effusion it may be present for a few days, then disappear and reappear when the fluid is absorbed or drawn off by paracentesis. In subacute or chronic cases the rub persists for some days or weeks, only disappearing as the layers of pericardium become adherent.

Disappearance of the rub may thus indicate (1) subsidence of the attack; (2) effusion into the pericardium; (3) formation of adhesion between the two layers of the pericardium.

**Friction fremitus** may be felt on palpation in well-marked cases over the area where the friction sound is best heard.

The action of the heart is excited and the pulse almost invariably accelerated, as a rule, before the friction rub becomes audible. Sometimes in children it may be irregular in rhythm for a time. After the friction rub has appeared, a peculiar triple cantering rhythm of the heart is frequently heard on auscultation at the apex, and is very characteristic. It is apparently due to reduplication of the first sound.

### Increase in the Area of Cardiac Dulness.

Increase in the area of cardiac dulness is usually one of the earliest physical signs. This is especially marked in children, in whom it is most easily mapped out on percussion. It is more rapid and extensive in proportion to the severity and acuteness of the attack. The dulness may extend upwards as far as the second left intercostal space, and outwards for an inch outside the vertical nipple line, and in the opposite direction for an inch or more to the right of the sternum, but it is usually not so extensive in adults as in children, and is less easily made out, because of the thickness of the chest wall and errors that may arise from pathological conditions in the lungs.

The view was held by Sibson* that this increase in the area of cardiac dulness indicates pericardial effusion, and that increase in effusion is indicated by extension of the cardiac dulness. In a certain proportion of cases this is undoubtedly true; but much evidence has been accumulated which tends to show that this is by no means the rule, and that the increase in dulness indicates in the large majority of cases of rheumatic pericarditis, increase in the size of the heart, or cardiac dilatation.

In 1895, in a monograph on "Adherent Pericardium,"

* Sibson's Works, edited by Ord.

I described a series of cases where marked increase in the area of cardiac dulness was found, post-mortem, to be due, not to effusion, but to cardiac dilatation. In two cases where the physical signs and symptoms seemed to point conclusively to considerable pericardial effusion paracentesis was resorted to, but in neither instance was fluid found, and the increase in dulness was found to be due to increase in the size of the heart.

Lees and Poynton * drew attention to the acute dilatation of the heart that occurs in the rheumatism and chorea of childhood. From an analysis of the post-mortem records of 150 cases of fatal rheumatic heart disease in children, they showed that cardiac dilatation is usually present, and marked excess of pericardial fluid rare; in only 12 cases out of 150 was there excess of pericardial fluid amounting to more than two ounces.

Out of 79 cases of paracentesis pericardii, collected by Dr. Samuel West,† only 11 were of rheumatic origin, and in only one of these eleven was the effusion large in amount.

Clinically, it is not an uncommon experience, even when the area of cardiac dulness is very much enlarged, extending to the right of the sternum, to hear a pericardial rub at several points over the dull area. This seems incompatible with the presence of fluid, and in many of these cases, at the post-mortem, no excess of pericardial fluid is found, but a dilated heart with the pericardium partially adherent.

**Effusion.**—In effusion the outline of the area of cardiac dulness tends to assume a pyramidal or pyriform shape, with the base or widest portion below. The transition from the dull area to the resonant lung is sudden and well-marked, and the extent and shape of the area of

* Trans. Med: Chi. Soc., June, 1898.

† West, S., "Paracentesis Pericardii," Trans. Med. Chi. Soc., vol. 66, p. 235.

cardiac dulness will vary somewhat with the position of the patient.

Sibson gave a series of diagrams to illustrate the shape assumed by the pericardial sac in the different stages of effusion, but it is doubtful how far these are of practical value for differential diagnosis, as they were not confirmed by post-mortem examination, and he appears to have taken it for granted that increase in the area of cardiac dulness invariably indicated effusion. It is, however, by no means an easy matter to decide by percussion alone, whether the increased area of dulness indicates effusion, cardiac dilatation, or dilated heart with the pericardium adherent.

There is much diversity of opinion as to the position assumed by the heart in effusion. Sibson maintained that it was usually pushed upwards and outwards, and the apex beat similarly displaced; but this is not invariably the case, and pericardial adhesions may fix the apex in various positions, and in effusion of any extent it is not as a rule palpable.

Bulging of the præcordial area as a whole, more especially of the intercostal spaces over this area, which is usually best marked in purulent pericarditis, is a more trustworthy sign of effusion.

Gradual enfeeblement of the apex beat from day to day, or even its eventual disappearance, together with increasing weakness and distance of the sounds heard at the apex, especially if there is at the same time an increase in the severity of the symptoms, and marked dyspnœa, are strongly suggestive of increasing effusion into the pericardium.

## SYMPTOMS.

The symptoms are partly local, due to the pericarditis itself, and partly constitutional, or due to a general toxæmia.

Pain in the præcordial region, increase in the pulse-rate, excited action of the heart, dyspnœa varying in degree, rise of temperature, restlessness at night, are symptoms usually well marked in acute pericarditis; but in the sub-acute variety, common in children, there may be little or no pain or fever, and very slight dyspnœa, though there is usually acceleration of the pulse. The symptoms, as a rule, precede the development of the pericardial rub, and are more marked when it appears. In children there may be premonitory symptoms of nervous origin, such as night terrors, crying out, and wandering in sleep, restlessness, and even slight delirium on first waking. Vomiting may set in, and is generally of serious prognostic significance. The face may be pale or flushed, the expression is often anxious or distressed, and the respiration hurried. There may be some pain or difficulty in swallowing from the proximity of the pericardium to the œsophagus, if the posterior aspect is inflamed, or if there is much effusion into the sac. The temperature ranges between 100° and 103°, and is usually higher in adults than in children, in whom the attack is commonly less acute and more insidious in its onset. The dyspnœa may become very considerable, not only in cases of effusion, but in cases where there is great cardiac dilatation and the pericardium is becoming adherent; the patient has to be propped up with pillows, and when there is much effusion or extreme dilatation of the heart, may find most comfort in leaning forward over a bed-board, with his head on his hands.

In severe cases, nervous symptoms may predominate, and there may be delirium, involuntary passage of motions and urine, great restlessness, or a state resembling collapse. Vomiting is always a serious symptom, and not infrequently ushers in the closing scene.

## Course of the Disease and Terminations.

The disease as a rule runs a somewhat different course in adults and in children. In adults it is usually acute, and the symptoms are more marked at the onset; in children it may from the first be sub-acute or chronic in character, and it results frequently in the formation of adhesions between the heart and pericardium. It must not be forgotten that the prognosis to a great extent depends on the degree to which the cardiac muscle is attacked by the inflammatory process. In very severe attacks death may ensue within two or three days from the time at which the disease is first recognizable by the pericardial rub. In such cases there is usually rapid increase in the area of cardiac dulness, and in the severity of symptoms, and sometimes attacks of vomiting. Post-mortem there is commonly little or no effusion beyond the lymph on the serous surfaces, but great cardiac dilatation, and it would seem as if the severity of the inflammation had caused paresis of the cardiac muscle, analogous to that which occurs in the muscular coats of the intestines in acute peritonitis.

In a mild case, though the symptoms at the onset may be severe, the friction rub persists for a few days only, perhaps not more than one or two; the area of cardiac dulness does not greatly increase, and rapidly decreases to normal when the friction rub has disappeared: convalescence is soon established. In the more severe type of acute cases, effusion may occur, and require removal by paracentesis.

In the sub-acute type, common in children, the onset is insidious, and the symptoms are ill marked. The friction rub may persist for some days or weeks, the area of cardiac dulness becomes greatly enlarged, and remains so permanently, and eventually, when the friction rub disappears, the pericardium is left partially or universally adherent to the heart. The child, even after convalescence is established, remains pale and thin, is short of breath, and incapable of exertion, as the heart with its muscle damaged by myocarditis and hampered by pericardial adhesions, remains permanently crippled.

In another class of sub-acute cases where the inflammatory process persists for some months, or repeated attacks in close succession ensue, dropsy may supervene, the liver becoming enlarged and the cardiac dilatation extreme, the patient dying with all the symptoms of cardiac failure from extensive damage to the cardiac muscle by myocarditis.

As an illustration of the life history of such a case, the following may be quoted:—

H. D., æt. 9, was admitted to the Children's Hospital, Great Ormond Street, 11th December, 1893, with a history of pains in the joints, fourteen days previous to his admission. When first seen, his heart was considerably dilated, and a mitral systolic murmur was audible at the apex. Five days after admission a pericardial rub was heard, which persisted for about a week, during which time the cardiac dilatation increased. A week later he began to improve, and the area of cardiac dulness gradually decreased. On the 15th February, 1894, two months after the onset of the pericarditis, the area of cardiac dulness was almost normal in extent, and he was sufficiently recovered to go to a convalescent home. A month later, he had a fresh attack of rheumatism with an eruption of nodules, and was readmitted 15th March; there was slight œdema of the legs, and rheumatic nodules were present on the elbows; the area of cardiac dulness was again greatly enlarged, and he suffered from severe dyspnœa. From this time he steadily got worse, the œdema of the legs rapidly increased, the liver became greatly enlarged, the veins of the neck distended and pulsating, and he died on the 21st April, with extreme symptoms of venous engorgement and right ventricle failure. At the post-mortem all the cavities of the heart were greatly dilated; the pericardium was universally adherent by recent adhesions, the muscle was soft, and showed evidence microscopically of myocarditis; there was no serious valvular lesion, though a few vegetations were present on the mitral valve, and its orifice was much dilated. Myocarditis and adherence of the pericardium to the dilated heart were thus responsible for his death. The symptoms were those of venous engorgement and right ventricle failure, as the right ventricle with its comparatively thin walls was more rapidly rendered helpless by the myocarditis, and more hampered by the adherent pericardium than the left, with its greater thickness of muscular tissue.

Effusion of any extent is rare in the sub-acute rheumatic cases in children, adhesions, partial or universal, between the heart and pericardium being the most common termination. Effusion is more likely to occur in acute attacks in adults, especially those associated with pneumonia or Bright's disease, and effusion of blood into the pericardium is common in scurvy.

## Diagnosis.

Till the pericardial friction rub is heard, a certain diagnosis of pericarditis cannot be made. Usually, however, in acute attacks there are premonitory symptoms, such as pain in the præcordial region, restlessness, dyspnœa, acceleration of pulse, and rise of temperature which enable us in some measure to anticipate the appearance of the friction rub. These symptoms may in some cases appear to be only exacerbations of those already existing, as the result of rheumatism, pneumonia, or, possibly, scarlet fever, but as the patient is then confined to his bed, we shall be on the look-out for cardiac complications, and are not likely to miss the first definite signs of pericarditis.

The sub-acute attacks so common in children are, on the

contrary, as a rule, very insidious in their onset, and the child may be going about with pericarditis, especially in the event of a second attack, before the symptoms are so severe as to attract attention to the child's condition, and cause the parents to seek medical advice, or the physician to examine the heart. Much damage may thus be done to the heart before the existence of pericarditis is discovered.

The articular manifestations of rheumatism in children are, moreover, slight, as a rule, while the heart is commonly attacked. It is important, therefore, not to neglect the slightest evidence of rheumatism in children, and if we have reason to suspect its existence, to keep a careful watch over the child, and examine the heart at frequent intervals.

## Differential Diagnosis.

A friction rub due to pleurisy in the neighbourhood of the heart will be readily distinguished by the fact that its rhythm is synchronous with the respiratory movements, and not with those of the heart. Some difficulty may, however, arise when, from friction between the pericardium and the pleura overlapping or adjoining it, the rhythm is of a to-and-fro character corresponding to the beats of the heart. A friction rub arising from this cause will be intensified by the respiratory movements, and will usually be extinguished when the breath is held in deep inspiration. It will, as a rule, be heard only at the left border of the heart over the ventricles, and not at the base of the heart, or to the right of the sternum. Moreover, as the pleurisy will seldom be confined to the præcordial region, a well-marked respiratory friction rub will usually be heard in the adjoining area.

Endocardial murmurs differ so completely in their character from pericardial friction sounds, that confusion will seldom arise. They will not, of course, be modified by pressure with the stethoscope.

## Prognosis.

Pericarditis is always a disease of considerable gravity owing to the myocarditis which usually accompanies it. In acute attacks, associated with rheumatism or pneumonia, death may take place within the first few days, but this is not a common occurrence. In a large proportion of rheumatic cases the immediate prognosis is favourable, though the liability to repeated attacks, the probable damage to the heart by myocarditis, and the formation of adhesions between the heart and pericardium, render the ultimate chances of long life unfavourable. When associated with Bright's disease, the prognosis is usually bad, and the chance of recovery small.

In sub-acute and prolonged cases the prognosis seems to depend on the degree to which the myocardium is affected by the inflammatory process. If the inflammation is of short duration and the changes in the muscle are slight, the heart may rapidly contract down again to its normal size, and be little the worse; if the inflammation is protracted and severe, involving great destruction of the myocardium, the heart is unable to recover for some time, and in the process of repair fibrous tissue takes the place of the damaged muscle, so the heart is permanently weakened. The pericardium may also become adherent to it.

Children, once attacked, are liable to repeated and prolonged attacks of cardiac inflammation, both pericardial, myocardial, and endocardial. They seldom grow up to maturity; or, if they do, it is with hearts so crippled that they do not survive many years.

Adults attacked by pericarditis usually fare better than children, for though the symptoms are usually more acute at the time of the attack, its duration is short, and the heart often seems to escape without serious damage.

## TREATMENT.

In the *treatment* of pericarditis various local applications, such as ice-bags, leeches, or blisters over the præcordial area, have been advocated. Of these, ice-bags are the most useful, as they relieve pain in acute pericarditis, and, according to Lees, modify the inflammation and limit the dilatation of the heart. Leeches are often of service at the outset of pericarditis, and may be followed by ice-bags; blisters are better suited for the later and more chronic stages. The administration of salicylates, which in the acute articular rheumatism of adults are given with such marked beneficial results, is of doubtful service. If the pain is severe, opium or morphia may be given with marked benefit; if stimulants are required, brandy, ammonia, and ether, or strychnine, may be given. Digitalis, and similar cardiac tonics, should not be given during the acute stage. As a general tonic, an effervescing mixture, containing quinine and bicarbonate of potash, is perhaps as useful as any. Nothing, however, in severe cases seems to arrest or exert any controlling influence on the course of cardiac inflammation in children, when once it has gained a firm hold. It is, therefore, of the first importance that any indications of danger threatening the heart should be recognized as early as possible, and due precautions taken. If, then, a suspicion of rheumatism is aroused by complaints of stiffness in the joints or pains in the limbs, in a child who comes of a rheumatic stock, or who has previously suffered from chorea or some other rheumatic manifestation, more especially if rheumatic nodules are present, the patient should be kept under careful observation, and the heart examined every two or three days for some weeks. Any exposure to chill should be guarded against, and exercise should be limited in amount for some time after all apparent symptoms have subsided.

**Effusion.**—If extensive effusion into the pericardial sac takes place, its removal by paracentesis may be necessary, and it is important that this should not be long delayed, as death from syncope is liable to occur from embarrassment of the heart by the pressure of the fluid. It is, however, frequently a difficult matter to determine whether the symptoms of cardiac embarrassment and the increase of cardiac dulness are due to cardiac dilatation or to the presence of effusion, and not infrequently the right ventricle has been punctured by mistake. I have seen two such cases in which blood was withdrawn from the right ventricle but no ill results followed. I have, however, known of two cases in which death from hæmorrhage resulted from a similar procedure where cardiac dilatation was mistaken for effusion. The best site for puncture when aspiration is decided on, is in the fifth left intercostal space, about one inch or one and a half inch external to the border of the sternum, outside the course of the internal mammary artery. Some advocate that this puncture should be made in the angle between the xiphoid cartilage and the costal margin, as this would penetrate the lowest part of the sac. A small aspirating needle should be used, and previous to its insertion, an incision should be made down through the skin to the intercostal muscles. Any bulging of the intercostal space can then be seen, and any risk of wounding the intercostal arteries be avoided by keeping close to the upper border of the rib.

The above description applies to the type of pericarditis which is met with in association with rheumatism or pneumonia, and it will be necessary here to briefly allude to the form it may assume in Bright's disease.

In *Bright's disease* pericarditis occurs most commonly as a complication of subacute parenchymatous nephritis or of the chronic interstitial variety. Statistics vary as to its frequency, from 3 to 14 per cent., according to different authors.

The onset of pericarditis in Bright's disease occurring, as it usually does, in debilitated subjects, may be insidious and unattended by any marked symptoms of local reaction. There may be little or no rise of temperature, no præcordial pain, and little beyond increase in the pulse-rate and slight exacerbation of pre-existing systems, such as dyspnœa and restlessness due to uræmia, to call attention to its presence. A friction rub is usually present and is well marked. A pleuritic friction rub may accompany it, and in some cases a pleuro-pericardial rub alone is heard, between which and a true pericardial rub it may be difficult to distinguish. The prognosis is always very grave and the treatment must be directed to the primary disease.

It is important, therefore, that the heart should be examined as a matter of routine, or the onset of pericarditis may easily escape notice.

## ADHERENT PERICARDIUM.

By the term "adherent pericardium" is implied the existence of adhesions between the visceral and parietal layers of the pericardium, the result of pericarditis.

**Morbid Anatomy.**—The adhesions may be limited to fibrous bands stretching across the pericardial cavity, or they may be universal, in which case the pericardium and heart are so intimately connected that the pericardial cavity is entirely obliterated. Adhesions may also exist between the chest-wall or pleura and the pericardium, as a result of so-called mediastino-pericarditis. The adhesions if of old standing are tough and fibrous, so that the pericardium cannot be stripped from the heart without tearing the heart-substance. There is also commonly some fibroid change in the heart-wall due to substitution of fibrous tissue for muscle fibres damaged by previous inflammation. In the case of recent adhesions or lymph undergoing organization into fibrous tissue, the two layers of pericardium on being separated will present a honeycomb or bread-and-butter-like appearance, owing to the layer of thick, sticky lymph which coats the surface.

## Physical Signs.

The physical signs differ according as the adhesions exist only between the two layers of the pericardium, or between the pericardium and chest-wall, or adjoining pleura as well. In the latter case they are more numerous and distinctive. Among them are the following:—

**Fixation of the apex beat**, so that it does not alter its position in deep inspiration and expiration or in change of posture of the body.

**Systolic depression** of one or more intercostal spaces to the left of the sternum, or of the lower end of the sternum and the adjoining costal cartilages, which may be caused by the heart dragging on them at each systole, through the agency of the pericardial adhesions. The systolic recession of spaces alone is, however, not a trustworthy indication, as it may be due to atmospheric pressure, more especially when the heart is much hypertrophied. When the costal cartilages or lower end of the sternum are dragged in there can be little doubt as to the diagnosis, as this could not be effected by atmospheric pressure.

**Systolic recession** of the site of the apex beat is an important sign when a definite apex beat can be felt; when there is no palpable apex beat, systolic pitting over its site may be due to atmospheric pressure.

**A diastolic shock** may sometimes be felt on palpation with the flat of the hand over areas on the chest-wall where systolic recession is present. It is due to the elastic recoil of the chest-wall at the commencement of diastole as soon as the pulling force exerted during the systole ceases.

**Systolic retraction** of the lower portions of the posterior or lateral walls of the thorax may indicate the presence of a universally adherent pericardium. Such retraction may, however, be seen though the pericardium is not adherent to the heart, but only to a larger extent than normal to the central tendon of the diaphragm and the muscular substance on either side, and to the chest-wall as well. In such cases the heart is usually greatly enlarged and hypertrophied from old valvular disease. The explanation seems to be that the portion of the diaphragm to which the pericardium is adherent is dragged upwards at each systole of the heart, so that the points of attachment of the digitations of the diaphragm to the lower ribs and costal cartilages are dragged inwards and retracted.

The descent of the diaphragm in inspiration may be interfered with by pericardial adhesions between the heart and diaphragm, more especially if the pericardium is adherent to the chest-wall in front as well. This will be shown by impaired movement in respiration of the upper part of the abdominal wall in the epigastrium and left subcostal region.

The area of cardiac dulness will be increased, and will remain unchanged in inspiration and expiration, where there are extensive adhesions between the pericardium and chest-wall, as the lung, which normally overlaps part of the heart, will have been pushed aside, or perhaps have become involved in the adhesions, and be collapsed.

**Enlargement of Heart.**—It is common with adherent pericardium to find the heart, more especially the right ventricle, considerably enlarged, in the absence of valvular disease or other obvious cause to account for it.

It seems probable that such enlargement may be indirectly due to pericardial adhesions as follows: The heart becomes dilated during an attack of pericarditis, and, before it recovers its tone or can contract down again to its normal size, the pericardium becomes adherent and fixes it in this condition of dilatation, the right ventricle suffering more than the left, owing to its thinner walls, as well as for other reasons.

Hypertrophy and dilatation of the heart, more especially of the right ventricle, may therefore, in the absence of other obvious causes, such as valvular disease, high arterial tension, etc., to explain it, be a physical sign of considerable importance.

**Diastolic collapse** of cervical veins was held by Friedreich to be of great diagnostic value when accompanied by systolic retraction of spaces; but I have never found it to be of service.

Systolic emptying of veins on the surface of the thorax may sometimes be observed, due to suction action, induced by the walls of the internal mammary veins being dragged apart by pericardial adhesions during systole of the heart.

When there are no adhesions between the pericardium and chest-wall the physical signs that may be present will be limited in number. There will be no recession of spaces except as the result of atmospheric pressure, no fixation of apex beat, no diastolic shock. As the pericardium is normally attached by fibrous bands to the central tendon of the diaphragm and to the muscular substance on either side of it, there may be some interference with the movements of the diaphragm in respiration. There may also be considerable enlargement of the heart, but in these cases a diagnosis will usually have to be made from other indications than physical signs alone.

**Symptoms.**—The symptoms in themselves are not in any sense characteristic. They are usually such as arise from cardiac embarrassment, more especially from the giving way of the right ventricle, such as œdema of the extremities, enlargement of liver, ascites, dyspnœa, etc.

## Diagnosis.

The physical signs or symptoms of adherent pericardium, few of which may be present, are often in themselves insufficient to allow of a diagnosis being made, or even to arouse suspicion of its presence; but valuable help may be derived from careful consideration of the physical signs and symptoms together, and by balancing the former against the latter, so that the question is raised, "Do the physical signs present afford evidence of sufficient disease to account for the symptoms that have arisen?" When the symptoms are those of right ventricle failure, and are more severe than the physical signs present would lead one to expect, and have not been induced by undue exertion or imprudence, adherent pericardium must be thought of as being possibly responsible. For it is the right side of the heart more especially that is seriously hampered by pericardial adhesions, so that their presence may account for the unexpected breakdown of the right ventricle when the physical signs indicate that the valvular lesion is slight. It must also be borne in mind that the heart-wall has in all probability been weakened by the substitution of fibrous tissue for muscle fibres destroyed by inflammation at the time of the attack of pericarditis.

When with symptoms of right ventricle failure there is an absence of cyanosis, or of pulmonary congestion or lung mischief, this is further evidence in favour of adherent pericardium as a possible cause of the breakdown of the right ventricle. If by these means a suspicion of the presence of adherent pericardium has been aroused, confirmatory physical signs should be carefully sought for.

The above remarks apply to the question of diagnosis in cases where, with or without valvular disease, there is no history of pericarditis, and the adhesions are of old standing.

In cases of pericarditis, which can be kept under observation after the attack, there will be less difficulty in arriving at a diagnosis, and the indications which would lead one to suspect that the pericardium was becoming adherent are as follows:—

1. Prolongation of the attack of pericarditis evidenced by a harsh friction rub over the præcordial area, which may persist for some weeks. When at the margins of the area of

cardiac dulness a pleuro-pericardial friction is also heard, it will indicate that adhesions are probably taking place between the pericardium and adjoining pleura or chest-wall as well.

2. Permanent enlargement of the area of cardiac dulness to a marked extent after the subsidence of the pericarditis.

3. The occurrence of symptoms of right ventricle failure after a period of temporary improvement, there being no apparent exciting cause for the breakdown of the right ventricle. Damage to the cardiac muscle by fresh myocarditis may, however, be responsible, and should be first excluded.

## Prognosis.

When the heart remains normal in size, and there are no adhesions between the pericardium and chest-wall, the universal adherence of the pericardium to the heart may not in an adult tend to materially shorten life. When the heart is enlarged, or when the pericardium is also adherent to the chest-wall, the prognosis is more serious. When adherent pericardium exists as a complication of valvular disease, it is still more likely to prove fatal eventually, by so hampering the right ventricle as to prevent its recovery when once compensation has broken down. The detection of adherent pericardium has also an important bearing on prognosis, inasmuch as it affords presumptive evidence of fibroid change in the heart-wall, and therefore renders the outlook even more unfavourable.

## Treatment.

The discovery of adherent pericardium, when present, is important from the point of view of treatment, not because anything can be done to remedy or remove the pericardial adhesions, once they are formed, but because, when it is present, it will be necessary to impose additional restrictions on the patient, so that no undue risks may be run of upsetting the compensatory balance, which would only be [re]stored with great difficulty.

## SUPPURATIVE PERICARDITIS.

Purulent pericarditis may occur as part of a general pyæmic or septicæmic condition, or in association with empyæma or some pneumococcal infection, abscess of the lung, suppuration of mediastinal or cervical glands, or of other adjacent structures. Sometimes no apparent cause can be found.

The inflammatory process is almost invariably septic from the onset, and is attended by effusion of pus into the pericardium: seldom, if ever, does a serous effusion of rheumatic origin become purulent.

The outset of the disease is, as a rule, insidious, and the discovery of pus in the pericardium is often not made till the post-mortem examination.

The micro-organisms which have been found are the staphylococcus pyogenes aureus, albus, and citreus, the streptococcus, and the pneumococcus.

**Physical Signs.**—There is seldom any definite friction rub to announce the onset of the attack.

The physical signs present will be those of pericardial effusion, which have already been discussed. Chief of these is increase in the area of cardiac dulness, and the difficulty of distinguishing whether this be due to cardiac dilatation or effusion will be intensified when no friction rub has been heard to suggest the possibility of effusion. Furthermore, it not infrequently happens that the area of cardiac dulness is encroached upon by, or runs into, a large dull area due to empyæma.

Feebleness or loss of the apex beat, and weak or distant heart-sounds may be noted, but will not be of great value, unless the case has been watched from the outset, so that a standard of comparison could be formed. There may, occasionally, be œdema over the præcordial region.

**Symptoms.**—The temperature is usually that characteristic of some septic infection, but may sometimes be normal throughout. Rigors seldom occur unless as part of a general septicæmia, except in the somewhat rare event of a serous pericardial effusion becoming purulent. Pain is absent, as a rule, but there may be a feeling of oppression in the præcordial region. The pulse rate and respiration are accelerated, and there may be marked dyspnœa, especially on movement.

**Diagnosis.**—The diagnosis presents many difficulties, and is frequently not made during life.

In the absence of an antecedent friction rub effusion may not be suspected, and the intermittent pyrexia may be attributed to an empyæma, or suppuration elsewhere than in the pericardium.

If effusion is suspected, an exploring-needle may be employed. The skin should be incised parallel to the ribs, as described under paracentesis pericardii, and the intercostal muscles divided before the needle is inserted into the pericardium, so that any bulging of the space may be noted, and the needle be accurately directed.

**Prognosis.**—The prognosis is always very serious, but there are reasonable grounds for hope in cases where the suppuration is not part of a general septic infection, but is a sequela of an empyema or other localized abscess.

The earlier the diagnosis is made and surgical interference is sought, the better will be the chance of recovery. The percentage of recoveries is, however, very small.

**Treatment.**—Abscess in the pericardium must be treated like any other abscess. It should be opened and drained as soon as the diagnosis is made, by an incision in the fifth space, close to the sternum on the right or left side, wherein any bulging of the intercostal space is apparent.

**Hydropericardium.**—By hydropericardium is meant effusion of serous fluid into the pericardial sac, as the result, not of inflammation, but of passive dropsical transudation.

Effusion of such degree, as to be clinically recognizable, occurs most commonly as part of a general dropsical transudation from whatever cause, and is therefore most frequently associated with Bright's disease or morbus cordis. It is much less common than effusion into other serous cavities, and when present is a late feature in the disease, and is gradual in onset. It is said also to occur as the result of mechanical obstruction, to the return of blood from the pericardial and cardiac veins from some local cause, such as pressure by mediastinal tumours, enlarged glands, or fibrous adhesions, but this must be very exceptional.

**Symptoms and Physical Signs and Diagnosis.**—The symptoms are increasing dyspnœa and præcordial oppression with enfeeblement of the pulse, and the physical signs are those of pericardial effusion, increase of the area of cardiac dulness, with progressive enfeeblement of the apex beat and weakness of the heart-sounds. As there is no antecedent friction rub to call attention to the possibility of effusion, it may readily escape notice in the earlier stages. The diagnosis cannot be made unless the effusion amounts to several ounces, and when there is effusion into one or both pleural cavities as well it is very difficult, and may be impossible.

**Treatment.**—Practically the treatment is that of the original disease to which the general dropsy and hydropericardium are due. Relief may occasionally be afforded by aspiration of the pericardium when the diagnosis of effusion can be made with certainty; but it is rarely employed or called for, as the relief can but be temporary, and does not long delay the fatal result.

**Pneumopericardium.**—The presence of gas in the pericardial sac is rare. It may be due to penetrating wounds of the pericardium by a sharp instrument or a fractured rib, but is more commonly the result of ulceration, by which a communication is established between the pericardial sac and an air-containing cavity. Thus, an old phthisical cavity, an abscess in the lung, a pneumothorax, a subphrenic abscess that has made its way through the diaphragm, may open into the pericardium, or a communication may be established with the œsophagus by ulceration, giving rise in each instance to pneumopericardium. Pus may find its way into the pericardium with the air giving rise to pyo-pneumopericardium, or blood in the case of punctured wounds, when the condition is termed hæmo-pneumopericardium.

**Physical Signs.**—Uniform bulging of the præcordial area may be noted. The apex beat is usually absent or feeble, but can sometimes be felt when the patient bends forwards.

On percussion the note varies with change of position, being dull over the fluid and tympanitic, or high pitched over the air-containing cavity. The gas always rises to the highest part of the cavity with change of posture of the patient. The relations of the gas and fluid will be remarkably altered by changes of posture, and can be readily made out by percussion.

On auscultation the heart-sounds acquire a peculiar metallic character, and are unusually loud and clear, so that they may sometimes be heard at some distance off, and are a source of annoyance to the patient himself. Splashing sounds, and metallic tinkling, and a bell note with coins can usually be heard.

**Treatment.**—As pneumopericardium is usually a complication of some grave disease, treatment must vary accordingly. Aspiration may be required to remove the gas or fluid, or possibly free incision may be necessary to allow of the escape of pus.

**Tuberculosis of the pericardium** may occur as part of a general acute miliary tuberculosis, when miliary tubercles will be found scattered over its surface, post-mortem, or from direct infection by adjacent tubercular lung or pleura, in which case the onset is insidious and the progress of the disease is usually chronic. The two layers of pericardium become thickened and tend to become adherent, so that the physical signs are those of chronic mediastinitis, or adherent pericardium.

**New growth of the pericardium** is very rare, and when found is usually due to invasion of the pericardium by a new growth in adjacent structures.

# CHAPTER IV.

## SIMPLE ACUTE ENDOCARDITIS.

ACUTE endocarditis means, strictly speaking, an acute inflammation of the endocardium or lining membrane of the heart. The inflammatory process is, however, as a rule, chiefly manifested on the valves, so that by the term endocarditis is usually understood inflammation of the valves of the heart. The mitral and aortic valves are most commonly attacked; rarely are the valves of the right side of the heart affected except as a result of endocarditis occurring during intra-uterine life. It must be borne in mind that acute endocarditis is commonly accompanied by myocarditis of varying extent, which may seriously and permanently damage the walls of the heart.

On etiological and pathological grounds it is doubtful whether simple or rheumatic endocarditis should be differentiated from malignant or pernicious endocarditis, and this question is discussed fully in the chapter on the latter affection. Clinically, the two diseases are more or less distinct, and for that reason they are here considered separately.

**Morbid Anatomy and Pathology.**—On naked-eye examination of an affected valve it is seen to be studded along the free margin with small greyish-yellow or pinkish opaque bodies, the so-called "vegetations," as shown on the aortic valves in Fig. 7. Microscopically these are seen to consist of a superficial layer of coagulated fibrin and necrotic tissue, in the upper stratum of which are entangled leucocytes and a few red corpuscles deposited from the blood stream. Deeper down is a layer of simple fibrin free from corpuscular elements, and below this, again, is a layer of granulation tissue, formed by proliferation of the endothelial cells

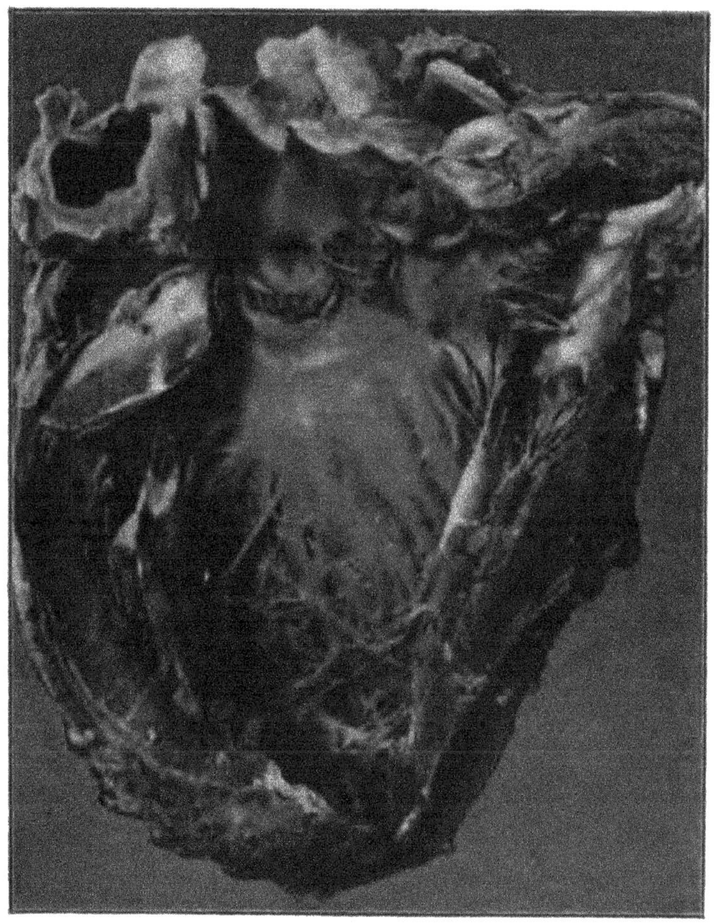

FIG. 7.

as a result of the inflammatory process. The inappropriately named "vegetations" are thus simply necrotic tissue, coagulated fibrin and leucocytes deposited from the blood stream on an inflamed surface. They may become partially absorbed, but, for the most part, the granulation tissue undergoes organization, and, later on, cicatricial contraction, so that the valves become puckered and misshapen, sometimes glued together at their margins, and incompetence or obstruction, or both combined, result. When the mitral valve is affected, the chordæ tendineæ are also, as a rule, more or less involved in the inflammatory process, so that they become shortened, thickened and deformed, and lose their flexibility. The shortening and fusing together of their fine subdivisions near the valves may be carried to such an extent that the margins of the valves seem to be directly attached to the papillary muscles.

**Etiology.**—Acute endocarditis is in the great majority of cases a complication, or rather an essential feature of rheumatism.

Of late years much evidence has been accumulated tending to prove that rheumatism is a disease of microbic origin, and that the valvulitis associated with it is a local manifestation of the activity of specific micro-organisms. The micro-organism in question is a minute diplococcus which has been isolated from the blood and pericardial fluid of patients suffering from acute rheumatism by various observers, Triboulet,* Wasserman,† Paine ‡ and Poynton, Shaw,§ Ainley Walker, Beattie, and others. This diplococcus, grown on suitable media and inoculated into rabbits, has in their hands produced arthritis, endocarditis, and valvulitis, and in early cases of rheumatic endocarditis minute diplococci can sometimes be demonstrated microscopically in the vegetations on the affected valves. Acute endocarditis occurring in association with chorea may be regarded as of rheumatic origin.

It is not uncommon as a *sequela* to scarlet fever. The type sometimes met with in smallpox, measles, and

* *Bulletin de la Soc. des hopitaux*, 1898, p. 93, *n*.

† *Berliner Klin. Woch.*, 1899, No. 29, p. 638.

‡ *Lancet*, Sept. 1900.

§ *Journal Path. and Bact.*, Dec. 1903.

pneumonia belongs rather to the category discussed in the next chapter.

Cole * has succeeded in producing valvulitis and arthritis in rabbits by inoculating them with different brands of streptococci obtained from cases of puerperal fever, septic peritonitis, and other sources, in which there was no history of rheumatism, the results being similar to those obtained by Paine and Poynton, Shaw, etc., by inoculation with the diplococcus isolated from cases of rheumatism. He therefore argues that there is no such thing as a specific rheumatic micro-organism, and the question is still to a certain extent *sub judice.* But, in view of the results obtained by Paine and Poynton and others, it scarcely seems fair to argue that because micro-organisms other than those associated with rheumatism can produce endocarditis in animals, as has long been known in the case of man, therefore there is no specific rheumatic organism. Moreover, rheumatism, whether in the child or adult, is such a definite clinical entity, that one would expect to find a specific organism, and would be confusing to vaguely classify it as a form of "septicæmia" in the ordinary sense of the term. We must hope that further work will be done on this subject, and that future investigators will be able to definitely settle the controversy.

It is most common in childhood and early adolescence, and is rare after middle age. It may also occur during fœtal life, when it is usually confined to the right side of the heart.

## Physical Signs.

The development of a valvular murmur, or, in the case of a second attack, of some change in the character of an existing murmur, is the only trustworthy indication of the presence of endocarditis. Evidence, however, of its existence is frequently found post-mortem in cases where no

* *Journal Infect. Diseases*, vol. i., No. 4, pp. 714-737.

murmur has been audible during life, so that it is probable that in many instances the inflammatory process may be active for some little time before a murmur is developed. It is important, therefore, to be on the look-out for other indications of its presence which may precede the development of a murmur, however indefinite and uncertain they may be. Of these the most significant is some alteration in the first sound, which may be reduplicated, prolonged and muffled, or rumbling in character, when the mitral valve is affected. The action of the heart may be tumultuous or irregular, and the area of cardiac dulness may become much enlarged, when the inflammatory process involves the muscular substance of the heart as well.

These indefinite signs are chiefly of value when present in cases in which an attack of endocarditis is to be anticipated, and it is therefore necessary that we should recognize such cases at the earliest possible moment. Of course, in a well-marked attack of rheumatism of the usual type in adults, we shall be on our guard; but in children, as pointed out by Cheadle,* the articular manifestations are usually slight, and may be confined to fugitive pains in the joints, while the heart is frequently attacked. The symptoms of rheumatism may thus be so ill-defined as to escape notice, and the onset of endocarditis may be very insidious.

To give an illustration of a case in point. Patrick D., æt. 14, employed at one of the large shops in London, walked up to the out-patient department at St. Mary's Hospital on 2nd January, 1897. He stated that he had vomited the previous day after having some pork for dinner, and complained of being rather short of breath. It was noticed that he was somewhat cyanosed, and was breathing rapidly, and the pulse rate was 132. On examining his chest, well-marked pulsation in the epigastrium, and in the third, fourth, and fifth left intercostal

* Harveian Lectures, 1889.

spaces, was noted. The apex beat was diffuse, and was visible in the fifth left space just outside the vertical nipple line. The area of cardiac dulness was enlarged and extended to the right, half an inch beyond the right border of the sternum; to the left, just beyond the vertical nipple line; and above, to the third space. At the apex a loud blowing systolic murmur was heard, conducted into the axilla, and at the base, over the aortic area, a soft diastolic murmur conducted down the sternum. There was no marked throbbing of the carotids, the pulse was not collapsing in character, and a distinct aortic second sound was audible at the base as well as the diastolic murmur; the pulmonic second sound was accentuated. The liver was somewhat enlarged, but there was no œdema of the extremities. Rheumatic nodules were present on the elbows and knees.

The history given by the boy was that, two months ago he had felt some stiffness in the knees, and had remained at home two days. He soon felt all right again, and up to the day on which he came up to the hospital he had been at work as usual. He was at once admitted, but got rapidly worse, suffering from great dyspnœa, and repeated attacks of vomiting; the diastolic murmur became more pronounced, and the pulse collapsing in character; the cardiac dilatation increased; the liver became more and more enlarged, and œdema of the lower extremities set in, and soon became extreme. He died on 17th February, six and a half weeks from the date of his admission.

The stiffness in the knees, two months before he came up to the hospital, seems to have been the only warning of the attack of rheumatism which gave rise to such serious cardiac mischief; and so slight were the symptoms, that the boy was undoubtedly going about his work with active endocarditis and myocarditis for some time before he sought medical advice, and by that time the heart had become dilated to an extreme degree. This case illustrates the insidious form that the rheumatism of early adolescence or childhood may assume, and shows how much damage may be done to the heart before any serious symptoms compel the patient to give in.

A history of pains in the joints or limbs, with slight febrile disturbance in children, should, therefore, put us on our guard, even though there be no appreciable swelling or tenderness of the joints, and the heart should be examined, not only when the patient is first seen, but from time to time for some weeks afterwards. A family history of rheumatism, or of a previous attack of chorea, should make us doubly suspicious of these ill-marked symptoms.

There are, however, certain unmistakable danger-signals for which we should be on the look-out, in children or young adolescents, when a suspicion of rheumatism is aroused. These are *rheumatic nodules*—small fibrous growths, commonly about the size of a split pea, sometimes much larger. They are found in the neighbourhood of joints over the bony prominences, and are attached by their base to the fascia, sheaths of tendons, or some underlying fibrous tissue. The skin over them is freely movable, and they are best seen by flexing the joint over which they are situated, so that the skin is rendered tense. They were first described by Barlow * and Warner; and Cheadle, in his book on the rheumatic state in children, has called attention to their evil prognostic significance. In themselves they are painless, and cause little or no discomfort to the patient, but they indicate that the rheumatism, to which they owe their existence, has got a firm hold on its victim, and where they are present in force, repeated attacks of cardiac inflammation are to be apprehended, though cases do occur in which the heart escapes. They are not present in all, or in the greater proportion of cases in which the heart is attacked, but a careful

* *Trans. Internat. Med. Congress.* London, 1881.

search for them should never be omitted, as they are of great clinical importance. They are seldom found in adults.

*Exudative erythemata*, of the type of erythema marginatum, or less commonly papular or urticarial in character, may occur in rheumatic subjects; they are not so frequently met with as nodules, but they may occur in conjunction with them, or alone.

In erythema marginatum, small raised patches about the size of a sixpence, with sharply defined margins, and of a dull red colour, make their appearance. The centre of the patch usually undergoes absorption, and becomes of a pinkish or pale colour, while the margins continue to spread as narrow raised red bands with irregular outline. The eruption is usually accompanied by some rise of temperature, and lasts a few days, gradually fading and leaving a slight brownish discoloration.

*Erythema nodosum* is sometimes looked upon as evidence of rheumatism, but it is by no means certain that it can be regarded as such.

## Symptoms.

The symptoms are not specially characteristic, and are, to a great extent, merged in those of the rheumatic affection of which endocarditis is a part. Dyspnœa, a tendency to sigh, a feeling of oppression in the præcordial region, restlessness, prolonged fever (the temperature not ranging high, as a rule, but from 99° to 101° F.), a fresh rise of temperature after a period of quiescence, increase of the pulse rate, are all symptoms which may give rise to a suspicion of endocarditis, and be present during an attack; but reliance cannot be placed on these alone for purposes of diagnosis.

## Prognosis.

During an attack of endocarditis, it is practically impossible to determine exactly the extent of the damage done to the valves attacked. It is not till some time after the inflammatory process has subsided and compensatory changes have in some degree developed, that we are able to estimate the extent of the lesion. If, in the course of an attack, a diastolic murmur develops over the aortic area, we may be certain that the aortic valves have been damaged, and a certain degree of aortic incompetence will permanently result. It does not, however, in the case of the mitral valve, necessarily follow, when a systolic murmur is developed at the apex, that the mitral incompetence which the murmur indicates will be permanent, though this may be the case. For the contractile ring surrounding the mitral orifice, and the musculi papillares may be temporarily thrown out of gear by the inflammatory process, so that the valves, though undamaged, do not come together at their margins, and some regurgitation takes place, or the murmur may be the result of dilatation of the ventricle. As the muscular fibres recover their tone after the inflammation has subsided, the valves may again become competent, and the systolic murmur disappear. If, however, the valves themselves, or the chordæ tendineæ, are seriously attacked, the former may become rigid and deformed, the latter puckered and shortened, and permanent incompetence results.

When the valves become thickened and glued together at their margins, stenosis of the orifice will ensue, which gradually increases as cicatricial contraction of the freshly organized fibrous tissue at the bases of the valves and round the mitral orifice takes place. Not infrequently incompetence and stenosis co-exist, the valves being thickened and depressed so that they cannot function effectively, while they are also adherent where they meet at their attachment to the margin of the orifice.

## Diagnosis.

When no cardiac murmur is present, a diagnosis of endocarditis is not possible. It is not always easy on discovering, for the first time, the existence of a cardiac murmur, to decide whether or not it indicates acute endocarditis. It may be due to a recent or old attack of endocarditis, to cardiac dilatation, or to anæmia. When hypertrophy or other compensatory changes of the heart are present, they will testify to a valvular lesion of old standing, but in such cases we must bear in mind the possibility and probability of a second attack, and watch carefully for any change in the character of the existing murmur, or for the development of a new murmur. The history of the case, the presence of nodules, articular pains, or other rheumatic manifestations, will be of assistance in arousing suspicion of acute endocarditis, and confirmatory evidence may be found in an irregular slightly raised temperature, or restlessness and dyspnœa, and other symptoms of cardiac disturbance. The murmurs of anæmia have been discussed elsewhere; the history of the case, the aspect of the patient, and the character of the murmur will usually enable us to distinguish these. Exocardial murmurs, whether due to pericarditis or pleurisy, are, as a rule, readily distinguished by their harsh grating or rubbing character, their position, and their relation to the cardiac rhythm.

The murmur caused by compression of a thin layer of lung between the heart and chest wall may be excluded by its occurring only during inspiration, and disappearing when the patient is told to make a deep expiration and hold his breath.

## Treatment.

Neither drugs nor local applications seem to be of avail to arrest the progress of endocarditis, or modify its course in an appreciable degree. Salicylates, alkalies, iodides, quinine, internally, and applications over the præcordial area of blisters, sinapisms, leeches, and ice-bags have been tried, but it is impossible to estimate with any degree of confidence their influence on the inflammatory process. Salicylates and salicin, while exercising an undoubted influence on the rheumatic condition, have no effect on the inflammatory process as such, and they weaken the heart when taken continuously for any considerable time. Alkalies are less open to objection, especially when given with quinine: citrates may lessen the tendency to deposition of fibrin on the valves by diminishing the coagulability of the blood, and thus perhaps prove of service. We shall do the best for the patient by keeping him in bed and treating symptoms as they arise, giving only an effervescing mixture of quinine and citrate of potash. At any rate, no active measures should be taken which could in any way impair his strength or increase his discomfort. The patient should be kept in bed, not only during the attack, but for some weeks or months after it has subsided, till sufficient time has elapsed for the heart to recover, and for compensatory changes to take place. In children who come of a rheumatic stock, a careful look-out must be kept for any of the premonitory symptoms of rheumatism or heart inflammation, and if any suspicion is aroused that the heart is being attacked, the child should be kept in bed till all doubt is over.

# CHAPTER V.

## "MALIGNANT" OR "PERNICIOUS" ENDOCARDITIS.

NOMENCLATURE OF THE AFFECTION—MORBID ANATOMY—ETIOLOGY—THE RÔLE PLAYED BY VARIOUS MICRO-ORGANISMS—PHYSICAL SIGNS AND SYMPTOMS—INFARCTION AND EMBOLISM—DIAGNOSIS—PROGNOSIS—TREATMENT. CHRONIC ENDOCARDITIS.

To this form of endocarditis various epithets have been applied to distinguish it from "simple or rheumatic" endocarditis: "infective" because of its microbic origin, "malignant" because of its fatal tendency, "ulcerative" because of the severity of the lesions in the valves attacked. In view of recent researches, which tend to prove that rheumatism is a disease due to a specific micro-organism which may be widely distributed in the body, the term "infective" is no longer appropriate, nor is "ulcerative" specially suitable, as ulceration of the valves, though frequent and extensive, is not an essential characteristic. We are left, then, with "malignant," which, though not a highly scientific effort, may be truthfully employed as expressing the grave nature of the malady; but, inasmuch as recovery undoubtedly occurs in some cases, it is not employed in quite the same sense as when we speak of "malignant" disease as a synonym for carcinoma. We would venture to suggest the term "pernicious" as a more appropriate epithet, used in the same sense as in "pernicious anæmia," which, while it denotes the serious nature of the disease, does not necessarily connote a fatal issue.

It is indeed difficult, if not impossible, to draw a hard-and-fast line between "simple or rheumatic" and "pernicious" endocarditis, and, as will be seen later in the section on etiology, there is convincing evidence in favour of the view that "pernicious" endocarditis, in a certain proportion of cases, is a virulent form of rheumatic endocarditis, and due to the same micro-organism.

Because simple endocarditis is not a fatal malady, we rarely find at autopsies the small bead-like vegetations on the valves supposed to be characteristic of this affection, unless the patient has succumbed to pericarditis or some intercurrent malady. But in children it is a common experience to meet with repeated and prolonged attacks of endocarditis, in which the temperature ranges from 99 to 101 degrees for some weeks, and the cardiac murmur changes in character, the child becoming progressively anæmic, but eventually recovering, with well-marked signs of mitral incompetence. Because there is no evidence of infarction, and the temperature is not high, and the child does not succumb at the time, it is customary to classify these as cases of simple rheumatic endocarditis, though probably they form an intermediate group between the two extremes. Again, when we meet with old cicatrized lesions of the valves, such as the "button-hole" mitral orifice, or great deformity of the aortic valves, in patients who succumb from the effects of these chronic valvular lesions, which from their very appearance must have been due to extensive damage and ulceration of the valves which have healed and cicatrized, we may justly infer that these were cases of ulcerative endocarditis at the outset, and they form another link in the chain between the mild and fatal varieties of acute endocarditis.

Gibson, in his treatise on the Heart, does not make any distinction in nomenclature between the various grades, but includes all varieties under the term "acute endocarditis."

It is, however, convenient for clinical purposes to differentiate two main groups, as we have done here, as there

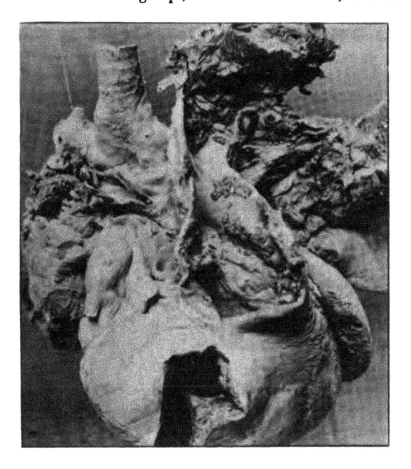

FIG. 8.—DESTRUCTION OF PULMONIC VALVES BY PERNICIOUS ENDOCARDITIS, AND VEGETATIONS ON THE PULMONARY ARTERY.

are certain clinical and pathological features which mark them off one from the other.

**Morbid Anatomy.**—The affected valves are usually masked by large, fungating vegetations readily detachable and extremely friable. On removal of these vegetations, the valve is frequently found to be partially or wholly destroyed by ulceration. The disease is often not limited to the valves, and vegetations or erosions may be present on the endocardium lining the cavities of the heart, especially the auricles, on the inner surface of the walls of the great vessels, as in Fig. 8, and along the chordæ tendineæ, which may be eroded or completely ulcerated through.

Microscopically, these vegetations are seen to consist of necrotic tissue, fibrin deposited from the blood stream in which may be entangled some red corpuscles and leucocytes, and in the deeper layers leucocytes and proliferating endothelial cells, or granulation tissue. Micro-organisms, usually micrococci in large masses, are invariably present in the superficial layers. *Vide* Fig. 9. The necrotic and amorphous appearance of the tissues in which the micro-organisms are embedded is very striking.

In certain of the more chronic cases the vegetations may assume a rounded, opaque, or verrucose form, and be of considerable size, consisting of pale, lobulated excrescences with smooth, rounded surfaces. Microscopically, it will be seen that the deeper layers consist of actively proliferating endothelial and connective tissue cells in process of organization into fibrous tissue, while the upper layers consist of fibrin and leucocytes more or less necrotic and amorphous, with few nuclei, staining very faintly. Micro-organisms are not present in large masses on the free borders, but may be undiscoverable or very difficult to find, and only revealed after careful search through many sections. If found, they do not take the stain well, and appear to be dead or moribund. Because of this absence or scarcity of micro-organisms, some observers have held that this was a special variety of simple rheumatic endocarditis, and have differentiated it under the name "verrucose endocarditis" (*vide* Fig. 10). These "verrucose" vegetations are, however, usually found in cases of long duration, and they are in all probability, from the pathological appearances, cases in which the disease has been wholly or partially arrested and repair is taking place, but the patient succumbs from exhaustion or from the effect of the valvular lesion.

Besides the cardiac lesions, there are commonly secondary lesions in the spleen, kidney, or brain, due to embolism from portions of the vegetations which are detached from the valves and lodge in the smaller arterioles. In the organs

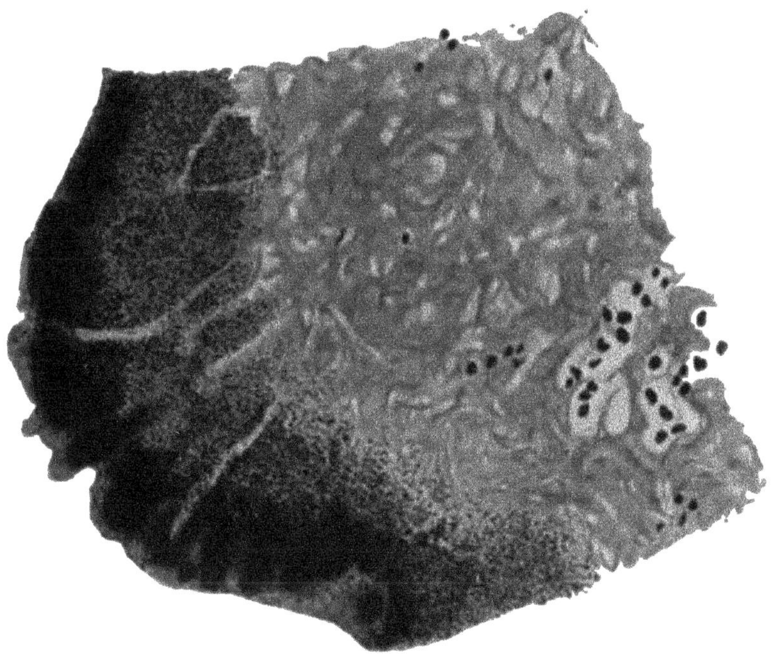

FIG. 9.—SHOWING MASSES OF MICRO-ORGANISMS IN THE VALVES (× 560).

above mentioned, the lodgment of an embolus in one of the terminal arterioles causes the death of the tissue supplied by that branch, as there is insufficient collateral circulation to nourish the part when its blood supply is suddenly cut off. The portion of tissue therefore undergoes coagulation necrosis, and the resulting condition is known as an "infarct." Infarcts in the kidney and spleen are usually wedge-shaped, but may be of irregular outline, and are almost invariably anæmic, *i.e.* of a pale, dead white colour, with a zone of congestion round the nerotic area, though occasionally in the spleen they are red or hæmorrhagic.

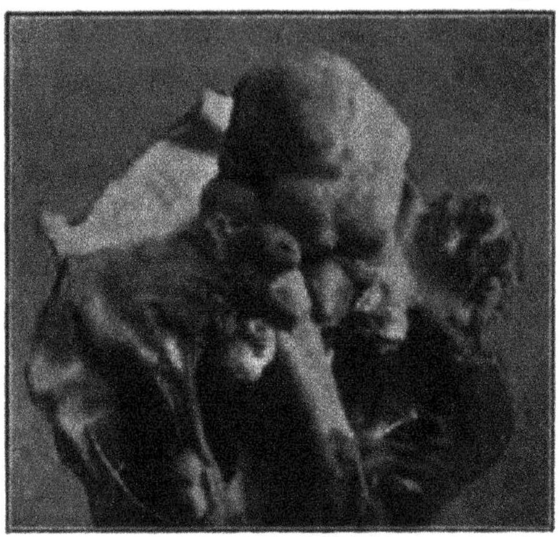

FIG. 10.—MITRAL VALVE, SHOWING "VERRUCOSE" VEGETATIONS.

**Etiology.**—Micro-organisms are almost invariably present in abundance in the vegetations on the affected valves, where they can be readily demonstrated by microscopic examination, and they can frequently be isolated in pure culture from the blood of the patient during life. They are usually micrococci. Some difference of opinion exists as to their nature, and as to whether any one specific micro-organism is the etiological factor in this disease. Previous to the isolation and identification of the diplococcus isolated in rheumatism, various observers had experimented with pure cultures obtained from the valves in malignant endocarditis. By injection of these into the jugular veins of animals, some experimenters with, and some without previous injury to the valves, had produced valvulitis, in some instances accompanied by metastatic infarcts. The organism found was not the same in all cases. Among the organisms which have been isolated from cases of malignant endocarditis are, the staphylococcus aureus and albus, and citreus, the streptococcus pyogenes, the pneumococcus, and the gonococcus, and the influenza bacillus.

In 1903,* Poynton and Paine read an important paper, in which they show that malignant endocarditis may be

* *Med. Chir. Trans.*, Vol. 85.

set up by a diplococcus, indistinguishable from that which they have isolated in rheumatic fever. They give an account of a series of cases of pernicious endocarditis, with a clinical history and an account of the post-mortem examination, in which they obtained from the affected valves a diplococcus, cultures of which, inoculated into rabbits, reproduced pernicious endocarditis in those animals. This diplococcus they considered to be identical with that which they have previously isolated in cases of pericarditis and endocarditis associated with rheumatic fever. By inoculating rabbits with an attenuated culture of this diplococcus obtained from a case of pernicious endocarditis, they showed that it might give rise to pericarditis without valvulitis, or to a disease indistinguishable from rheumatic fever. Conversely, by inoculating a rabbit with a culture of a diplococcus originally obtained from a case of rheumatic fever, the virulence of which had been raised by passage through several rabbits, they produced in the animal well-marked pernicious endocarditis.

In all the cases they describe in this paper there was a history of rheumatic fever at some period previous to the attack of pernicious endocarditis.

In view of these results, it is only fair to admit that pernicious endocarditis may in some cases, if not in a large proportion, be due to infection by the rheumatic diplococcus, and that it occurs either because the virulence of the micro-organism is great, or more probably because the resistance of the individual attacked is very low. Injury to the valve is probably an important etiological factor, for in the majority of cases pernicious endocarditis affects valves which have been damaged in a previous attack of rheumatism.

We must now consider the *rôle* played by other micro-organisms which have been met with in this disease.

1. **The Pyogenic Organisms.**—Numerous observers have testified to the presence of the streptococcus pyogenes, the

staphylococcus aureus and albus in the vegetations on the affected valve and in the blood, and cultures have been made from the blood during life and from the vegetations after death.

Of these, the streptococcus pyogenes is the most commonly found, and next in frequency the staphylococcus aureus. Combinations of two of these organisms are also frequently met with, *e.g.* of the streptococcus and staphylococcus aureus, or albus, or of the staphylococcus aureus and albus. If we admit the possibility of a specific rheumatic diplococcus being a cause of pernicious endocarditis, it is probable that it may frequently be one of the organisms in a mixed infection, but not be recognized, because it is a delicate organism and requires special culture media for its growth.

It is a remarkable fact that while many observers have succeeded in producing endocarditis in rabbits by inoculation of pure cultures obtained from a case of pernicious endocarditis in man, few have succeeded in producing this condition by inoculation of cultures of the streptococcus or staphylococcus pyogenes obtained from other sources, *e.g.* cases of pyæmia or septicæmia. Cole * has succeeded in doing so with cultures derived from puerperal fever and peritonitis, as already mentioned. Poynton and Paine † made several attempts with different brands of pyogenic organisms, and succeeded in some instances, but the usual result was septicæmia and the early death of the inoculated animal. Again, though ulcerative endocarditis is met with sometimes in cases of septicæmia, pyæmia, puerperal fever, erysipelas, osteomyelitis, etc., it is the exception rather than the rule, and we would expect it to be very common were the pyogenic organisms mainly responsible for the disease known as malignant or pernicious endocarditis. It is also remarkable that infarcts in this affection so rarely suppurate.

* *Journ. Infect. Diseases*, vol. i. No. 4, 1904.

† *Trans. Med. Chir. Soc.*, Vol. 85.

These considerations tend to support the view of Paine and Poynton that pernicious endocarditis may in some instances be a form of pernicious rheumatism.

**The Pneumococcus.**—Pernicious endocarditis is sometimes met with in association with pneumonia and pneumococcal meningitis, and the pneumococcus has been frequently isolated from the affected valves. Netter * has written several important papers on this subject, and has produced an ulcerative endocarditis in rabbits after injury to a valve by inoculation of cultures of the pneumococcus. Michaelis † has also produced the affection in dogs by repeated inoculation of cultures of the pneumococcus at frequent intervals. Osler, Weichselbaum, Huchard, and many others have published cases of pneumococcal endocarditis.

We must therefore admit the pneumococcus as one of the causes of pernicious endocarditis, though, when it is found, pneumonia or meningitis is usually the primary disease.

**The Gonococcus.**—That ulcerative endocarditis can be caused by the genococcus was first shown by Gluzinski. Schedler, His, ‡ Councilman,§ and others have confirmed his observations. Harris ‖ and Johnson have recently described two cases of gonococcal endocarditis, and in a paper read before the Pathological Society in April, 1905, Horder describes a case of malignant endocarditis, in which he isolated the gonococcus from the blood during life and from the affected valve post mortem.

**Pfeiffer's Influenza Bacillus.**—Some cases of ulcerative endocarditis due to this organism have recently been described.

Austin ¶ has published an account of three cases in which he found Pfeiffer's influenza bacillus in the affected valves. Horder ** has also published two cases which he attributes to this bacillus.

* *Soc. Anat.*, March, 1886; *Arch. de Phys.*, 1886, etc.
† *Med. Soc. of Berlin*, 1895.
‡ *Berlin Klin. Woch.*, 1892.
§ *Amer. Jour. Med. Sc.*, 1893.
‖ *Journ. Amer. Phys.*, 1902.
¶ John Hopkins' Reports, 1899.
** *Trans. Path. Soc.*, April, 1905.

Other micro-organisms which have occasionally been found in the affected valves in pernicious endocarditis are the bacillus endocarditis griseus of Weichselbaum, the bacillus capsulatus of the same author, and the bacillus coli.

Pernicious endocarditis may occur as a complication in scarlet fever and smallpox, and in erysipelas, puerperal fever, pyæmia, septicæmia, esteomyelitis, and pneumonia, as has already been stated.

**Modes of Infection.**—The ways in which the micro-organisms which attack the valves may obtain admittance to the circulation are manifold: by the skin, as in cases of open wounds; by the mucous membranes of the pharynx, especially the tonsils, or of the intestines; by the genito-urinary, and by the respiratory tracts. All, therefore, may be, at one time or other, exposed to the attacks of the pyogenic microbes, which give rise to this form of endocarditis, but in only a small proportion of cases are the endocardial tissues specially susceptible.

**Symptoms and Physical Signs.**—While it is difficult to draw a hard-and-fast line between simple and pernicious endocarditis, there are certain clinical features which may be said to distinguish the latter. These are prolonged irregular pyrexia of a septicæmic type, the occurrence of embolism, change in the character of the cardiac murmurs, progressive anæmia and loss of flesh. Rigors may occur, but are not common.

The age of the patient is also of importance. Malignant endocarditis appears to be a disease of young adult, or middle life, and is rare in young children. From an analysis of seventeen cases on which I made post-mortem examinations during the years 1900 to 1904 at St. Mary's Hospital, I find the average age works out at 34. Curiously enough, this almost exactly coincides with the average age arrived at by Dreschfield from an analysis of cases during a period of four years at the Manchester Infirmary, namely 34½.

The youngest of the patients in the St. Mary's cases was

16, the oldest 54, and no less than thirteen out of seventeen were between the ages of 22 and 45.

**The Temperature.**—This may vary considerably. Sometimes the onset is insidious and the temperature is little raised above normal, ranging from 99 to 100, with intervals of apyrexia for some days. Later on, as the symptoms become more pronounced, the temperature ranges high, and assumes a septicæmic type, running up to 102, 103, or 104 in some period of the twenty-four hours, and dropping to 99 or 100 at another. In the final stages, when the patient is exhausted by the disease, it is frequently subnormal in the morning and

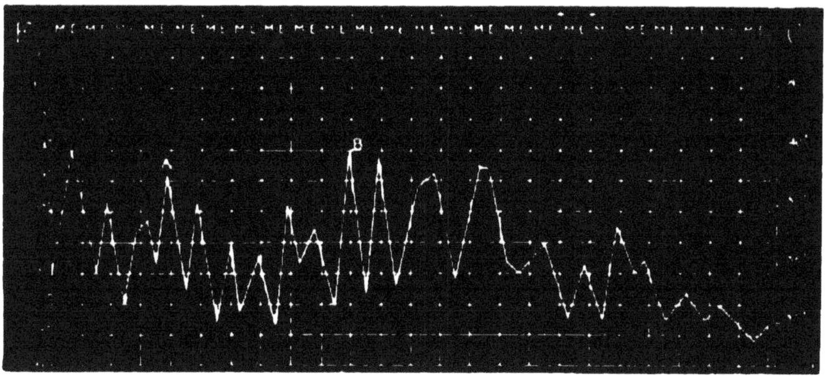

TEMPERATURE CHART FROM CASE OF PERNICIOUS ENDOCARDITIS

only slightly above normal in the evening. Exacerbations of temperature usually mark the occurrence of infarcts.

The above temperature chart, from the later stages of a severe case, shows the extreme irregularity of temperature that may occur.

There was evidence of infarction of the kidney and spleen respectively when the temperature rose to 103° and 104° F. at the points marked A and B on the chart.

**Infarction.**—Infarction of the spleen will commonly be attended with pain in the left hypochondriac region, with tenderness of and possibly some enlargement of the spleen. Infarct of the kidney is usually marked by pain in the loin, followed by hæmaturia and albuminuria, but these may sometimes be absent, and hæmaturia may occur as a result of nephritis without infarction.

Of the cerebral vessels, the middle cerebral artery is the most common seat of embolism, an embolus being especially liable to lodge where it divides into its four main branches opposite the island of Reil.

Hemiplegia may result with aphasia if on the left side; sometimes this may pass off in four to six days from shrinkage of the embolus or establishment of some collateral circulation. In a case of which the specimen is in the St. Mary's Hospital Museum, a man of 23, suffering from malignant endocarditis, suddenly became aphasic and lost all power in his right side. In five days he had completely recovered his speech and almost entirely the power in his limbs. Post mortem the embolus was found to have lodged in the left middle cerebral artery where it divides into its main branches. The embolus had apparently shrunk, and did not occlude two of the branches.

Embolism of the superior mesenteric artery may occur, giving rise to gangrene of the small intestine, with symptoms of collapse and shock followed by profuse melæna.

Embolism of the arteries of the extremities may cause pain and temporary numbness with pallor and coldness of the limb if a large vessel is blocked, but usually collateral circulation is established and the symptoms pass off.

Aneurysms are occasionally met with as a result of lodgment of emboli containing micro-organisms in an artery and the destructive action of the toxins of the organisms in the vessel wall. They may be multiple or single. In the St. Mary's Hospital Museum is a specimen with thirteen aneurysms of the coronary artery of the heart. I have seen two instances of aneurysm of the gluteal artery, and one of the femoral, and aneurysms of the cerebral and various other arteries have been described, so that it would appear that almost any artery may be affected.

Infarcts in the lung are exceptional, not merely because the disease is commonly confined to the left side of the heart, but because lodgment of an embolus in a small branch of the pulmonary artery, if the valves of the right side of the heart are affected, would probably not cause an infarct, unless there is in addition extreme pulmonary congestion from back working.

Sometimes numerous capillary embolisms occur, giving rise to petechiæ on the skin.

**The Cardiac Murmurs.**—The development of a murmur in association with a previously healthy valve will, of course, give a clue to the condition, but not infrequently the valve attacked is already the seat of a previous lesion, and a murmur may already be present. Change in the character of the murmur should be carefully watched for and noted; it may become softer and weaker, or louder and musical. The development of a fresh murmur at another orifice should also be looked out for.

**Anæmia** is usually pronounced and progressive, and the complexion assumes a waxy and sallow hue.

**The Appetite** may remain good and the tongue clean till a very late stage in the disease, and gastro-intestinal troubles are not usually marked, though diarrhœa is often present in the septicæmic types.

**Diagnosis.**—When a cardiac murmur of recent development is present, associated with pyrexia, a high range of temperature of an irregular or septicæmic type and the occurrence of embolism will usually enable a diagnosis to be made early in the course of the disease. The persistence of the irregular pyrexia, the progressive anæmia, the sallow complexion, loss of flesh, and occurrence of embolism, will afford confirmatory evidence of the malignant character of the endocarditis. In young children we frequently meet with prolonged subacute attacks of cardiac rheumatism, in which a valvular murmur may be present, associated with pyrexia, lasting many weeks; but in these cases recurrent attacks of pericarditis are the rule, and this, with the accompanying myocarditis leading to cardiac dilatation, is the more serious malady, and is readily recognised. It would, indeed, seem that in young children we have a type of pernicious pericarditis corresponding to the pernicious endocarditis of adults.

When no murmur exists, or when a valvular murmur of old standing is present, in association with pyrexia of unexplained cause, a differential diagnosis may have to be made from typhoid fever, septicæmia, and acute miliary tuberculosis. Typhoid can, after a week or ten days, be identified by the eruption of spots, abdominal symptoms, condition of the tongue, and Widal's reaction. Septicæmia, in the ordinary sense of the term, may be usually traced to some source of septic infection, but inasmuch as pernicious endocarditis is a septicæmia complicated by a valvular lesion, it is out of place to use the term "differential diagnosis" in this connection. In acute miliary tuberculosis, if we cannot discover any old tubercular lesion, we may have to wait till definite signs in the lungs or the onset of tubercular meningitis disclose its nature.

Change in the character of a pre-existing murmur, or the development of a valvular murmur, and the occurrence of embolism will usually, sooner or later, make clear the nature of the malady in pernicious endocarditis.

In the acute cases cultures of micrococii can frequently be made from 10 c.c. of blood withdrawn under aseptic precautions by a sterile syringe from the median basilic vein, and inoculated into suitable culture media.

It must be borne in mind that possibly the rheumatic diplococcus is responsible for a certain number of cases, and the culture media must be selected accordingly. These micro-organisms do not flourish in broth or on agar, though they may grow feebly, but, according to Poynton and

Paine, grow best in milk, so this, or blood agar, on which Shaw* finds they grow freely, should be included.

**Prognosis.**—The prognosis is, as the name implies, very grave. In the acute cases, when the temperature ranges high, and embolism takes place early, recovery is rare, and the disease may prove fatal in a few weeks. In the more chronic cases of insidious onset, unexpected recovery sometimes takes place after the lapse of two months or more, when the patient seems almost reduced to the last extremity. That a certain proportion of cases recover in which severe ulceration of the valves has taken place, attended with infarction of the kidney or spleen, is demonstrated from time to time by post-mortem examinations, in which greatly deformed cicatrized valves or cicatrices on the endocardium and old cicatrized infarcts are found some years later. In a large group of cases, in which there is no evidence of infarction, the lesions found in the valves indicate that extensive ulceration and destruction must have taken place during the attack of acute endocarditis. The two last-mentioned groups could scarcely be classified as "malignant," inasmuch as the acute disease did not prove fatal, though they were undoubtedly instances of "ulcerative endocarditis." The question of prognosis will therefore vary with the degree of virulence of the causative micro-organism and the resistance of the individual, as evidenced by the formation of protective substances in the blood, or the reverse.

**Treatment.**—Various drugs have been tried without any appreciable result. Salicylates are useless: salol, sulpho-carbolate of soda, and benzoate of soda have been freely given, but have not proved to be of service. Perchloride of mercury, administered freely, has seemed to be efficacious in some cases. General tonics, such as iron quinine and strychnine, are of most value, as they help to maintain the

* Etiology of Acute Rheumatic Fever, *Journal of Path. and Bact.* December, 1903.

strength of the patient, though they are not in any sense a specific remedy. Citric acid may be given with advantage, as it reduces the coagulability of the blood by combining with the calcium salts, and thereby lessens the tendency to formation of clot on the diseased valve and the chauces of embolism. Possibly thymus gland may be of service by stimulating the production of leucocytes.

Good results have been claimed from time to time by various authors from the injection of antistreptococcic serum. As the disease may be set up possibly by the rheumatic organism, possibly by streptococci, or pneumococci, or gonococci, it is obvious that the indiscriminate use of a so-called antistreptococcic serum is not rational or scientific, even if one were sure that the serum really possessed any antitoxic substances, and this we have as yet no accurate means of determining.

## CHRONIC ENDOCARDITIS.

Under this heading are comprised certain chronic degenerative changes in the valves which set in insidiously in later life, and are usually associated with degenerative changes in the aorta. They are to be distinguished from chronic valvular lesions, which are the result of cicatrization after an attack of acute endocarditis.

### Morbid Anatomy.

The valves become thickened and opaque and lose their elasticity. The aorta is usually dilated and atheromatous. The aortic valves are chiefly affected, and though there is no actual loss of substance, the rigidity of the cusps, together with the dilatation of the aorta, occasions a certain degree of incompetence. Sometimes calcareous plates may be present in the aorta at the root of the valves, and project into the cusps themselves. A certain degree of obstruction may result, giving rise to a systolic aortic murmur, but this may be due to roughening of the valves without actual stenosis. The mitral valve is affected to a less degree than the aortic, but becomes thickened and opaque, and slight incompetence may result.

**Etiology.**—Among the recognized causes of chronic degenerative valvular lesions are lead poisoning, gout, kidney disease, and what Murchison termed lithæmia, from excessive eating and drinking with defective elimination. These are conditions associated with high arterial tension, involving constant undue strain on the aorta and its valves.

Valvular change of like character is common in men following certain arduous occupations, such as those of the miner, collier, blacksmith, hammerman, and soldier. Here we have undue intermittent pressure within the aorta. As was pointed out by Clifford Allbutt, Fothergill, and others, in the occupations mentioned the undue pressure is created by effort in a constrained and cramped position, or by work of such a character as to require prolonged closure of the glottis and fixation of the chest by holding the breath, or by violent muscular exertion constantly repeated throughout the day.

**Heredity** is an important factor in connection with high arterial tension, due to gout or lithæmia, as the tendency may be transmitted through many generations.

**Age.**—Degenerative changes in the valves usually set in after middle life, from the age of 40 to 45 onwards, and are frequently associated with degenerative changes in the aorta or cerebral vessels.

In later life, apart from actual disease, there is a tendency to thickening, opacity, and loss of elasticity in the valves, which in some instances may give rise to a murmur.

**Syphilis** may be incriminated in a certain proportion of cases, especially where degenerative changes occur early in life.

The symptoms and physical signs vary according to the valve affected, and are discussed later in the chapters on the different valvular lesions.

## CHAPTER VI.

### ETIOLOGY OF VALVULAR LESIONS.

**Acute Endocarditis.**—This is by far the most common cause of valvular lesions. This has already been fully discussed in a previous chapter. The acute inflammatory process may rapidly impair the efficiency of the valve and render it incompetent. Subsequent cicatricial contraction of the fibrous tissue formed in the process of repair may still further impair its efficiency, or give rise to progressive stenosis, which may result, in extreme cases, in a narrow funnel-shaped rigid orifice less than half an inch in diameter.

**Chronic Endocarditis.**—Chronic endocarditis is an insidious affection occurring in middle or later life, usually due to high arterial tension, whether from gout, kidney disease, or other causes, and intimately associated with the degenerative change known as atheroma of the aorta. The valves become thickened, and lose their elasticity, and incompetence usually results from this in conjunction with dilatation of the aorta. Syphilis may be a cause, especially when atheroma of the aorta occurs early in life, associated with degenerative change in the valves.

**Rupture of a Valve.**—Rupture of a valve is of rare occurrence. It is usually the aortic valve which suffers, and, except as a result of direct violence, the rupture will nearly always have been preceded by disease in its structure, and by the cause of such disease, high arterial tension. The rupture usually takes place during some severe muscular exertion, and is attended by great pain in the region of the heart. It may be a complete or partial rupture of one of the cusps of the aortic valve, or may be a mere slit in it.

One or more tendinous cords of the mitral valve may be found ruptured when this valve has been the seat of disease; but this occurrence can rarely be dated by any recognized accession of symptoms, though it must give rise to a considerable increase in the derangement of the circulation.

**Dilatation of the Orifice of a Valve.**—Dilatation of the orifice may upset the functional efficiency of a valve while the valve itself has not undergone any material change. The aortic orifice is less liable to be stretched and enlarged than the mitral, as would be expected from the difference in the structures surrounding the two. It is only comparatively late in life that the strong fibrous ring at the root of the aorta ever yields, and it will then only take place as part of a general dilatation of the first part of this vessel, the result of atheroma or chronic degenerative changes. The usual result is more or less insufficiency or regurgitation; but, paradoxical as it may appear, there may actually be obstruction as well, the valves being rigid and projecting, even during systole, across the dilated mouth of the aorta.

Mitral insufficiency from failure of fairly healthy valves to close the orifice is not uncommon. Sometimes the orifice is very much enlarged, admitting four or five fingers instead of three. Frequently, however, there is no stretching of the opening, and the valves themselves are unaffected, although during life there has certainly been regurgitation. Various explanations of this fact have been offered. It has been supposed that irregular action of the papillary muscles interferes with the accurate adjustment of the valvular curtains; and, again, that the papillary muscles, being carried by dilatation of the ventricle so far from the valvular ring that the tendinous cords are dragged down too far, do not allow the margins of the valves to meet during the systole.

The real cause of the imperfect closure of the valves is that originally suggested by Donald McAlister.* He pointed out that an important factor in the valvular mechanism is the active contraction of the mitral orifice with the systole of the ventricle. We are accustomed to imagine that this opening, like the aortic, is surrounded by a strong fibrous ring, maintaining its form and patency under all circumstances; but this is not the case, as was shown by Sibson in dissections and specimens, which I had the pleasure of assisting him to prepare; for it was demonstrated that the mitral ring of fibrous tissue, taking its origin from the central fibro-cartilage of the heart, gradually thins out till at the opposite side of the orifice it is practically non-existent. There is nothing, therefore, to keep the mitral orifice rigid, or prevent it from altering its shape; hence we find that, during systole, the transversely circular fibres of the cardiac muscle, by their contraction, cause a narrowing of the mitral orifice, and partially close it independently of the valves. Such a closure is in effect a part of the general obliteration of the ventricular cavity during systole. When, therefore, there is dilatation of the ventricle, this active constriction of the auriculo-ventricular opening is imperfectly performed, and the valve fails to cover the whole area of the orifice.

Mitral regurgitation caused in this way, may occur at any period of life, and under very different conditions. The cardiac dilatation may be the result of imperfect nutrition in advancing years, or of debilitating influences, or it may be induced by acute disease, such as enteric fever or acute rheumatism. Perhaps the most common and important cause is anæmia; it is most important because of its frequency in young adults, and because, though curable, it

* *British Medical Journal*, August, 1882.

is yet liable to be rendered permanent by imprudence and neglect. George Balfour has rendered good service by calling attention to this condition under the head of "Curable Mitral Regurgitation." Now, although weakness of the cardiac muscular fibres, or want of energy in their contraction, is perhaps an essential condition in the production of dilatation, another factor plays an important part, namely, high arterial tension. We should not expect anæmia to be attended with any such state of the circulation, but this is very frequently the case in the ordinary type.

Pernicious anæmia, however, is less commonly attended with high arterial tension, perhaps because of the frequent intercurrent attacks of pyrexia; for pyrexia, as is well known, relaxes arteries and lowers the arterial tension.

It may be remarked in passing, that the low arterial tension which accompanies pyrexia probably renders the occurrence of dilatation of the ventricle much less frequent in acute disease than we should expect as a result of the debilitating effect of the accompanying myocarditis or "cloudy swelling" of the muscular walls of the heart.

Mitral incompetence may, further, be a secondary consequence of aortic incompetence, through the dilatation of the left ventricle. But, unless cardiac debility have a share in the production of this dilatation, a comparison between it and the dilatation just spoken of is illusory. The one is the result of asthenia, the other of over-distension of the ventricular cavity; in the one, the contraction of the ventricle is never completed; in the other, it is carried through energetically.

**Congenital Valvular Affections.**—Lesions of one or more of the valves of the heart are sometimes found at birth. They may be the result of a congenital malformation, or of endocarditis occurring while the fœtus was in utero. In the former case the pulmonic valve is most commonly at fault, the lesion being usually constriction of the orifice, and frequently the valvular defect is associated with a malformation of some other portion of the heart. In the latter case the valves of the right side of the heart usually suffer, but those of the left side may also be affected, the aortic more commonly than the mitral.

# CHAPTER VII.

## VALVULAR LESIONS.

POINTS TO BE CONSIDERED IN STUDYING A CASE OF VALVULAR DISEASE—THE PHYSICAL SIGNS—CARDIAC MURMURS, THEIR SIGNIFICANCE AS REGARDS THE SEAT AND AS REGARDS THE EXTENT OF THE LESION—MODIFICATION OF HEART-SOUNDS—THE PULSE, ITS IMPORTANCE IN DIAGNOSIS.

DISEASES of the heart are classified as structural and valvular, according as the morbid change affects the muscular walls or the valves. There are, again, functional derangements which must be included among the affections of the heart.

The valvular lesions will be first discussed: they are what is usually understood by heart disease, and are most important because most numerous. We know more about them, and can be more certain of their diagnosis, thanks to the murmurs to which alterations in the valves give rise. We are also in a better position to estimate the extent of the lesion, and to give an accurate prognosis in valvular disease than in structural. The estimation of the obstruction produced by a certain degree of narrowing of one or other orifice, or of the amount of reflux resulting from incompetence of a given valve, is a problem of hydrostatics capable of solution, but no such definite conclusion can be arrived at, when in structural disease we have to form an opinion as to the contractile power and durability of muscular fibres in a certain stage of degeneration.

## The Clinical Study of Valvular Disease.

In studying a case of valvular disease of the heart, the following are the points which must be taken into consideration:—

1. The valve affected, and the relative danger attaching to the particular lesion.
2. The actual condition of the orifice and valve—the degree of obstruction or amount of regurgitation to which the lesion has given rise.
3. The origin of the lesion, whether due to acute rheumatism, degenerative changes, or other causes.
4. The degree of soundness and vigour, functional and nutritional; firstly, of the muscular substance of the heart itself; secondly, of the tissues generally. How far, in fact, and for how long compensatory changes can be counted upon. In considering this question, family history will have an important place.

## Localization of the Valvular Disease.—Significance of the Cardiac Murmurs.

The chief guide in localizing disease in the valves of the heart is a murmur, produced, either by obstruction to the current of blood when one or other orifice is narrowed or roughened, or by regurgitation of the blood when a valve no longer closes perfectly. The term stenosis or constriction is employed to denote the condition of an orifice which is narrowed, the result of the narrowing being obstruction: the term insufficiency or incompetence is employed to characterize the state of a valve which fails to close the opening it ought to protect, while regurgitation or reflux expresses the functional effect. It is well, as far as possible, to observe the distinction between the names indicative of structural change and those expressive of functional derangement resulting therefrom, but the terms "obstruction" and "regurgitation" are in such familiar use that they are frequently employed when "stenosis" and "insufficiency" would be more exact.

By means of the murmurs we learn definitely which valve is affected and what is the nature of the affection—whether such as to produce obstruction or regurgitation—but they fail altogether by themselves to indicate the amount of damage which a valve has sustained. A loud murmur may be produced by a very slight change, and a murmur which is scarcely audible may be indicative of extensive destruction of valves. Some information, however, may be gathered from a careful study of murmurs.

## Different Characters of Murmurs: their Value as regards Estimation of the Extent of the Valvular Lesion.

Murmurs may be compared or contrasted in several respects: in intensity, they may be loud or soft; in duration, they may be long or short; they may be blowing, or musical, or mixed, rough and vibratory, or smooth. Again, they may begin with an accent, or rise gradually to a maximum intensity.

A loud murmur is, on the whole, of less serious import than one which is weak and soft. It is, at any rate, indicative of force in the heart's action, and of vigour in the movement of the blood; and weakness of the heart constitutes the greatest of all dangers. Then, again, although a rough edge to a large opening in aortic or mitral incompetence may generate vibrations which will produce a loud murmur, a mere slit in a membranous valve, or a shred of fibrin hanging by one end, is more likely to have such an effect.

In a case seen with Dr. Parrott of Hayes, a systolic mitral murmur, of such intensity as to be heard distinctly across a billiard-table, had been present for fifteen or twenty years without giving rise to symptoms, until dilatation of the heart was induced by extreme over-exertion. Another very loud murmur which came under my notice was attended with no important symptoms for the several months during which the patient was under observation. It was systolic aortic, and could be heard half a yard or more from the chest, through the man's clothes. In another case, a murmur almost as loud was found, after death, to be due to a delicate fibrinous thread at the free margin of one of the aortic valves.

On the other hand, cases are met with in which the pulse may indicate serious aortic regurgitation while no diastolic murmur can be heard, and a murmur gradually develops itself as the patient gains strength and recovers from a state of extreme prostration; and it is common in mitral stenosis for murmurs to disappear with the supervention of serious symptoms, and to reappear as these are abated by treatment. It must not be concluded that a soft or weak murmur is necessarily indicative of either a failing heart or greatly damaged valve; but a diminution in the intensity of a murmur, gradual or sudden, may confirm unfavourable indications given by symptoms.

The character of a murmur—its roughness or vibratory character or smoothness—may have diagnostic significance, as will be pointed out later, but it does not give any information with regard to the extent of structural change or functional derangement. A musical murmur would seem to require for its production either a very fine chink with thin margins, or a thin membrane capable of vibrating like a string, and would therefore seem to be inconsistent with serious disease; but this cannot be laid down as an absolute rule. A musical note is often heard in the midst of a blowing murmur or at the beginning or end of such a murmur. A long murmur, except in the case of mitral or aortic stenosis, is usually indicative of early and comparatively slight disease and of efficient action of the heart. A short murmur may be innocent of prognostic import, but it is very frequently an indication of ruined valves and of a failing heart: it may, for instance, indicate that the orifice is so patent, say, in aortic insufficiency, that the refluent blood passes through it rapidly and with little hindrance; or in mitral disease, that the systole is brief and imperfect, the heart being on the point of breaking down.

The accent at the beginning of a murmur is chiefly observed in the regurgitant diastolic murmur of aortic insufficiency where it represents the second sound, and it is important as showing that the valves still act as a check on the reflux of blood from the aorta. It has the same significance in a minor degree as persistence of the aortic second sound—a very important fact, which will be fully explained later, in the chapter on aortic regurgitation.

It will thus be seen that the murmurs, while pointing out distinctly and certainly what valve is affected, afford also some information as to the extent of change which has taken place, though only of a vague character.

## Modification of Heart-Sounds.

The heart-sounds may be modified by murmurs in various ways. A mitral systolic or an aortic diastolic murmur may accompany, replace, or follow the sound with which it is associated in the cardiac cycle. Generally speaking, when the heart-sound is distinctly heard as well as the accompanying murmur, the lesion is slight: when, on the contrary, it is entirely replaced by the murmur, the lesion is probably severe.

When a mitral murmur follows the first sound at a brief

but appreciable interval, constituting a "retarded systolic" murmur, it seems to show that the valves come together accurately at first, but fail to remain in apposition throughout the whole period of the ventricular contraction. It indicates, therefore, that the changes in the valves, and consequently the amount of leakage, can only be slight. A "retarded diastolic" aortic murmur is sometimes met with, but it has not the same favourable significance.

The first sound in association with the presystolic murmur of mitral stenosis may be greatly modified. It is not replaced by the murmur, but is usually altered in character, becoming short, sharp, and high-pitched.

## The Pulmonic Second Sound.

This is usually accentuated to a varying degree in mitral affections, owing to increase of pressure in the pulmonary circulation. There are two factors instrumental in causing this increase of pressure—obstruction to the outflow of blood from the pulmonary veins into the left auricle, due to the mitral lesion; and increased driving power of the right ventricle, the result of compensatory hypertrophy. The degree of accentuation of the pulmonic second sound depends on the degree of pressure in the pulmonary circulation: it will thus afford important evidence as to the amount of reflux or obstruction caused by the mitral lesion, and also as to the state of efficiency of the right ventricle. For instance, if in a case of mitral disease the pulmonic second sound is greatly accentuated, it will tend to show that the mitral lesion is one of some severity, and, as confirmatory evidence, we should expect to find hypertrophy of the right ventricle. Bronchitis, or any intercurrent lung trouble, increasing the obstruction to the flow of blood through the lungs, will ıd to cause still greater accentuation of the pulmonic second sound, provided that the right ventricle does not break down under the strain. If in a severe case of mitral disease the pulmonic second sound, from being greatly accentuated, becomes feeble or much diminished in intensity, it will indicate, not, of course, that the valvular lesion is less, but that the right ventricle is beginning to fail.

The aortic second sound will be accentuated when the tension in the systemic circulation is high from any cause; it will be altered in intensity and pitch in aneurysm, or in dilatation of the aorta.

## Reduplication of Heart-Sounds.

**Reduplication of the second sound** heard at the apex of the heart indicates that the pulmonic and aortic valves do not close synchronously. It is of common occurrence in mitral disease, especially in mitral stenosis, when it indicates that the pressure in the pulmonary circulation has become so considerable as to cause the pulmonic valves to close before the aortic.

**Reduplication of the first sound** heard at the apex indicates that the two ventricles do not accomplish their systole simultaneously, owing to the fact that one is beginning to give way under extra strain imposed on it. It is not infrequently met with in advanced aortic stenosis, or in cases of high arterial tension, such as results from kidney disease; it will then show that the left ventricle is beginning to fail.

## Alterations in the Cardiac Rhythm.

**Intermission** is less frequent than irregularity as a result of valvular disease. The particular affections in which this deviation from the normal rhythm is most liable to occur are aortic incompetence, when it indicates a faltering of the heart's action, and certain functional disturbances due to a reflex from gastric troubles. Irregularity is very common as a result of mitral incompetence, when it is not of serious import. It may also occur in association with fibroid degeneration of the heart walls in conjunction with general arterio-sclerosis, when the prognosis is grave, as death may occur from a syncopal attack, or hemiplegia result from rupture of a cerebral vessel.

## THE PULSE.

### INFORMATION TO BE GATHERED FROM THE PULSE AS TO THE NATURE AND EXTENT OF VALVULAR LESION.

In aortic stenosis the artery will be somewhat small, and full between the beats; the initial percussion-wave will be slight and gradual, and the pulse-wave prolonged. This modification of the pulse is due to the fact that the blood has to pass through a narrowed orifice on its way from the left ventricle into the aorta. Hence the impact of the systole upon the column of blood in the aorta will be diminished, and more time will be required for the passage of the contents of the ventricle into the arterial system.

In aortic incompetence we have the well-known collapsing or water-hammer pulse; the artery is large, and empty between the beats; the pulse-wave is sudden, forcible, short, and ill-sustained, and its cessation is very abrupt.

In mitral stenosis the artery is small, full between the beats, with higher tension than would be expected, and the pulse-wave is long.

In all these three forms of valve-lesion the pulse is regular till the heart begins to break down.

In mitral regurgitation, on the other hand, the pulse is usually irregular, both in force and frequency, if the lesion is at all severe. The pulse-wave is also short, and passes the finger rapidly.

The characteristics of the different types of pulse, as brought out by the sphygmograph, are shown in the accompanying tracings.

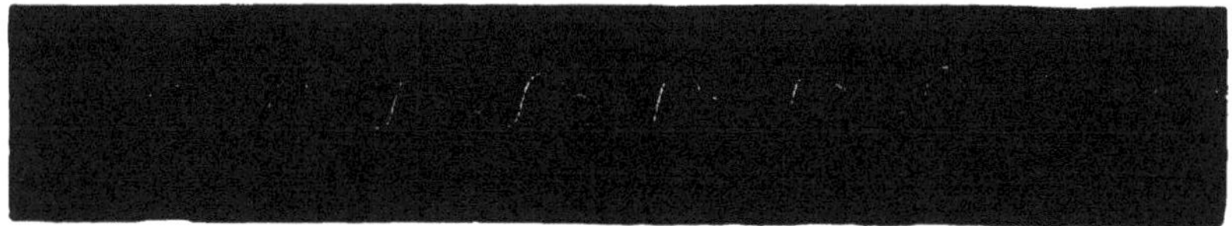

FIG. 11.—AORTIC STENOSIS.

FIG. 12.—AORTIC INCOMPETENCE.

FIG. 13.—MITRAL STENOSIS.

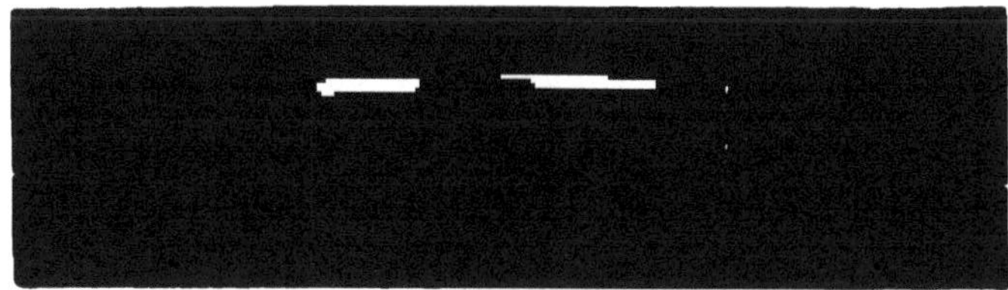

FIG 14.—MITRAL INCOMPETENCE.

In Fig. 11, the pulse of aortic stenosis, it will be seen that the wave is of little altitude, and has a sloping upstroke, with a rounded top and a gradual descent; that is to say, the wave is small, and attains its maximum gradually, is persistent or long, and subsides slowly. There is no dicrotic wave, as the conditions necessary for its production, great fluctuation of the blood-pressure and rapid contraction of the ventricle, are absent.

In Fig. 12, the pulse of aortic incompetence, the upstroke is high, perpendicular, has a sharp top, and falls rapidly; that is, the wave is large, owing to the size of the artery, is sudden and rapidly attains its maximum, is very short and rapidly falls. Dicrotism is not altogether absent, but, owing to want of the fulcrum formed by the aortic valves, it is much less marked than might be expected from the violence of the fluctuations and the rapidity of the systole.

In Fig. 13, the pulse of mitral stenosis, the upstroke or percussion-wave is short, and soon attains its maximum; the wave is long, and is slowly extinguished. Dicrotism is absent.

In Fig. 14, the pulse of severe mitral incompetence, the tracing shows that the pulse is very irregular both in force and frequency; the wave is short and small, and ill-sustained. When, however, the amount of regurgitation is slight and compensation is good, the pulse will usually be regular.

The character of the pulse, therefore, affords important information as to the nature of the lesion; while the degree in which the special peculiarities are developed, in each instance gives some clue to the extent of the valvular mischief. The pulse, however, may be modified in various ways; for instance, where aortic stenosis co-exists with regurgitation, the collapsing and sudden character of the regurgitant pulse will, to a great extent, be lost. Such modification, when present, is in itself a valuable help to diagnosis, as it enables us to say with certainty that there is real aortic stenosis, and not merely roughening of the aortic valves, either of which might be indicated by the presence of a systolic basic murmur.

Much information may thus be gained from the pulse; but the character of the pulse, even when taken in connection with the murmurs, is not sufficient to enable us to estimate the degree of obstruction or the amount of regurgitation in a given case. Further indications are to be obtained, firstly, from the effects on the cavities and walls of the heart produced by the mechanical difficulties resulting from the valvular imperfections; secondly, from the evidences of obstructed circulation in the lungs or system.

## CHAPTER VIII.

THE IMPORTANCE OF HYPERTROPHY AND DILATATION OF THE HEART AS A MEANS OF ESTIMATING THE EXTENT OF A VALVULAR LESION—POSSIBLE OBJECTIONS TO THIS VIEW DISCUSSED—EXPLANATION OF THE WAY IN WHICH THE DIFFERENT VALVULAR LESIONS GIVE RISE TO HYPERTROPHY AND DILATATION: (1) AORTIC STENOSIS; (2) AORTIC INCOMPETENCE; (3) MITRAL REGURGITATION; (4) MITRAL OBSTRUCTION—COMPENSATION.

THE most important indications as to the extent of a valvular lesion are to be gathered from its effects on the walls and cavities of the heart, resulting in hypertrophy of the former and dilatation of the latter. These changes are due to the efforts of the heart to overcome the mechanical difficulties in the circulation occasioned by the regurgitation or obstruction to which the valvular lesion has given rise.

Hypertrophy and dilatation must be looked upon as caused by the valvular lesion, and as affording a measure of its extent. The degree of these structural changes is ascertained by the increased area of deep cardiac dulness, by the displacement and modification of the apex beat, by the situation and character of the impulse, and by associated changes in the character and rhythm of the heart-sounds; the more pronounced these changes, the greater is the mechanical difficulty in the propulsion of the blood, and the more grave is the prognosis.

Not that a given degree of hypertrophy or dilatation,

or of the two combined, is indicative in all cases of the same extent of valvular change. Each kind of valvular disease has its own special form and degree of structural change, and comparisons, to be valid, must be made between like cases; a degree of hypertrophy and dilatation, which would have little significance in aortic insufficiency, might indicate a serious amount of mitral regurgitation; and again, mitral stenosis, which has reached a dangerous degree, may be attended with less conspicuous structural change than a degree of mitral insufficiency which gives rise neither to danger nor to inconvenience. It will be well, indeed, to exclude mitral stenosis while the general question under consideration is argued out. Numerous other modifying influences are also in operation, so that, while it is generally true that the greater the dilatation and hypertrophy, the greater the functional imperfection of the valves, the converse statement, that the less the hypertrophy or dilatation, the smaller the valvular damage, must not be taken without important qualifications. This statement is indeed usually true in the absence of serious symptoms, but sometimes the very failure of the heart to undergo the changes required for the compensation of valvular inefficiency canses severe embarrassment of the circulation, and gives rise to an early fatal termination.

It is stated by Walshe, and is undoubtedly true, that no direct ratio constantly holds good between the amount of hypertrophy and valvular change, as ascertained by post-mortem examinations. This, however, is capable of explanation, if we take into account the various circumstances that may modify the development of the hypertrophy.

*Firstly.* The age of the patient at the time when the lesions of the valves take place is an important factor. The enormous hypertrophy and dilatation sometimes met with are produced almost exclusively in early life, when the heart is still developing and its muscular substance is capable of active growth; later, the heart loses its adaptive capability in great measure, and thus a valvular lesion which, at the age of fifteen or twenty, would be survived with enormous hypertrophy, would at forty or fifty prove fatal with very little change.

*Secondly.* Time is an important element in the development of hypertrophy, which may take years to reach its maximum growth; and it is often very difficult to assign a date to the origin of a given morbid condition. For instance, of two cases in which the extent of the valvular mischief, as seen by post-mortem, is apparently the same, in one the heart may be found to be considerably hypertrophied, because the patient did not at once succumb to the injury; in the other there is perhaps little hypertrophy but great dilatation, because the difficulty of carrying on the circulation increased more rapidly than the power of the heart to cope with it, so that death occurred quickly.

*Thirdly.* We must take into account the fact that different affections of the valves have inherently and mechanically different degrees of tendency to the production of structural alterations. For instance, aortic incompetence gives rise to enormous hypertrophy of the left ventricle, whereas mitral incompetence gives rise to very moderate hypertrophy, and uncomplicated mitral stenosis to atrophy rather than hypertrophy.

*Fourthly.* The mode of life, whether active and accompanied by considerable muscular exertion, or sedentary and unattended by anxiety and excitement, will be an important consideration. The amount of work the heart is called upon to do will vary in each instance, and the hypertrophy will vary in direct proportion.

Again, the presence of high tension in the vascular system will tend to increase the degree of hypertrophy to a considerable extent.

*Fifthly.* The period after the occurrence of the valvular

change at which active exertion is undertaken, allowing or not allowing the heart to adapt itself gradually to this change, will have great influence on the condition of its walls and cavities. For example, after endocarditis, which has given rise to damage of the aortic or mitral valve, one patient has prolonged rest, care, comforts, and change of air, so that dilating influences are postponed by the rest while the heart is weak and liable to yield, and the muscular walls are enabled, by a good state of nutrition, to resist dilatation; another must return to work, or is allowed to exert himself before the heart has recovered from the effects of the illness, and its badly nourished fibres give way and permit of dilatation, which will be followed later, if the patient lives, by hypertrophy.

We have in the above conditions the quota of causation, beyond the mechanical difficulty at the valves, which explains the variation observed; and it will be evident, from these considerations, that an unvarying direct ratio between the valvular and structural changes is not to be looked for, and that its absence furnishes no valid objection to their standing in the relation of cause and effect.

## Mechanism of Causation of Hypertrophy in the Different Valvular Diseases: its Beneficial Effects.

**Aortic Stenosis.**—Taking first the most simple case. If the constriction of the aortic orifice is sufficient in amount to give rise to mechanical obstruction to the flow of blood through it, there must either be increase in the propulsive power of the heart, or a slowing of the circulation; for it is obvious that the same force will not propel the same amount of blood in the same time through a narrowed orifice as through one of normal size. We find, however, that the rate of circulation is maintained, the increased power necessary to drive the blood through the narrowed orifice at a more rapid rate being gained by hypertrophy of the heart, which takes place to a degree necessary to overcome the obstruction. This is a simple illustration of the physiological law, that increased functional activity gives rise to increase of structure. If the hypertrophy did not take place, there would be a slowing and finally a standstill of the circulation.

**Aortic Insufficiency.**—In this lesion a certain proportion of the blood driven into the aorta at each systole returns into the ventricle through the leaking valves; consequently, in order that the same rate of circulation may be maintained, there must be either an increase in the number of heart-beats per minute, or an increase in the quantity of blood expelled by the ventricle at each contraction. Mere augmentation of the force of the systole would not answer the requirement: for instance, if five ounces of blood are driven into the aorta at each systole, and one ounce returns, the normal supply of blood would obviously not be maintained by propelling the five ounces more forcibly; what is needed is that six ounces of blood should be driven into the aorta, so that when one ounce has regurgitated into the ventricle, five ounces would still remain in the arterial system. This requirement is met by an increased capacity of the left ventricle, which is the primary compensatory change taking place in aortic insufficiency. Increased capacity is, in other words, dilatation. In this instance, therefore, dilatation of the left ventricle, which under other conditions is injurious, is actually a beneficial and conservative change when reinforced by hypertrophy, and this we shall see is a natural sequence.

It is true there is no direct provocation to hypertrophy in the shape of increased resistance to the blood-flow; but there is a call for increased exercise of force in the additional quantity of blood to be projected from the ventricle into the aorta at each systole. Further, the total internal area of the walls of the ventricle is greatly increased owing to the increase in its capacity, while the same pressure is exerted on each square inch during systole, hence the amount of force to be exercised by the muscular walls of the heart must be proportionately augmented. These two causes give rise to the hypertrophy present in so remarkable a degree in aortic regurgitation.

It must not be supposed that, because the dilatation which takes place in aortic regurgitation is compensatory and necessary, this is a sufficient explanation of its occurrence. It is produced in the following way: During diastole, the most defenceless period of the heart in the cardiac cycle, when the muscular fibres are in a state of relaxation, the ventricle is exposed to a double distending force. Firstly, the entry of blood from the left auricle and pulmonary veins; secondly, the backward rush of the blood from the aorta: the greater the amount of the regurgitation, the greater will be the distending force, and consequently the greater the dilatation of the left ventricle. This dilatation, however, is a totally different thing from the dilatation which is sometimes met with as the result of structural change and degeneracy of the muscular walls of the heart: in the latter case, the walls yield because they are inherently weak, and the effect on the circulation is disastrous, a gradually increasing stagnation from deficient *vis a tergo*; in the former case the walls yield, not because they are weak, but because they are subjected to an abnormal distending force while in a condition of relaxation and least able to resist it; ultimately, when this dilatation is backed by hypertrophy, the effect on the circulation is beneficial, since it neutralizes, more or less completely, the tendency to stagnation produced by the regurgitation.

When, however, aortic regurgitant disease is set up late

in life from degenerative changes in the valves, there is frequently also degeneration and consequent weakening of the muscular substance of the heart; then, owing to the inherent weakness of the walls of the heart, the dilatation due to the aortic regurgitation will be excessive, unless the case is cut short by sudden death, and, as there is little chance of sufficient compensatory hypertrophy taking place, the condition will be one of distress and danger, if the regurgitation is extensive.

### Mitral Regurgitation and Mitral Obstruction.

In affections of the mitral valve the effects of the derangement of the circulation due to the lesion no longer fall mainly on the left ventricle, but primarily on the left auricle and lungs, and eventually on the right ventricle. The left auricle in mitral lesions corresponds in its relation to the current of blood to the left ventricle in aortic lesions; hence, by analogy, in mitral regurgitation, we should expect to find hypertrophy and dilatation, and in mitral obstruction marked hypertrophy of the left auricle. This is what occurs to a certain extent, but as the auricle is thin walled and poor in muscular substance, it is impossible for it to take on hypertrophy and compensate for the mitral lesions in the same way that the ventricle does for aortic lesions; it may, indeed, be distended so as to form a thin walled sac of considerable size. The result is that the burden of the work of compensation is thrown on the right ventricle by back pressure through the pulmonary circulation, which thus becomes the channel through which the effects of the mitral regurgitation or obstruction are transmitted from the left auricle to the right ventricle. We find, therefore, that the right ventricle undergoes hypertrophy and dilatation as a result of mitral lesions, while the pressure in the pulmonary circulation, the connecting channel, is enormously increased.

It thus comes to pass that the right ventricle, by the additional force it gains from hypertrophy and the additional capacity it gains from dilatation, aids in supplying the left ventricle with blood, and in neutralizing the disturbing effects of mitral lesions on the circulation; for the increased pressure in the pulmonary system and left auricle will send the blood more rapidly through a constricted orifice in case of mitral stenosis, and will resist the regurgitation in mitral incompetence.

## Dilatation of the Left Ventricle in Mitral Incompetence.

A certain limited amount of dilatation and hypertrophy of the left ventricle, as well as of the right, takes place in mitral incompetence, the explanation of which is as follows:—

During diastole, in consequence of the increased pressure in the pulmonary circulation and left auricle, the blood will rush through the mitral orifice with greater force and rapidity than normal; hence the pressure on the walls of the left ventricle will be greater than normal, and the muscular fibres, being relaxed and defenceless, readily yield to the extra distending force: in this way some degree of dilatation results. Then as the dilatation increases the area of ventricular wall exposed to pressure, it increases also the amount of work to be done in systole, and thus creates a demand for hypertrophy, which also takes place to a moderate extent.

In mitral stenosis, though there is increased pressure in the pulmonary circulation which would tend to cause dilatation of the left ventricle during diastole in the same way as in mitral incompetence, the mitral orifice, being narrowed, does not allow a volume of blood, sufficient to exert a distending force, to pass through; indeed, in severe cases, the constriction may be so great that the ventricle has never time to fill during diastole, so that it tends rather to decrease in size than dilate, and there will be no demand for hypertrophy.

In incompetence of the mitral valve, therefore, the amount of hypertrophy and dilatation of the right ventricle and the degree of pressure in the pulmonary circulation are among the most important indications of the extent of the lesion.

In mitral stenosis this holds good up to a certain point, but the changes in the right ventricle are not so safe a guide, since the dilatation and hypertrophy sometimes appear to be restricted in extent by the absence of accompanying changes of a similar character in the left ventricle, which remains very small.

## Compensation.

It has thus been seen that dilatation and hypertrophy of the left or right ventricle or of both are a necessary consequence of valvular disease of any severity, if the patient lives, and the mechanism of their production has also been discussed. These changes in the cardiac walls are spoken of as compensatory, that is, they are changes which must take place to enable the heart to cope with the extra work thrown upon it as a result of the valvular lesions; in the case of aortic disease it is the left ventricle, in the case of mitral lesions the right ventricle, more especially, which undergoes compensatory changes. Compensation is said to be established when the hypertrophy and dilatation, the former especially, have so far developed that they neutralize the disturbing effects on the circulation which the valvular lesions would otherwise produce, and enable the patient to live his ordinary life without discomfort, and without any marked symptoms.

When compensation is imperfect, the symptoms incident to the valvular disease from which the patient is suffering will present themselves more or less readily under moderate exercise or exertion, their severity varying inversely with the degree of compensation established.

For instance, a boy who is allowed to go about immediately after he has contracted a valvular lesion of some severity, and is suffering, say, from aortic incompetence, will be extremely short of breath, and incapable of walking any distance, will have attacks of severe pain in the præcordium, and perhaps fainting fits, one of which may prove fatal; whereas the same patient, if he is kept at rest till the compensatory changes have had time to develop, will be able to take moderate exercise comfortably and go about his work free from pain or respiratory distress, though he may be incapable of any prolonged or violent exertion.

In mitral disease dyspnœa, cyanosis, and œdema of the lower extremities are among the earlier symptoms of failing compensation. In the later stages one of the most important guides as to the state of compensation is the size of the liver. When this organ becomes engorged and enlarged, owing to obstruction to the flow of blood from the inferior vena cava to the right auricle, it will indicate that the right ventricle is unable to cope efficiently with the increased pressure in the pulmonary circulation caused by the mitral lesion, and consequently that compensation is imperfect. A further indication will be pulsation and fulness of the veins of the neck, which may sometimes be seen to fill from below. The liver may attain a considerable size, extending below the umbilicus, and may eventually pulsate when tricuspid regurgitation has become established.

# CHAPTER IX.

## AORTIC STENOSIS.

MORBID ANATOMY AND ETIOLOGY—THE MURMUR OF AORTIC STENOSIS—CONDITIONS OTHER THAN AORTIC STENOSIS WHICH MAY GIVE RISE TO SYSTOLIC AORTIC MURMURS—DIFFERENTIAL DIAGNOSIS OF MURMURS—ESTIMATION OF EXTENT OF LESION BY MEANS OF THE MURMUR, THE CHANGES IN THE HEART AND THE PULSE—PROGRESS OF THE DISEASE: SYMPTOMS—PROGNOSIS—TREATMENT.

THE first valvular change to be considered will be aortic stenosis. This is the least common of the valvular affections of the left side of the heart, as shown both by post-mortem statistics and clinical experience.

### MORBID ANATOMY AND ETIOLOGY.

narrowing of the mouth of the aorta is almost
to changes in the valves, the cusps of which
and rigid from cicatricial contraction of fibrous
endocarditis, with rounded and thickened
condition which does not permit them to fall
the sinuses of Valsalva before the current of
ead, therefore, of a circular orifice of the same
vessel beyond, there is a roughly triangular
reduced area, formed by the edges of the
sequent calcification may render the valves

still more rigid and deformed. Sometimes adhesions take place between damaged valves at the angle in which they meet, so that a narrow funnel-shaped orifice results. This condition may be left by endocarditis, whether rheumatic or occurring in the course of scarlet fever or other bacterial, infection of the valves. Or the valves may be deformed by atheroma or chronic degenerative changes, which destroy their flexibility, cause puckering and contraction of their margins, and lead to calcareous deposits in their substance.

It is also possible that by dilatation of the ring at the root of the aorta, a slight and unimportant obstruction may be produced; valves, not themselves greatly diseased, being so put on the stretch that they cannot fall back, but remain as an obstacle to the stream of blood.

### Physical Signs.

The characteristic physical sign to which aortic stenosis gives rise is a murmur systolic in time which usually has its maximum intensity in the second right intercostal space close to the sternum, in the so-called aortic area. All systolic murmurs heard over this area do not, however, necessarily imply actual obstruction of the aortic orifice, but may have other significance.

**The Murmur.**—The systolic aortic murmur, as is indicated by its name, is heard during the systole of the left ventricle, and is produced by the rush of blood through the obstructed aortic orifice from the ventricle into the aorta. Its commencement coincides in time with the first sound of the heart, and may either accompany or replace it, and it may begin with a burst or accent, or gradually. The duration of the murmur varies; it is usually long, sometimes occupying the entire interval between the first and second sounds, which interval may be prolonged, but it may be short. It is audible over the sternum at the level of the third intercostal space, but is most distinct just outside the right edge of the sternum in the second space, or sometimes over the third costal cartilage, at which point on the surface the aorta comes from under the pulmonary artery, and nearly touches the anterior wall of the chest. It is conducted upwards, as the phrase is, along the right side of the sternum to the right sterno-clavicular articulation, where it is distinctly audible, and it is also heard over the carotids in the neck and occasionally over the thoracic aorta along the spine. It is frequently heard along the right margin of the sternum lower down, sometimes to the fourth or fifth space right or left of the sternum, more especially when the aorta is dilated and elongated, and it may have its maximum intensity over the sternum near its left edge at the level of the third rib or space, *i.e.* immediately over the aortic valves. This, however, is not common, as the root of the aorta is deeply seated in the chest, and has, between it and the surface, the conus arteriosus of the pulmonary artery. The murmur is lost over the right ventricle, but is again audible, as a rule, at the apex, being conducted to this point by the wall of the left ventricle. This murmur may be loud—sometimes extremely loud—and when this is the case, it may be heard all over the chest behind, as well as in front, or it may be comparatively soft; it is often rough and vibratory, more rarely, croaking in character, but it may be smooth and blowing, or musical. Occasionally it is accompanied by a systolic thrill felt in the second or third right space, or in both close to the edge of the sternum.

**Causes other than Aortic Stenosis which may give rise to a Basic Systolic Murmur.**—Such a murmur in one or other of its varieties may be due to several causes, which will now be enumerated.

1. Anæmia may be mentioned first. It is not well understood how it is that this condition gives rise to murmurs, but the fact is exemplified by the venous hum

heard in the neck, by pulmonic and mitral murmurs, and also, though less commonly, by a systolic aortic murmur. This murmur is rarely rough or loud, but it is often distinct and audible along the edge of the sternum upwards to the sterno-clavicular articulation, and in the neck. It accompanies the first sound, and does not substitute itself for it. Hæmic murmurs are commonly multiple, which renders their diagnosis more easy.

With the hæmic aortic murmur may be grouped the murmur of similar character, sometimes accompanying or following acute febrile disease of long duration, such as rheumatic fever and typhoid fever, although it is not certain that the causation is exactly the same. A systolic mitral murmur is more common, and is usually present as well as the aortic murmur. Such murmurs may perhaps be attributed to a temporary loss of tone of the heart and vessels. They usually disappear as the patient regains health and strength.

2. Mere roughening of the orifice or valves, or impaired flexibility of the latter, slight congenital malformation, fenestration of one or more of the cusps, a shred of fibrin hanging from the edge of a valve, may give rise to a loud systolic murmur without offering any appreciable obstruction to the course of the blood.

3. An aortic murmur may be produced by acute or subacute aortitis, a rare and obscure disease which may be suspected when, with a murmur not previously known to be present, there are irregular pyrexia, dull sub-sternal pain, and rapid and apparently unaccountable failure of the heart.

4. Dilatation of the aorta just above the valves, the orifice and valves remaining unchanged, produces a murmur. The fibrous ring at the root of the aorta, which gives attachment to the muscular fibres of the ventricle, and supports the semilunar valves, is extremely strong, so that it does not readily give way and allow the orifice to be enlarged,

but the aorta just above the ring is prone to dilatation, and the blood passing through an opening of normal size into a larger cavity beyond is thrown into eddies, the vibrations attending which produce the sound heard as a murmur.

In none of these conditions is there stenosis of the orifice, or obstruction to the stream as it issues from the heart; the condition last mentioned has dangers of its own, but they do not arise from aortic obstruction.

**Differential Diagnosis of Basic Systolic Murmurs.**—It is clear that the first point to be ascertained when a systolic murmur is present is, whether it indicates the existence of obstruction or not. In this we shall be greatly assisted by the history, aspect, and age of the patient. We should, for example, suspect that the murmur was hæmic, and not produced by obstruction if the patient were a young and anæmic girl, or if it were first heard during convalescence from an acute illness, more especially if similar blowing murmurs were heard at other valves as well.

The history of an attack of rheumatic fever would, on the other hand, favour the conclusion that the orifice was actually narrowed.

A systolic murmur over the aorta, appearing after middle age, or in advanced life, or discovered for the first time at this period, will seldom be due to actual narrowing of the orifice, but will be caused by roughness or rigidity of the valves, or by dilatation of the aorta above the valves with perhaps atheromatous irregularities in its walls. Fortu-[illegible]ly the aortic second sound is of very great assistance [illegible] determining the point. Under the condition just [illegible]posed it will almost certainly be unduly loud and [illegible]uated from co-existing high arterial tension, while [illegible] diminishes the intensity of the second sound in two [illegible] by the changes present in the valves impairing their [illegible]ility, and by the less sudden recoil which follows [illegible]lower distension of the arterial system. Prolonged observation of cases of high arterial tension from gout, lead poisoning, renal disease, or other causes in advanced life,

al attendant the
nce and gradual
n addition to the

ur, or the extent
does not give us
usually soft and
hich are due to
some that when
oth and rounded
iderable narrow-
on can scarcely
le blood against
terates sonorous
passage of the
le channel. A
e ventricle and
ay render the
l enfeeblement
c murmur may
dest murmurs,
ost frequently
r more of the
lve, or some-
a part of the
that all loud
fer is that a
icular systole

alone it may
rtic stenosis,
striction.
by Degree of

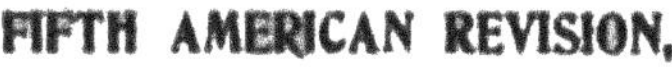

but the aorta just above the ring is prone to dilatation, and
the blood passing
larger cavity bey
attending which

In none of t
orifice, or obstru
heart; the condit
but they do not a

Differential D
is clear that th
systolic murmur
existence of obstr
assisted by the
We should, for
hæmic, and not
were a young an
during convalescen
similar blowing m

The history of
the other hand, fa
actually narrowed.

A systolic mur
age, or in advanc
this period, will s
orifice, but will b
valves, or by dila
perhaps atheroma
nately the aortic
in determining
mentioned it will
accentuated from
stenosis diminishe
ways: by the cha
flexibility, and b
the slower disten

observation of cases of high arterial tension from gout, lead poisoning, renal disease, or other causes in advanced life, will not unfrequently afford the medical attendant the opportunity of noting the first appearance and gradual development of a murmur over the aorta in addition to the accentuated second sound.

The loudness or character of the murmur, or the extent to which it is conducted along the aorta, does not give us much help. Hæmic aortic murmurs are usually soft and smooth, but so also may murmurs be which are due to extreme narrowing. It has been stated by some that when the margins of the thickened valves are smooth and rounded there may be no murmur in spite of considerable narrowing; but if the fact be true, the explanation can scarcely be accepted, since it is not the friction of the blood against the valves as it passes over them which generates sonorous vibrations, but the eddies produced by the passage of the blood through a small orifice into a large channel. A more probable explanation is weakness of the ventricle and languid propulsion of the blood which may render the murmur weak or inaudible; thus the gradual enfeeblement and ultimate disappearance of a systolic aortic murmur may be a serious prognostic indication. The loudest murmurs, such as have already been mentioned, are most frequently produced by rigidity or deformity of one or more of the cusps or by a calcareous deposit in the valve, or sometimes by a delicate band stretched across a part of the orifice, but it would not be safe to conclude that all loud murmurs are harmless. All we can safely infer is that a long, loud murmur indicates a vigorous ventricular systole which is a good prognostic element.

It is thus evident that from the murmurs alone it may be impossible to make a certain diagnosis of aortic stenosis, and still less to estimate the amount of the constriction.

**The Heart: Estimation of Degree of Stenosis by Degree of**

**Cardiac Hypertrophy.**—We turn, then, to the condition of the heart. If there is actual obstruction its existence will be betrayed either by the changes in the walls and cavities which are required in order to overcome it, or by some evidences of derangement in the circulation.

The change by which aortic obstruction will be overcome will be more or less pure hypertrophy of the left ventricle. This does not bring the heart to the gigantic size which it reaches as a consequence of aortic regurgitation. The apex beat will be lower than the normal position by an intercostal space, or perhaps more, but it will not be greatly displaced outwards; it will be a well-defined and deliberate push of no great violence. The first sound here will be dull and prolonged, and not very loud; perhaps accompanied by a murmur which may be mitral, but most commonly is, in the early period of the disease, the aortic murmur conducted to the apex by the walls of the left ventricle. The other sounds will present nothing remarkable, except that the aortic second sound will be weak. If we get such evidence of hypertrophy of the left ventricle as this, *i.e.* the downward displacement and definite push of the apex with a prolonged first sound, in a young person without kidney disease, together with a systolic aortic murmur, there can be no hesitation in inferring stenosis of the aortic orifice. At and after middle age it would be necessary to consider whether the hypertrophy might not have been produced by long-continued, antecedent resistance in the peripheral circulation and high arterial tension; but in this case the apex would usually be less defined, the first sound louder and less deliberate, and the aortic second sound much accentuated. When aortic incompetence has preceded the stenosis, as is often the case when it is due to acute endocarditis, the left ventricle will attain a greater size by reason of the previous dilatation to which hypertrophy has succeeded.

**The Pulse.**—Almost more important than the hypertrophy of the left ventricle will be the character of the pulse. The orifice being narrowed, the blood discharged from the ventricle will require more time to pass through it, and the pressure in the arterial system will not at once rise to its maximum; in other words, the so-called percussion element of the sphygmographic trace will be weakened and the pulse wave will be long and slow, not striking the finger or lever abruptly and vigorously, but raising it gradually. The artery will, for the most part, be small and full between the beats of the pulse. A large sudden pulse is incompatible with aortic stenosis unaccompanied by regurgitation, and when it is a question whether or not an aortic systolic murmur is due to obstruction at the orifice, the pulse becomes the most certain criterion to which we can appeal; if there is an apparent contradiction between the indications of the heart and those of the pulse, the latter must dominate.

For instance, if with a systolic and diastolic aortic murmur and a hypertrophied heart, the pulse is large, sudden and collapsing, we shall infer that there is no real stenosis of the aortic orifice; if, on the other hand, the pulse lacks these features characteristic of aortic incompetence, we shall conclude that there is aortic stenosis which has interfered with their development; and we shall estimate the degree of stenosis from the extent to which it has modified the pulse.

A systolic murmur heard over the aortic valves and along the aorta will not, in the absence of cardiac hypertrophy and the long, small pulse described above, indicate stenosis of the aortic orifice, and even when there is hypertrophy, if the pulse is large, short and abrupt, there can be no real narrowing.

## EFFECTS OF THE DISEASE: SYMPTOMS.

When the constriction is moderate in amount and is a result of endocarditis, in a young subject the heart will usually undergo hypertrophy sufficiently to overcome the obstruction, and no serious or troublesome symptoms will arise. In severe cases there may be dyspnœa and anginoid pains. There is a tendency for the constriction to increase, and when this is so considerable as to have given rise to great hypertrophy of the left ventricle, the latter is sure to give out sooner or later. As a consequence of the deficient propulsive power resulting therefrom, there will be a tendency to systemic stagnation, and as a result of the incomplete emptying of the ventricular cavity in systole, there will be insufficient room for the whole contents of the left auricle in diastole, and consequent back pressure through the left auricle and pulmonary circulation. Mitral incompetence may ensue as a result of the giving out of the left ventricle, but there will also be other injurious influences at work which may give rise to regurgitation in the following way: The pressure in the ventricular cavity will be greatly increased owing to the powerful contraction of the muscular walls, which is necessary to overcome the obstruction at the orifice; as a consequence of this, there is a constant and severe strain upon the flaps of the mitral valve and the chordæ tendineæ, so that eventually they become stretched or give way, and mitral incompetence results, or chronic degenerative changes may take place, leading to thickening and contraction of the valves and cords. It will thus be seen that in aortic stenosis of any severity there is little chance of the mitral valve escaping damage in the long run, and if it has at the outset been injured by the same attack of endocarditis which gave rise to the aortic mischief, the outlook is far more serious. The barrier formed by the mitral valve being thus broken down, the door is open to backward pressure through the auricle, which will take effect upon the pulmonary circulation and right ventricle. It has been said by some that timely yielding of the mitral valve acts as a safety valve, as tricuspid regurgitation is supposed to do for the right ventricle, preventing sudden death through over-distension and consequent paralysis of the left ventricle. This view does not commend itself to my judgment, and must, in the nature of things, be purely hypothetical. There can be no doubt that the establishment of mitral regurgitation marks a downward step and renders the prognosis grave. The obstacle to the outflow of blood from the ventricle, which has given rise to the whole train of consequences, remains irremovable, and the setting in of mitral symptoms marks the failure of compensation.

## Prognosis.

Nearly all authors concur in making aortic stenosis the least dangerous of the valvular affections, and on *a priori* considerations such would seem to be probable; but this conclusion will scarcely seem quite secure if the cases of systolic aortic murmur without actual narrowing of the orifice are eliminated. Just as the inclusion of all cases in which a systolic aortic murmur is heard makes aortic stenosis apparently the most frequent valvular disease, while on post-mortem evidence it is seen to be the least common, so the dilution of the death-rate by the cases in which no real narrowing exists makes it appear to be the least fatal. The relative danger of real stenosis cannot be estimated with confidence, but it is certainly greater than has been supposed, and though, perhaps, it is not so serious as aortic incompetence or mitral stenosis, it is more so than mitral incompetence. The average age of the cases of this disease in the post-mortem statistics referred to in the chapter on prognosis was about forty, and would have been higher had deaths by intercurrent independent disease been excluded. The age of the oldest patient among these, however, was fifty-three; this would bear out the above statement that aortic stenosis must be looked upon as more dangerous than mitral incompetence, of which numerous examples are known to have reached the age of seventy.

There is no risk of sudden death as in aortic incompetence, and there is little danger as long as the patient is free from symptoms; but when once dropsy has set in from back pressure due to dilatation of the left ventricle, there is a smaller possibility of recovery than in other valvular affections. For when the left ventricle has given way under the resistance it encounters, it has little chance of regaining its normal condition, since the resistance persists undiminished, and there is no other compensatory influence which can be called upon. Further, if the break-down occurs after middle life, it is probable that degenerative change is taking place in the hypertrophied left ventricle, which will render the prognosis still more unfavourable.

In regard to this it must be borne in mind that at and after middle age, a systolic aortic murmur appearing for the first time may be indicative of degenerative change, and obstruction is the smallest of the dangers to which degenerative change in or about the root of the aorta may give rise. The loss of flexibility in the valve which gives rise to obstruction may permit of regurgitation. Again, the degeneration may affect one of the sinuses of Valsalva and produce aneurysm here, or may implicate the orifice of the coronary arteries, and by cutting off the supply of blood lead to fatty change in the walls of the heart. Any murmur at the aortic orifice, then, in an elderly person, must be looked upon as a possible forerunner of serious disease, though I have known of cases in which a rough systolic murmur has been present for upwards of ten years without any serious symptoms arising.

## TREATMENT.

In regard to the treatment of aortic stenosis, there is little to add to what has been said on the treatment of valvular disease in general. We cannot hope to rectify the constriction which has already taken place, and can do little to modify the process of narrowing, which may be going on as a result of cicatricial contraction, or adhesion of the valvular curtains, after acute endocarditis has subsided. When, however, the valves are being damaged by a chronic inflammatory process due to syphilis, benefit may be sometimes obtained by the administration of large doses of iodide of potassium.

Supposing the contraction of the aortic orifice to have reached a certain point and become stationary; the dangers likely to arise out of this condition will be, at an early period, an imperfect degree of compensatory hypertrophy and later degeneration of the hypertrophied muscular wall, with, in both cases, secondary dilatation of the left ventricle. From this, mitral incompetence may result, and subsequently right ventricle failure with its train of symptoms of venous obstruction.

The hypertrophy is usually sufficient in the first instance, as the contraction of the orifice takes place slowly, so that the structural increase can keep pace with it, provided that the patient is a young subject. A moderate degree of constriction may therefore exist for years without apparently affecting the health or well-being, or interfering with ordinary occupations, giving rise to no symptoms except perhaps shortness of breath and præcordial pain on too great exertion. Even considerable stenosis is not incompatible with moderate exercise and work and apparent health.

Exceptions occur when the patient is weak and anæmic, either as a result of protracted illness, or from other causes, and nutrition being poor, the hypertrophy is inadequate and accompanied by dilatation. In such cases prolonged rest may be of great service.

Secondary dilatation and break-down of the left ventricle is to be averted by carefully avoiding over-exertion, fatigue, and anxiety, and by attention to general health. Moderation in food and drink is necessary, as the amount of exercise which can be taken is limited, and anything that may lead to high arterial tension and increased peripheral resistance is especially to be guarded against. Tonics may be given when required, and anæmia is to be combated by all means in our power. The protracted administration of digitalis is of very questionable utility. When the left ventricle has begun to give way, and symptoms of backward pressure through the lungs and embarrassment of the right ventricle supervene, then digitalis and similar remedies will be of service. If, however, these symptoms have come on insidiously, and are not traceable to over-exertion, chill, or any definite cause, drugs will rarely be able to improve materially the condition of the patient or postpone for long the fatal termination.

When the hypertrophied walls of the heart have begun to undergo degeneration, and there is præcordial pain and oppression, the administration of nitro-glycerine and nitrites, or the nitrates of erythrol and mannitol, by diminishing the arterio-capillary resistance, and thus relieving the stress on the left ventricle, will often afford the heart distinct relief, and produce a general amelioration of symptoms. These drugs may be given at the same time with digitalis.

On the other hand, I have more than once known aconite, given with a similar object, completely overthrow the compensation established by hypertrophy, and cause rapid cardiac dilatation, with frequent weak and small pulse accompanied by pallor and cold sweats.

# CHAPTER X.

## AORTIC INCOMPETENCE.

ETIOLOGY — PHYSICAL SIGNS—THE DIASTOLIC MURMUR: DIRECTIONS IN WHICH IT IS CONDUCTED—PRESYSTOLIC MURMUR, ITS SIGNIFICANCE — MODIFICATION OF THE AORTIC SECOND SOUND—PULSATION OF ARTERIES—CAPILLARY PULSATION — THE COLLAPSING PULSE — PULSUS BISFERIENS — IRREGULAR PULSE—ESTIMATION OF THE AMOUNT OF REGURGITATION FROM THE CHARACTER OF THE MURMUR, OF THE AORTIC SECOND SOUND, OF THE PULSE, AND THE CHANGES IN THE HEART—AORTIC INCOMPETENCE DUE TO SYPHILIS AND CAUSES OTHER THAN ACUTE ENDOCARDITIS—SYMPTOMS —PROGNOSIS—TREATMENT.

### ETIOLOGY.

THE commonest cause of this affection in childhood and early adult life is acute endocarditis. As the clinical features of aortic incompetence which develops in later life from other causes, differ materially, discussion of these will be deferred till later on in this chapter.

### PHYSICAL SIGNS.

**The Diastolic Murmur.**—The diagnostic sign of this condition is a murmur produced by the backward rush of the blood from the aorta into the left ventricle during its diastole. Two forces will be at work in its production—the suction action of the ventricle, and the pressure in the arterial system generally and in the aorta in particular, due to the elastic recoil of the walls of the great vessels. The cause of the murmur is not necessarily roughness or irregularity of the valves or orifice ; it may be due partially or entirely to the vibrations generated by the passage of liquid through a constricted point in a channel, into a large cavity beyond.

The seat of production of the murmur being the valves which encircle the root of the aorta, the point on the surface of the chest immediately over and nearest to the origin of the sound will be close to the left margin of the sternum at the level of the third cartilage ; but it is not always here that the murmur is best heard, as the conus arteriosus of the pulmonary artery is interposed between the aorta and the chest wall.

The murmur is conducted in various directions, and the seat of its maximum intensity differs in different cases. It is, with rare exceptions, audible in the so-called aortic area just outside the right edge of the sternum in the second intercostal space, or over the second costal cartilage, and is usually conducted upwards from this point along the sternal margin as far as the sterno-clavicular articulation, though losing rapidly in intensity the while. It can frequently be followed downwards along the side of the sternum to the fourth space, or even lower, sometimes with increasing intensity over one or two ribs ; it is also frequently heard along the sternum itself, or to the left of it, the seat of maximum intensity being frequently in the fourth or fifth spaces near the left edge of the sternum, where it may be audible when not heard over the aortic area. It may again be audible at the apex after having been lost over the right ventricle, but it is usually weakened here, and is not at its loudest. Another point at which it may be heard is the third left space exactly over the pulmonic valves or artery.

**Cause of the Conduction of the Murmur.**—In a certain degree we may say that the distribution of the murmur described is explained by its conduction downwards by the current of the regurgitant blood, and this must be held to account for the difference between obstructive and regurgitant aortic murmurs, in regard to the points on the chest wall where they are best heard. But the direction which the blood takes will be towards the apex, and if the current carried the murmur, it would be at the apex that we should hear it most distinctly, which is not the case. The truth is that we are apt to lose sight of the fact that much more blood enters the ventricle from the auricle than from the aorta—any other state of things would be incompatible with onward movement of the blood in the systemic arteries, and therefore with life—and also that the regurgitant stream through the valves is comparatively small if rapid. We are also perhaps given to figure in our imagination, this stream as falling into an empty vessel, whence has arisen such an explanation as the collision of the blood with the ventricular wall, to account for some abnormal sound or other. The ventricle is never an empty cavity into which blood can fall with violence as into a bottle or jar; there is no large and powerful stream rushing straight from the aorta down to the apex; during diastole, in a case of aortic insufficiency, there must be complicated cross currents in the ventricle, rendering conduction of sound in any definite direction impossible. The vibrations, then, must be conveyed by the walls of the ventricles, and not by the contained blood, or at any rate the blood thrown into sonorous eddies will communicate the vibrations to all parts of the ventricular wall indifferently, and not impinge upon any special point carrying thither the sound.

**Presystolic Murmur.**—Sometimes, more usually when there is stenosis as well as incompetence of the aortic orifice, a presystolic murmur is heard in the region of the apex, resembling very closely that of mitral stenosis, which does not, however, denote constriction of the mitral orifice. This is sometimes termed the Flint murmur, as it was first described by him. It is, of course, possible that mitral stenosis may co-exist with double aortic disease; but in some cases in which a presystolic murmur has been audible at the apex, together with a systolic and diastolic murmur in the aortic area, the mitral orifice has been found to be normal at the autopsy, and the only lesion has been constriction and incompetence of the aortic orifice. The following explanation of the origin of this murmur has been suggested. The mitral and aortic orifices are in close apposition, and it is probable that the regurgitant stream from the aorta impinges to a certain extent on the anterior or aortic flap of the mitral valve. It is conceivable that the murmur may be due to this flap of the mitral valve being thrown into vibration by the regurgitant stream from the aorta, the vibration being conducted to the apex by the chordæ tendineæ and papillary muscles, or, on the other hand, that the backward rush of blood from the aorta prevents the complete falling back of this flap of the mitral valve, so that some actual obstruction of the mitral orifice results, giving rise to a presystolic murmur.

**Violent Arterial Pulsation.**—One of the most striking features in aortic regurgitation is the sudden, abrupt, and violent pulsation of the arteries throughout the body, most conspicuous in the carotids. So marked is this that one can often make a diagnosis at sight. The pulse is visible at the wrist, the brachials at the bend of the elbow throw themselves into violent curves, the femoral and anterior tibial arteries are scarcely less visible; the temporals, facials, and labials may be seen beating; even the digital arteries may be seen as well as felt to an unpleasant degree. As was first pointed out by Sibson, the radial pulse is audible when the hand is raised, a sign more interesting perhaps than valuable.

The arteries, as may be easily seen in the radial at the wrist, are large, because the entire contents of the left ventricle, expanded to two or three times its normal capacity, are launched into the arterial system, distending it momentarily to a corresponding degree.

**Capillary and Venous Pulsation.**—Another interesting effect is capillary pulsation, a pulsatile reddening of the skin, which is sometimes observed in the palms of the hand when warm, especially when pyrexia is present, and a similar phenomenon may at any time be provoked at various parts of the surface, most conveniently perhaps on the forehead, by bringing out a red patch or line by friction, the margins of which will be seen alternately to extend and fade, synchronously with the pulse. This is due to the extension of the arterial relaxation into the capillaries, and when it is general the pulsatile movement of the blood may even reach the veins. To render this visible the hand should be so held as to drop at the wrist when the veins on the dorsum will fill, and sometimes will be seen to pulsate, not with the sudden beat of the artery, or like the rapid flush of the capillaries, but with a gentle and deliberate movement followed with difficulty, but which a filament of sealing-wax across the vein will render visible.

Capillary pulsation, however, is not a phenomenon peculiar to aortic incompetence, as it may be produced sometimes in pneumonia, or phthisis, or enteric fever, or other conditions associated with a pulse of low tension.

**The Pulse.**—This is the well-known collapsing or water-hammer pulse, sometimes named after Corrigan, who is believed to have first called attention to it. The artery at the wrist is large. In the intervals between the pulsations it is empty and allows itself to be completely flattened against the bone; then the wave comes with a sudden violent rush, filling the vessel and lifting the fingers forcibly. It is as short as it is sudden, and the artery at once collapses again under the pressure of the fingers. In order that all these features may be fully realized, the hand must be above the level of the heart and above the shoulder or elbow. When the patient is lying in bed, the act of giving the hand for the pulse to be felt brings about this condition, but when he is sitting, as during an interview in the consulting-room, or standing with the arm hanging down, although the artery may be large and the beat sudden, the collapse will not take place.

The cause of the collapse is, that in consequence of the loss of the support of the aortic valves, the column of blood is not sustained, and therefore drops out of any vessel which is above the level of the heart in obedience to gravity. If, then, the hand is hanging down, the radial artery remains full, having above it a column of blood up to the arch of the sub-clavian.

The collapsing character of the pulse is indispensable as an evidence of aortic regurgitation, though certain complications, which will be enumerated later, may interfere with the degree of collapse.

In cases of pulmonic regurgitation, which are rarely met with, the absence of the collapsing pulse and of undue carotid pulsation will be the most important distinguishing features. Similarly their presence, in cases where the diastolic murmur is heard loudest or exclusively over the pulmonic area, will clear up all doubts as to diagnosis.

The evidence afforded by the collapsing pulse is corroborated by conspicuous pulsation in the carotid arteries. This is visible not only at the root of the neck, where pulsation is often seen, but can be followed upwards along the entire course of the artery in front of the sterno-mastoid and between this muscle and the ramus of the jaw, also in front of the ear.

egurgitation is
an appreciably
at of the heart
which varies
e. This delay
' state of the
heir large size
ial system has
.unching of a
re the vessels
lse-wave to be
;icle on Aortic
seems to him
siological and
nt later on in
elay, as shown
ford, the delay
cardiac systole.
hich he claims
re is no delay.
e may be that
es. Mackenzie
of incompetence
conditions one
converted into
ity would tend
to do away with
ls of the great
linical evidence
as to bring out
hereas in instru-
pulse wave, the
f the shoulder,

*Ibid.*, p. 965.

so that the column of blood in the arm does not fall back towards the heart, tending to empty the vessel, but is ready to transmit the systolic pressure.

The **pulsus bisferiens** is sometimes met with in aortic incompetence, more commonly when there is concomitant stenosis. It is a peculiar double beat, best felt when the fingers exert a moderate pressure on the artery, less than is necessary to bring out fully the collapsing character of the pulse, but more than is employed to appreciate dichrotism. It can be readily demonstrated by the sphygmograph. It is produced by a double systolic effort, which can sometimes be felt or heard in the heart itself, and which frequently gives rise to a double rush of blood audible in the carotids.

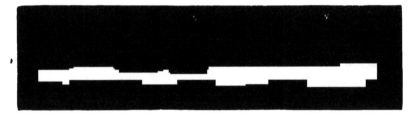

FIG. 15.—PULSUS BISFERIENS.

According to D'Espine, of Geneva, the normal systole of the heart is à deux temps, or a double contraction, of which this is an exaggeration. The pulsus bisferiens can not uncommonly be induced by an effort, which throws additional work on the heart; for instance, in one case it was not present while the patient lay quietly in bed, but was brought out when he held up both his hands.

**Irregularity of Pulse.**—Though the pulse of aortic incompetence is for the most part regular in force and frequency, in advanced cases, especially when the heart is beginning to fail, irregularity of pulse is not uncommon. The irregularity, which may be described as faltering, is first manifested by the occurrence of a short and rapid pulsation of less force and amplitude than the ordinary wave, and occurring at irregular intervals. It succeeds the previous beat very quickly, and is followed by a longer interval than usual. It would seem to indicate an effort of the heart to supplement an inadequate and inefficient preceding contraction, or to be an abortive systole. Later on, the irregularity, both in force and frequency, becomes more general and more marked, though the pulse is still recognizable as that of aortic regurgitation.

## Estimation of the Extent of the Lesion.

The amount of blood which returns into the ventricle is a matter of the first importance in estimating the prospects of life and comfort before the patient, and we have now to consider the different sources of information on this point.

**The diastolic murmur** itself affords but vague indications. As has been already mentioned, it may be loud or feeble, rough or smooth, long or short. It usually begins with an accent. Speaking generally, a long loud murmur shows that a considerable degree of pressure is kept up in the aorta, which is a desirable thing in itself, and a proof that the heart is acting with vigour, and also that the leakage of the valves is not excessive; it is usually, therefore, among the favourable auguries. On the other hand, a weak short murmur indicating an opposite state of things may be a note of impending danger or death. But there are so many exceptions to the rule hinted at that it is not to be relied upon.

**Aortic Second Sound.**—A very important auscultatory sign, however, is the presence or absence of the aortic second sound. We must listen for this, not at the apex or in the aortic area, but in the neck. A second sound of some kind, probably the pulmonic conducted, is often heard at the apex or base, but it has not the same favourable significance. The point of the sign is this: the aortic second sound is produced by the sudden tension of the aorta and its semilunar valves at the moment of closure of the valves; it is not their clicking as they meet, or the tension of the valves alone under the column of blood, but the vibration or sudden strain on the entire ascending aorta. If, then, the incompetence is considerable, there cannot be the sudden check to the column of blood which sets the aorta vibrating, and the diastolic murmur takes the place of the second sound; if, on the contrary, the leakage is only small, the required check or shock is given by the closing valves, and the second sound is distinct, although there may be a murmur. It is not the murmur, which may be loud or feeble, that drowns the second sound and prevents it being heard. In listening in the neck over the carotid artery, we have the advantage of being out of reach both of the diastolic murmur and of the pulmonic second sound, and the tension in the aorta must be real in order that the second sound may be heard here. A second sound, therefore, heard in the neck indicates that the regurgitation is small in amount and is consequently a favourable prognostic element. The second sound is usually loud and ringing when the incompetence is the result of dilatation of the aorta involving the orifice, but this is not of favourable prognostic significance, as the lesion is due to degeneritive change and is likely to be progressive.

**The Pulse.**—The degree of collapse in the pulse is an important factor in the estimation of the amount of the regurgitation. The greater the regurgitation, the more pronounced will be the collapsing character of the pulse. In the absence of any marked collapse in the pulse, a diastolic murmur, whatever its character, would not indicate any serious degree of incompetence. While this may be taken as a general rule, three important exceptions must be mentioned:

1. Concomitant aortic stenosis may interfere with the suddenness and completeness of the collapse, when the amount of regurgitation would have to be estimated by other means than by the pulse.

2. In the last stages of aortic regurgitation, when the heart is failing, there may not be sufficient force in the cardiac systole to produce the collapsing pulse.

3. In aortic disease, acquired in later life from dilatation of the aorta or degenerative changes in the valves, the

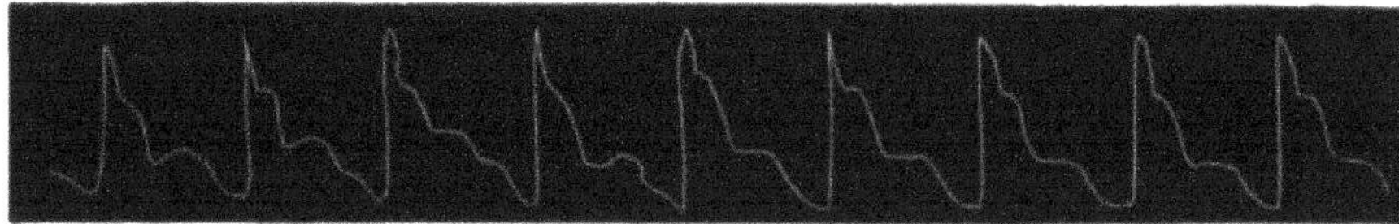

FIG. 16.—COLLAPSING PULSE OF AORTIC REGURGITATION DUE TO ACUTE ENDOCARDITIS.

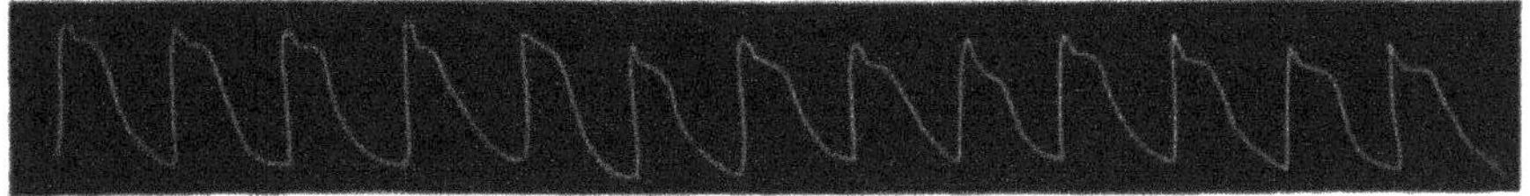

FIG. 17.

FIGS. 18.—LOSS OF COLLAPSE IN PULSE OF AORTIC REGURGITATION DUE TO DEGENERATIVE CHANGES.

pulse has not the typical sudden and collapsing character. (Figs. 17 and 18.) This absence of collapse in the pulse is partly due to the rigidity and loss of elasticity in the vessels, partly to the fact that the incompetence is not great, as in such cases life is rarely prolonged if the regurgitation becomes considerable.

The difference between the pulse of aortic incompetence, due to degenerative changes in the valves, and the ordinary collapsing pulse is well brought out by a sphygmographic tracing.

**The Heart.**—Other evidence as to the amount of regurgitation is obtained from the changes which it has induced in the heart. It has already been pointed out that if the normal amount of blood is to be propelled through the systemic arteries, while a certain proportion of that sent by each systole into the aorta is returned into the ventricle, an increase in the capacity of the ventricle is necessary. In other words, it must be dilated. We are not arguing that, because the necessity exists, therefore the provision is made, but showing that the dilatation always found is not injurious but useful, inasmuch as increased force in the ventricular contraction would not alone meet the difficulty.

The process by which the dilatation is effected is the distending influence of the backward pressure from the aorta, during the diastole of the ventricle, when the muscular fibres are relaxed and unresisting. Finally, hypertrophy results from the excessive functional activity imposed upon the walls of the ventricle by the mechanical conditions present. It is in aortic incompetence that the extremes of dilatation and hypertrophy of the left ventricle are met with, and we have the apex beat displaced downwards to the sixth, seventh, or eighth space, and carried beyond the nipple or, in exceptional cases, up to or beyond the anterior axillary line. The apex beat may be well defined, or spread over a large area, and will be powerful. Sometimes the wall of the chest between the apex and the sternum is visibly lifted by the forcible contraction of the left ventricle. Very frequently two or three spaces, between the nipple line and the sternum, will be depressed with the systole, and this systolic recession of intercostal spaces has been supposed to prove the existence of adhesion between the pericardium and heart. It is, however, frequently only the result of atmospheric pressure contributing to fill up the space left by the great diminution of volume of the heart during systole.

## Estimation of the Extent of the Lesion by Degree of Dilatation and Hypertrophy of the Heart.

The dilatation and hypertrophy being the effects, are also, with certain qualifications, the measure of the regurgitation, in the absence of symptoms such as conspicuous breathlessness on very slight exertion, or faltering action of the heart and tendency to fainting or giddiness. The most important qualification is that arising out of the inability of the heart to take on these compensatory changes late in life; so that when aortic insufficiency develops for the first time after the age of thirty, an opinion as to its degree, and as to the danger attending it, can only be arrived at after prolonged observation and repeated examination. It is an interesting and important question up to what age effectual compensation for serious aortic regurgitation is possible. In my own experience all really satisfactory examples have been among those in whom the valvular lesion has been established under the age of twenty. Cases have come under my observation in hospital practice in which the valves have been extensively damaged between the age of twenty and thirty, and the patients have remained under observation for some time afterwards, without developing symptoms of cardiac failure; but such cases are too soon lost sight of for trustworthy conclusions to be based upon them.

The amount of dilatation attending a given degree of incompetence will also vary according to the amount and duration of the care bestowed upon the patient during the first few months of its existence. If he has been allowed to leave his bed too early and engage in exercise, or has undertaken work before the heart has fully recovered from the effects of acute disease, the dilatation will have gone further than would have been the case if due precautions had been observed till the strength was fully restored.

Dilatation, moreover, may be increased during subsequent illness attended with pyrexia or anæmia. In all such cases, however, if the extent of the changes in the cavities and walls of the heart does not accurately correspond with the degree of change in the valves, it indicates the extent to which the functional efficiency of the heart is endangered.

## Aortic Incompetence due to other Causes than Acute Endocarditis.

In the account just given of the physical signs of aortic incompetence, reference has been made from time to time to differences observed when the valvular disease is established during or after middle life, and from causes other than rheumatism. Such causes are syphilitic affection of the valves and the wall of the aorta, degenerative changes included under the general term atheroma, and rupture of a cusp of the valve.

**Syphilis** may be suspected as the cause of aortic incompetence, which comes on in early adult life or middle age, and is not traceable to rheumatic endocarditis or to gout or high arterial tension. It is usually associated with degenerative changes and dilatation of the aorta. Aneurysm is indeed more common than aortic incompetence as a result of syphilis. The regurgitation may rapidly become considerable, and as regards the murmur and the character of the pulse, there will be no important deviations from the description given. The principal difference will arise from the fact that the heart-walls and cavities do not so readily take on compensatory changes; consequently the relation between the degree of dilatation and hypertrophy which makes the latter approximately a criterion by which to estimate the former, no longer holds good. There may, therefore, be considerable regurgitation with comparatively little enlargement of the heart.

**Atheroma of the Aorta.**—Atheroma may involve the aortic valves or give rise to dilatation of the aorta, including the aortic orifice, and thus produce insufficiency. When the incompetence is the result of such degenerative changes, there will be hypertrophy and dilatation of the heart, not, however, induced by and compensatory of the valvular defect, but developed antecedently to it by the high arterial tension which has given rise to the aortic disease. The pulse will exhibit only partially and imperfectly the collapsing character; the artery will be large, and the wave sudden and brief; but when the hand is held up the vessel does not collapse, but can be rolled under the finger throughout the diastolic interval. It will be visible, not however from the sudden filling of the previously collapsed artery, but from the artery being thrown into curves. Further, there will not be the marked loss of time between the apex beat and the pulse at the wrist. The second sound is usually heard in the neck, and has the low pitch and ringing character indicative of dilatation of the aorta and high arterial tension. Very frequently the diastolic murmur is audible across the manubrium, along the course of the aorta.

The insufficiency in such cases is produced, not simply by changes in the valve, but by concurrent dilatation of the aorta implicating its orifice, which is sometimes, indeed, so stretched that the valves, even when retaining their normal size, fail to close it, and the actual amount of regurgitation can never become considerable without producing fatal syncope.

**Rupture of Valve.**—Rupture of a valve is always a very serious lesion. It may occur as the result of severe exertion when the valve has been weakened by degenerative changes. The valve affected is usually the aortic, and the sudden and severe strain on the heart, which has no time to accommodate itself to the altered conditions of the circulation, leads to dilatation of the left ventricle and the consequent onset of severe symptoms when the rupture of a cusp is complete. The patient may be seized by a syncopal attack, which will at once prove fatal. He may, however, appear to progress favourably for some time, but will rarely recover sufficiently to be able to go about again as usual, for the accident usually takes place at a time in life when degenerative changes are already beginning to take place in the walls of the heart, and it is incapable of undergoing sufficient hypertrophy to compensate for the valvular lesion. Hence the ultimate cause of death, if the patient survives, is a gradual stasis of the circulation, the premonitory indications being a rapid increase in the size of the liver, with dilatation of the right ventricle following on that of the left, and later the onset of œdema of the extremities. It may be some weeks or months after the accident before the fatal termination ensues.

The early symptoms, however, are not necessarily so severe.

In a case that was under my care at St. Mary's Hospital in 1893, the patient, a man aged fifty-two, walked up to the casualty room, complaining that he could not use his right arm, and saying that he thought he had sprained it while lifting a heavy weight. The history of the accident was that he was carrying a heavy bag on his shoulder; and when throwing it off his shoulder he tried to prevent it falling with too much violence on to the ground by catching hold of it with his right hand. He then felt a sudden pain in his arm and chest, and was violently sick. He walked up to the hospital, apparently without much discomfort. He was somewhat pale, but was not suffering from dyspnœa, and complained chiefly of his right arm. On examination, the right radial pulse was found to be absent owing to thrombosis of the brachial and axillary arteries. The pulse in the left radial was 98, regular in force and frequency, slightly collapsing; respirations, 18.

On examining the heart, the apex beat was found to be in the fifth space, just inside the nipple line; a faint systolic and diastolic murmur were audible at the apex, and a diastolic murmur was also heard at the aortic cartilage and down the sternum. The liver was not enlarged.

He remained in hospital from April 22 till May 13, when he left at his own request. During this time no serious symptoms had developed, and he had been up and walking about the ward without any discomfort beyond a little shortness of breath.

Rather more than a fortnight later, on May 30, he came back to the hospital complaining of extreme shortness of breath and swelling of the legs. The pulse was then 116, the respirations 34. The legs were œdematous, and the face was very pale and anæmic. On examining the heart, it was found to be much dilated, the area of cardiac dulness extending up to the third rib above and inwards to the middle of the sternum, outwards for half an inch outside the nipple line.

The apex beat was not visible or palpable, but the sounds were best heard in the seventh space, half an inch outside the nipple line. A systolic and long soft diastolic murmur were audible at that point, and the diastolic murmur was heard down the sternum. The aortic second sound was almost entirely replaced by the murmur, and the first sound was very feeble. The liver was much enlarged, extending down to within two inches of the umbilicus, and was pulsating.

Rest and treatment failed to improve his condition, which got steadily worse, the symptoms increasing in severity till he died on August 9, some ten weeks later. At the autopsy it was found that the anterior flap of the aortic valve was ruptured, and that there was extensive incompetence. There was considerable dilatation of the cardiac cavities, and little or no compensatory hypertrophy.

## Symptoms.

The symptoms in well-marked aortic regurgitation are those of deficient and unsustained blood supply in the systemic circulation. The patient is pale, anæmic, short of breath on slight exertion, and liable to fainting or syncopal attacks, one of which may prove fatal. Pain, or a sense of oppression in the cardiac region, may be present, amounting in severe cases to angina pectoris. There may be sleeplessness or paroxysms of severe dyspnœa, and vomiting is sometimes persistent in severe cases where compensation has not been established or suddenly breaks down.

The above may be termed "aortic" symptoms, as distinguished from the train of symptoms which set in when the mitral valve has given way under the strain and mitral incompetence is established. The burden of compensation then, as in mitral disease, falls on the right ventricle, and we get a train of "mitral" symptoms in addition to the already existing "aortic" symptoms.

There will be back pressure in the pulmonary veins with congestion of the lungs, increased dyspnœa, and perhaps cyanosis. Dilatation of the right ventricle eventually occurs, and enlargement of the liver and dropsy supervene.

Secondary mitral symptoms are less common in aortic regurgitation than stenosis, as if the lesion is severe the patient is liable to sudden death from syncopal attack. When stenosis supervenes in a severe case of regurgitation, it appears to have a beneficial effect, and limits the amount of reflux, so that the patient has a better chance of surviving for a time; and it is in cases of double aortic lesions that we usually meet with the train of secondary mitral symptoms, when the patient eventually succumbs from right ventricle failure.

## Prognosis.

When, with a diastolic murmur, the aortic second sound is distinctly audible in the neck, the pulse exhibits the collapsing character only in a moderate degree, and the dilatation and hypertrophy of the heart are inconsiderable; that is, when the physical signs indicate that the lesion is slight in extent, the patient may enjoy life and do hard work untroubled by symptoms for many years, provided that the lesion is due to acute endocarditis and not to degenerative changes.

This may be illustrated by an example. A medical man, aged forty, called on me in October, 1883, whom I had known and examined sixteen or eighteen years previously, when he was under Dr. Sibson's care as a student at the hospital. He had had aortic incompetence ever since an attack of acute rheumatism at the age of fourteen, so that its duration was twenty-six years. The following is an account of the physical signs, they were identical with those present when he was at the hospital: "Apex beat in sixth space not much below and very little to the left of the normal situation, being a good push, but not violent or extensive; the first sound good, the second sound also distinct. A systolic murmur, probably conducted from the aorta, is audible at the apex. At the right second intercostal space a weak systolic murmur is audible, and along the right edge of the sternum, from the third cartilage downwards, over the lower part of the sternum and over the left costal cartilages, a very distinct, long, smooth diastolic murmur is heard. There is a good second sound, audible at the right second space and sterno-clavicular articulation and in the neck. The pulse is short and is felt in the fingers as well as at the wrist, but is scarcely collapsing; the carotid pulsation is marked, but the pulse at the wrist and in the temporals is not visible." He had gone through his medical studies with distinction, and had ever since carried on a hard-working country practice, with all its incidents of night-work and exposure and excessive fatigue. He could walk uphill or run upstairs without experiencing any inconvenience, and it was not for any cardiac symptoms that he consulted me in 1883.

Aortic incompetence sufficient to abolish the second sound in the neck, and to give rise to considerable dilatation and hypertrophy and to well-marked collapsing pulse is serious, though it may for many years be compatible with apparent health and strength. The patient will be capable of ordinary work and exercise, but will be sooner out of breath on going uphill or from any unusual exertion than a man in health, or may feel suddenly faint and giddy instead of losing his breath; emotion again will more readily induce palpitation. The future in such circumstances must be estimated on the principles laid down in the chapter on general prognosis. After calculation of the degree of valvular inefficiency, we must consider the tenacity of the family constitution and the vigour of the individual, as well as his age, habits, occupation, and circumstances, bearing in mind always that even in the most favourable cases the nutrition of the enlarged heart will not be well maintained after middle age, and that as years go on there is a tendency to increased resistance in the peripheral circulation. We must look, therefore, for failure of the heart and accession of symptoms sooner or later, at best long before the natural term of life. There is also the possibility that the compensatory equilibrium may at any time be dangerously disturbed or finally overthrown by imprudent exertion or anxiety or acute illness of any kind.

The **Age** of the patient at the time when the lesion is acquired is a most important consideration in prognosis, and a case may be quoted to show how long a severe lesion may be survived even under unfavourable circumstances, when the patient is young, and the heart can take on compensatory changes. The patient, a boy of fifteen, came under my observation in 1868, when he was admitted to St. Mary's Hospital, complaining of shortness of breath. His condition on admission was as follows: "Heart impulse extensive and violent, apex beat in the fifth and sixth spaces just outside the nipple line. Loud systolic and diastolic murmurs, audible over all the cardiac area, especially at the lower end and down the right border of the sternum. Pulse large, sudden, and collapsing; no second sound audible in the neck." The patient was a greengrocer, and continued to do his work, but frequently attended the hospital as an out-patient. Five years later, a mitral systolic murmur first developed, and by that time the heart was of great size; the apex beat was in the seventh space in the axillary line, and was a forcible thrust, which could be seen through his clothes. Dilatation and elongation of the aorta had carried the outer side of the ascending arch beyond the right edge of the sternum, so that, pressed into the second, third, and fourth spaces, the fingers came upon marked pulsation and thrill. He was still able to do his work, and a year later, at the age of twenty-one, he married and set up in business for himself. He had now to go to the early market regularly instead of occasionally, and had more work. This he did pretty well for a time, but he soon had to spare himself, and his business fell off. In 1875, seven years from the time he was first seen, he was ill at home with rheumatism, and then lived in a basement. In 1880, when again attacked by rheumatism, he consented to enter the hospital as in-patient, which he had refused to do previously. He was again in the hospital for sub-acute rheumatism from March 5 to May 8, 1882. The rheumatism quickly subsided, and there was no pain after March 18; he had, however, a severe cough. During his convalescence, the kind of irregularity of pulse and heart beat characteristic of cardiac failure in aortic regurgitation was manifest; after three or four regular and fairly equal beats, a weak supplementary beat would follow too quickly, or while perceptible at the heart would be missing at the wrist, or the irregularity might go further than this; sometimes also the pulse would reveal two distinct efforts of the ventricle in its systole, and have the "bis feriens" character. Occasionally he had a severe attack of dyspnœa. He improved, however, and after being up and about the wards for some time, was sent to a convalescent hospital, where after doing well and gaining strength, he died suddenly, fourteen years after he was first seen. A post-mortem examination revealed old-standing extensive disease of the valves, which had in effect ceased to exist as valves, great general dilatation of the aorta, some thickening of the mitral flaps and shortening of the tendinous cords, extreme dilatation and hypertrophy of the left ventricle, some dilatation and hypertrophy of the right ventricle without any affection of the valves of this side of the heart. The weight of the heart was forty-two and a half ounces.

But even in young subjects, as soon as marked symptoms begin to present themselves, danger is at hand; when they are not habitually present, the readiness with which they are induced by exertion serves as a dynamic test of great prognostic value. Some years since, I examined, within a short time of each other, two boys with very extensive aortic incompetence, attended with almost the maximum degree of dilatation and hypertrophy. The physical signs could only tell us that there was great incompetence, and great compensatory change in both, but in the one the heart was readily put off its balance, and serious symptoms were induced by slight exertion; in the other, this was not so. The prognosis was, therefore, widely different in the two cases. The former died suddenly three years after I first saw him, while the latter did not die till ten years later.

In aortic regurgitation, acquired late in life, the prognosis is rarely favourable. Even if the lesion be the result of acute endocarditis, and therefore stationary, the heart is unable to undergo adequate hypertrophy, and efficient compensation will not be established. But after middle age acute endocarditis is of rare occurrence, and the incompetence will usually be due to degenerative changes in the valves; the lesion will therefore be progressive, especially if the arterial tension, the primary cause in all probability of the trouble, is not carefully kept down by suitable treatment. The prognosis is still more unfavourable if the affection is due to syphilitic disease of the aorta invading the valves.

## Prognosis in Aortic Regurgitation with Stenosis.

When aortic stenosis gradually becomes established in a case where aortic incompetence already exists of such severity that symptoms are readily and easily induced, it may act to a certain degree as a palliative agent, by limiting the amount of regurgitation and making the circulation more equable and regular. As the stenosis makes its effects felt, the pulse will lose to a great extent its collapsing character, and the artery will not empty so completely between the beats. The heart will undergo further hypertrophy, and the risk of undue dilatation will be diminished. Dyspnœa will be less readily induced, and the patient will be less liable to syncopal attacks.

I have seen several cases in which a patient, after being in imminent danger from aortic regurgitation, has, on the supervention of aortic stenosis, been enabled to enjoy a life of comparative comfort for many years. It does not follow that the onset of aortic stenosis is of favourable prognostic import in all cases of incompetence; it is only when the aortic valves are severely damaged and are incapable of checking the regurgitant stream in any effectual degree that this holds good, and when the patient is still young enough for further cardiac hypertrophy to take place.

## TREATMENT.

Perhaps more can be done to prolong life and postpone suffering in aortic regurgitation than in any other form of valvular disease; at any rate, it is in this disease that the greatest difference can be made by care on the one hand and imprudence on the other. A patient may die suddenly from a single rash act who might have lived twenty years, or condemn himself by a single imprudence to a short and suffering existence when fair health and many years of life were possible for him. It is more especially shortly after the occurrence of the lesion, before full compensatory hypertrophy has had time to take place, that such accidents are likely to happen. Hence it is especially important when aortic regurgitation has been recently established in acute rheumatism that prolonged rest should be insisted upon.

Six or eight weeks in bed, and after this rest in the recumbent posture for another month or six weeks, is advisable, and the boy should not go to school, or the young man to business for another six, eight, or twelve months, according to circumstances. It is even possible that a diastolic murmur may completely disappear, and with it all symptoms of aortic incompetence, when due care of this kind has been taken.

Not uncommonly incompetence of the aortic valves is discovered unexpectedly at an interval after an attack of rheumatism during which endocarditis had not been suspected, or had not been revealed by murmurs. It is a most important and useful precaution, therefore, to examine the heart at intervals for some time after rheumatic fever and it is an imperative duty to do so when there has been cardiac complication of any kind or degree.

In children, as the articular manifestations of rheumatism are usually so slight, and the heart is so frequently attacked, an examination of this organ should never be omitted: there may be nothing to suggest the presence of endocarditis: but a history of transient pains in the joints with febrile disturbance should at once arouse suspicion, and the presence of rheumatic nodules is almost pathognomonic of cardiac mischief present or to come. Irreparable damage to the heart not infrequently results from a child being allowed to go about with unsuspected endocarditis.

Caution and rest are necessary, not only after an attack in which there has been endocarditis setting up aortic regurgitation, but also after a febrile attack of any kind complicating cases of aortic incompetence. Dilatation is easily induced in a heart weakened by fever under the continual strain to which the left ventricle is exposed, and there is special liability to sudden death during the period of convalescence from acute illness.

On the other hand, provided care and complete rest are insisted on, the heart may actually regain lost ground from the diminution of resistance in peripheral circulation due to the arterio-capillary relaxation attending pyrexia. In a severe case of aortic regurgitation, I have known an old-standing mitral regurgitation from secondary dilatation of the left ventricle, disappear for some time under these circumstances.

The risk of sudden death makes it imperative that the patient suffering from aortic disease should be specially warned against over-exertion and hurry, such as running to catch a train or running upstairs, or excessive mental excitement of any kind. The fatal event does not always take place during the exertion or excitement, but may be postponed till the next day. Periods of rest from time to time may be of striking service. Whenever exaggeration of the short and sudden character of the pulse is observed, especially if there is a faltering in the beat now and then, and still more when the apex of the heart is found to be receding outwards, and the beat is becoming diffuse, the recumbent posture should be enforced for some two to six weeks.

As compensation fails and symptoms become more continuous and severe, they will arise from and take their characteristics from one of two causes: either (1) failure on the part of the left ventricle to maintain a sufficient movement of blood in the capillaries, or (2) backward pressure in the veins, the result of right ventricle failure secondary to that of the left. In the former case, sudden death from syncope with little warning or apparent cause is liable to occur; failing that, there may be sleeplessness of a peculiarly harassing kind, or painful dyspnœa, unexplained by any interference with the entry of air into the lungs, or by want of aëration of the blood. The face will be pale and have an anxious and suffering expression; the patient will be very restless and weary. Dropsy, if present, will be slight, though there may be some fluid in the pleural cavities with œdema of the bases of the lungs.

Under these circumstances the object of treatment is to sustain the failing heart by nourishment, stimulants, and such remedies as may contribute to this end—nux vomica or strychnia, with ammonia and ether, to which belladonna or atropin often makes a valuable addition; sometimes digitalis may be of service, but it must be used with caution; or strophanthus, which theoretically ought to be safer as having less contractile influence on the arterioles. Morphia hypodermically is often of the greatest possible benefit, giving quiet sleep, which is not only an inexpressible comfort to the sufferer, but frequently recruits the strength, and, by rendering the recumbent posture possible, so far relieves the heart that it proves the starting-point for a temporary recovery. Occasionally, however, a patient, after a good night's rest procured in this way, will say he feels better, sit up in bed, and suddenly fall back dead. This danger of syncopal attacks should be explained to patients and friends, so that watchfulness and care on their part may guard against any imprudent effort or sudden movement which might be attended with such fatal consequences. Morphia or opium administered by the mouth is much less effectual, bromides are mostly useless, chloral is positively dangerous.

Angina pectoris may complicate this form of heart failure. It is usually relieved by nitrite of amyl or nitro-glycerine, and patients suffering from anginoid pain complicating aortic regurgitation may come to take the latter remedy in extraordinary doses. When relief cannot be obtained in any other way, morphia may be given hypodermically. Whatever tends to strengthen the heart or relieve it from work will tend to prevent the onset of anginoid symptoms, and when such threaten, treatment must be directed to these two points.

Arsenic, and more especially phosphorus, have had in my hands a very beneficial influence as cardiac tonics in such cases.

When the preponderating character of the symptoms is that of venous obstruction, the jugular veins being distended and pulsating, the liver enlarged, and dropsy present; when, in fact, we have with aortic physical signs mitral symptoms, the line of treatment is quite different to that just described.

Purgatives should be given in full doses, but judgment and caution must be exercised in their administration, as unfavourable effects may develop abruptly. Digitalis may then be given, usually with great benefit, and when there is much dropsy, diuretics in addition to the digitalis will often have a marked effect. It is under such conditions that digitalis finds its opportunity in aortic regurgitation, and justifies the statements of those who find this remedy of the same service in aortic as in mitral disease.

If the administration of digitalis is persisted in after the recovery from dropsy and the more severe symptoms of venous stasis, it is not uncommon for patients to die suddenly, sometimes before leaving bed, more frequently when they have begun to get up and move about. There are grounds for suspicion that digitalis contributes to this, but sudden death may occur whether it has been left off or not. In the absence of mitral symptoms, it is rarely that digitalis is called for in aortic incompetence or is of service, and it may undoubtedly do harm. It may set up sickness, which is an ominous symptom in this form of disease, and induces a condition of asthenia difficult to remedy.

Venesection, even when the venous stasis is severe, is rarely to be contemplated. It is true that the relief to the right ventricle so afforded might enable it to regain control over its contents and increase the supply of blood to the left ventricle and the amount available for distribution to the arterial system, but before this occurs there may be a momentary faintness, leading to a fatal attack of syncope.

## CHAPTER XI.

# MITRAL INCOMPETENCE OR REGURGITATION.

ETIOLOGY AND MORBID ANATOMY—PHYSICAL SIGNS—THE MURMUR OF MITRAL INCOMPETENCE—THE PULSE—EXPLANATION OF IRREGULARITY OF PULSE—MITRAL INCOMPETENCE DUE TO ENDOCARDITIS—ESTIMATION OF EXTENT OF LESION, FROM CHARACTER OF MURMUR AND FIRST SOUND AND FROM COMPENSATORY CHANGES IN THE HEART—SYMPTOMS—PROGNOSIS—MITRAL INCOMPETENCE WITHOUT DAMAGE TO VALVES — ITS CAUSATION AND EXPLANATION—DIFFERENTIAL DIAGNOSIS—TREATMENT.

### Etiology and Morbid Anatomy.

The causation of mitral incompetence is most varied. It may be due to actual damage to the mitral valve by acute or chronic endocarditis, or to imperfect apposition of the valves or stretching of the orifice from dilatation of the left ventricle. The former group, where the valves have been injured by an inflammatory process, will be first considered.

The kind and degree of deformity produced by endocarditis may vary greatly. The edges may be thickened and shrunken, presenting, instead of the translucent, thin, flexible curtain, an opaque, inelastic, rounded border, in which the delicate marginal ramifications of the tendinous cords are swallowed up and lost. A considerable area of valve may still be available for closing the orifice, although the apposition may not be accurate. In a more advanced state of change, the body of the cusps may be opaque, thickened, and contracted so that a considerable gap must remain, allowing of great reflux even when their approximation is greatest; and sometimes this is carried so far that, as valves, they are practically non-existent, especially when the chordæ tendineæ are greatly shortened, which they may be to an extent which brings the margins of the flaps close to the apices of the papillary muscles.

Chronic endocarditis or degenerative change may produce some opacity, thickening, and deformity, giving rise to insufficiency, and calcification is not uncommon.

## Physical Signs.

**The Murmur.**—The evidence of regurgitation through the mitral orifice is a systolic murmur heard in the region of the apex, and very frequently beyond the apex in the fifth or sixth space towards the axilla. It is often audible also at the back of the chest, between the scapula and the spine, at about the middle of the posterior border of the scapula. The murmur reaches the surface at this point, not by extension round the thorax from the axilla, but by an independent route, being conducted by the vertebræ from the base of the ventricle, the shoulder of which rests upon the spinal column. Occasionally the murmur of mitral regurgitation is heard more loudly in the fourth or even in the third space in the vertical nipple line or just outside it, than at the apex. When this is the case, an impulse is usually to be felt at or near the same point.

**Murmurs which may be mistaken for Mitral Regurgitant Murmur.**—The only murmurs likely to be mistaken for this are, a systolic aortic murmur conducted to the apex, a systolic and therefore regurgitant tricuspid murmur, and the spurious murmur produced by compression of the edge of the lung by the ventricular systole. A pulmonic systolic murmur is also occasionally heard almost at the apex. A question which frequently arises when a systolic murmur is heard both at the base and at the apex, is, whether it is one and the same, in which case it will be aortic, or whether it arises from two independent sources. It is only when the murmur is loudest over the aorta that there can be any uncertainty, and as a rule it is not difficult to decide. Any marked difference in the tone or character of the apex murmur, as compared with that heard at the base, or a superadded musical element in it, would be sufficient to show that it was not the conducted aortic murmur, and where such evidence as this is lacking, if the apex murmur is longer than the aortic, and especially if it is conducted outwards for any distance, or is heard in the left inter-scapular space, there can be no doubt. It must be remembered, however, that a loud, rough, aortic murmur may be heard as a smooth murmur of a different tone at the apex, the thick muscular wall of the ventricle not lending itself to the propagation of coarse vibrations, which are, in fact, vibrations of the aorta itself. A loud aortic murmur, again, may be audible all down the thoracic spine.

With regard to the tricuspid murmur a special warning may be of service, as it is not unfrequently set down as mitral. The tricuspid area, so called, is over the lower costal cartilages, near the ensiform appendage, but a systolic tricuspid murmur is often heard as far out as the apex, and occasionally has its maximum intensity just to the inner side of the apex. When a murmur heard at the apex is lost immediately to the left of the beat, while it is audible between the apex and the lower end of the sternum, its seat of production is at the tricuspid, and not at the mitral orifice.

An imitation of a systolic apex murmur is not unfrequently produced by movement of air in the lungs overlapping the heart as it is compressed by the systole of the heart, and it is sometimes loud enough to be heard by the subject. The imposture is easily detected, by the fact that it is only audible, as a rule, during inspiration, or is, at any rate, much more distinct then, and that its distribution does not coincide with the conduction of the true mitral murmur, but follows the line of the thin edge of the lung across the pericardium from the neighbourhood of the apex towards the sternum.

The sources of error just mentioned being eliminated, a systolic murmur audible at and to the left of the apex, is mitral in origin, and indicates incompetence in the valve and reflux of blood into the left auricle. There is not the same doubt as to its significance as there is with regard to the constant association of obstruction with an aortic systolic murmur; a mitral systolic murmur means regurgitation. It does not, however, necessarily imply that there is actual disease of the mitral valve, as there are other causes, enumerated later, which may give rise to mitral regurgitation from dilatation of the left ventricle or stretching of the mitral orifice.

**The Pulse.**—The distinguishing characteristic is irregularity, both in rhythm and in force. In advanced cases no two beats are alike; a few fairly strong, full pulsations, at something like proper intervals, will be followed by a number of feeble, hurried beats, these again perhaps by a single good stroke, after which there is a pause and then renewed hurried action. Little difference of opinion exists as to the association of mitral incompetence with irregularity of pulse. It would not be true to assert that there can be no considerable regurgitation without irregular action of the heart, but it is a safe working hypothesis that a mitral murmur is not attended with serious reflux while the pulse remains regular. What, then, is the cause of the irregularity? We find similar irregularity occasionally attending dilatation of the heart, and it might be suggested that, as mitral insufficiency is not unfrequently the result of dilatation of the ventricle, the irregularity of the pulse is symptomatic of the dilatation, and not of the regurgitation; but the irregularity accompanies incompetence caused by rheumatic damage of the valves, quite as constantly as it does the insufficiency due to dilatation.

Irregular heart action and pulse, again, may be among the final symptoms in any form of valvular disease, though they are rarely quite of the same character as in mitral regurgitation; but in this latter disease the irregularity supervenes early, and is not inconsistent with fair compensation and apparent health for many years.

It is probable that the varying pressure to which the heart is subjected in inspiration and expiration may account for it. The variations of intrathoracic pressure in ordinary respiration have no obvious effect on the action of the heart; but we can at any time slightly disturb the rhythm of the heart and pulse by taking and holding a very deep breath. When again there is incipient irregularity careful observation will almost always show that the break in the rhythm occurs at the moment when there is a change in the intrathoracic pressure at the beginning and end of inspiration or expiration. This is best seen, perhaps, in cases of bronchitis and emphysema with dilated right heart. The thin-walled auricles will be all the more susceptible of this change of pressure when distended and dilated, while it will scarcely affect the ventricles.

The heart works habitually under a negative pressure due to the elastic traction of the lungs, and is only subjected to positive pressure, strictly speaking, when the chest is filled and the glottis closed in effort. The aspiration resulting from the negative pressure is greatest in inspiration, and aids the circulation by drawing the blood into the auricles, which then carry it on into the ventricles. In expiration the auricles are more or less compressed as the chest walls collapse.

When the left auriculo-ventricular valves are incompetent, the pressure on the auricle during expiration will aid in resisting the systolic reflux from the ventricle, and in driving the blood into the ventricle during diastole; at the moment when the positive pressure of expiration is exchanged for the negative pressure of inspiration, the resistance to the reflux of blood into the auricle is suddenly diminished, so that more will be allowed to regurgitate, and less will be carried into the aorta, and there will be no compression of the auricle to aid in filling the ventricle. Corresponding differences of an opposite kind will attend the end of inspiration. The varying supply of blood to the ventricle thus induced, cannot fail to produce a tendency to irregularity.

**Estimation of the Extent of the Lesion.**—Our first inquiry will be as to the physical signs and symptoms by means of which we may approximately infer the degree of impairment of the valves, and the amount of regurgitation which takes place.

The murmur affords, in some cases, important information. When it is not conducted much beyond the situation of the apex beat, the apex itself not being greatly displaced, and is not audible in the back, the regurgitation is usually slight. But an exception to this statement may be found at the opposite extreme, when the orifice is gaping and the ventricle weak. Under such circumstances the murmur may be short and scarcely audible; symptoms, however, will at once distinguish between the two conditions.

The persistence of the left ventricle first sound is evidence that there is no advanced change in the valves, more especially when the murmur is retarded. This is an important point to note. If the regurgitation is considerable, the murmur takes the place of the first sound, and is said to hide it; but it is not a mere question of loudness, there is a true substitution of the murmur for the sound. When, therefore, the first sound is distinctly heard heading the murmur, some difference exists. It would be going too far to say, as in the case of the aortic valves, that the sound indicates sufficient check to the refluent blood to produce tension of the valves and cords, and of the ventricular wall, but the inference tends in that direction. With regard to the retarded-systolic mitral murmur, when the murmur follows the first sound at a distinct though very brief interval, it would seem that there is, in the first instance, complete closure of the valves, but that during the contraction of the ventricle, the apposition is deranged so that leakage occurs. Such leakage can scarcely be other than slight. These inferences are confirmed by the fact that the persistent first sound and the retarded systolic murmur are most common in the curable or temporary regurgitation of anæmia, and the conclusions based on this observation may be extended to other cases than those of early life. One caution is necessary, that is, to beware of taking the modified short, sharp, first sound of mitral stenosis, when there is both obstruction and regurgitation, for the normal second sound.

The general statement made in the first chapter that a loud and long murmur is usually significant of a lesser degree of structural damage and functional imperfection than a short and weak murmur, is another point to be borne in mind. Loudness implies strength of contraction, and length shows that the ventricle goes through with its systole, and also that it is not quickly emptied, as it would be were there a large escape into the auricle. The murmur of worst significance is a short, weak whiff, varying in intensity and duration in successive beats.

It is the mitral systolic murmur which is most frequently musical; very commonly, but not perhaps always, the musical murmur indicates a narrow chink, and therefore little reflux. The musical note may be high-pitched or low, nearly always it is accompanied by a blowing murmur, and, according to my experience, has never the pure tone sometimes produced at the aortic orifice. It does not always begin at the same time with the blowing murmur, but may be interpolated into it, beginning later and ending sooner.

As the action of the heart is frequently irregular, the intensity, character, pitch, and length of the murmur may vary from one beat to another.

For further evidence we must trace the effects of regurgitation through the mitral orifice. The immediate effect of reflux of blood into the left auricle will be to distend this cavity, but, lying deeply as it does, the physical signs of an early stage of dilatation are not such as can be relied upon for definite information; but another result which follows early is obstruction to the free outflow of blood from the pulmonary veins into the auricle, and this soon makes itself felt backwards through the capillaries of the lungs, and gives rise to high pressure in the pulmonary artery. Here we come upon audible evidence; the increased tension brings down the semilunar valves with greater force, and gives rise to accentuation of the pulmonic second sound. It is not easy to say what degree of intensification of this second sound is required as proof of obstruction to the flow of blood through the lungs. The aortic second sound has to be taken as a basis for comparison, and while most observers say that the aortic is the louder of the two, my own conclusion is that the pulmonic is usually louder than the aortic. Again, the pulmonic second sound may be accentuated by resistance arising in the lungs themselves, as in bronchitis and emphysema. Marked and persistent intensification of the pulmonic second sound, when a mitral systolic murmur is present, must, however, be taken as evidence of sufficient reflux to increase the pressure in the pulmonary artery by the obstruction to which it gives rise.

**Changes in the Heart.**—From this follow hypertrophy and dilatation of the right ventricle. The call upon the right ventricle for increased force in propelling the blood through the lungs results in a combination of dilatation and hypertrophy, of which the physical signs are displacement of the apex outwards or to the left and undue right ventricle impulse, felt when the hand is placed over the lower costal cartilages to the left of the sternum, and seen, and perhaps felt, in the epigastrium and below the left costal margin. The right ventricle in effect comes to the aid of the left; the heightened pressure maintained by its means in the left auricle resists the reflux of blood from the ventricle, and since life is often sustained when the valves are practically non-existent, the intra-auricular pressure must in such cases almost, if not quite, equal the pressure in the systemic arteries. Further, the same force which resists the reflux must, on the relaxation of the left ventricle, drive the blood violently into it, taking it, so to speak, at a disadvantage, and distending it in the same way, though not to the same degree, as aortic regurgitation, giving rise thus to dilatation, which is accompanied or followed by more or less hypertrophy. In proportion as the left ventricle is enlarged, the apex will be carried downwards and its beat become conspicuous, and the hypertrophy of the right ventricle pushing it outwards and sometimes upwards, the ultimate displacement of the apex will be the resultant of the changes in the two ventricles. There will also be dilatation of the auricles. The volume of the heart as a whole will thus be increased, giving rise to a corresponding extension of the area of deep dulness.

These changes, the necessary result of the incompetence of the mitral valve, traceable directly to the mechanical difficulty produced by it, become the measure of the difficulty and of the incompetence. A systolic mitral murmur without increase in the area of cardiac dulness, without much displacement of the apex, and without marked accentuation of the pulmonic second sound, without, again, symptoms indicative of disturbance of the circulation such as might be due to failure in the compensatory changes, is not attended with any considerable regurgitation, and is not a source of present danger. Unless there is reason to look upon it as the beginning of progressive damage, it may practically be disregarded. As the signs of pressure in the pulmonary circulation and of changes in the walls and cavities of the heart increase, we infer increase in the amount of reflux, for they indicate greater difficulty in neutralizing its injurious effects. We, therefore, calculate on diminished stability of the compensatory balance and on less power of regaining a working equilibrium of the circulatory forces if it is once overthrown.

To sum up the indications by which the extent of the lesion may be surmised:

While it may safely be said that if the pulse remains regular the reflux is slight, the degree of irregularity of the pulse will not be any criterion as to the extent of the reflux. More is to be learnt from the degree of vigour of the beat, and the length of the pulse wave.

Further information will be derived from the character of the murmur, and the extent to which it replaces the first sound, and again from accentuation of the pulmonic second sound; but the amount of dilatation and hypertrophy of the heart, more especially of the right ventricle, will afford a more accurate basis for the estimation of the degree of incompetence. The symptoms must also be concurrently taken into consideration.

### Symptoms.

No symptoms will be present in cases of slight regurgitation even on moderate exertion. In more severe cases, or when compensation is beginning to fail, shortness of breath, a tendency to cyanosis, and slight pitting of the legs at night will be among the earliest symptoms. The dyspnœa and cyanosis will become more marked and persistent as time goes on, and are due to congestion and passive hyperæmia in the lungs from back pressure in the pulmonary circulation, which gives rise to the secondary changes in the lungs described in the chapter on mitral stenosis. The pressure in the pulmonary circulation, however, is not so high as in mitral stenosis, and hæmoptysis does not occur in pure mitral incompetence, nor is the condition of brown induration so definitely established. The tendency is rather to congestion and œdema of the bases of the lungs than to fibrosis, and cough is often a troublesome symptom, the more so as the patient is especially liable to attacks of bronchitis. Œdema of the legs is a comparatively early symptom, but is at first readily amenable to treatment by rest in bed and suitable medicaments. The liver enlarges as the right ventricle is unable to cope efficiently with the effects of the mitral lesion, and its varying size is therefore an important indication as to the efficiency of compensation. It will pulsate when tricuspid incompetence is established, but, as a rule, it feels less firm and hard than in mitral stenosis, and ascites is less common.

The morbid anatomy of the secondary changes in the lungs and liver in mitral disease are described in the chapter on mitral stenosis.

### Prognosis.

The range of possibilities as regards duration of life in mitral regurgitation, due to actual damage of the valve by acute endocarditis, is more extensive than in any other form of valvular disease. It is the least serious and the most amenable to treatment of all the valvular affections.

When the lesion is slight the patient may live to old age without experiencing inconvenience from the results of the leakage, and may be capable of much hard work and pass through serious illnesses. In moderately severe cases, with reasonable precautions, he may live many years without serious symptoms declaring themselves. Women with mitral regurgitation may bear children with impunity.

In endeavouring to forecast the further course of a case of mitral incompetence when the regurgitation is inconsiderable, or when compensation has been established, one of the most important considerations will be the degree of arterial tension. Everything, so to speak, will depend upon the amount of resistance in the peripheral systemic circulation, and this may vary extremely. If with a given degree of mitral incompetence, we have undue arterial tension, the force of the regurgitant stream will be great, the back pressure in the auricle and pulmonary circulation high, the demand upon the right ventricle severe, all of which are circumstances tending to the production of structural changes; if, on the other hand, the arterial tension is low, the conditions are reversed.

The case of a patient, whom I have known to have mitral regurgitation for at least thirty-five years, may illustrate this. When first seen there were disquieting symptoms, a sense of constriction and oppression at the chest on moderate exercise, and liability to slight fainting attacks. Finding with such symptoms the pulse extremely short, soft, and compressible, it was at first feared that there were degenerative changes in the heart, but the family pulse, as exhibited by several children and grandchildren, was one of extremely low tension, and this was found to be the explanation of the patient's weak pulse.

There can be no doubt that the absence of resistance in the systemic arterioles and capillaries had an important share in the prolonged immunity from structural changes which he has enjoyed in spite of work of the most trying and arduous kind.

One or two other examples of prolonged survival may be mentioned. Two gentlemen, in whom I found mitral regurgitation more than twenty years since, were, when I last saw them, more than forty years of age and in active work. The murmur was loud and long in both, and in one there was considerable hypertrophy of the right ventricle and marked irregularity of the pulse. Another gentleman, whom I have repeatedly examined, and found to have a mitral systolic murmur, was, thirty-five years before I saw him, condemned to life-long inactivity, and I learnt from the family medical man that there had been a continuous history of valvular disease for that length of time; he rebelled against the sentence, and was still at the age of sixty-four doing strenuous work. Nothing is more common than to find a mitral systolic murmur after the age of seventy, but we cannot say how long it has been present, as it is not often that we can date it. Mitral regurgitation is the disease which sends patients into hospital time after time, often with advanced dropsy or severe pulmonary complication, from which they recover so completely as to resume work for a while. It is again the affection most commonly met with in out-patient hospital practice, while among in-patients and in the post-mortem room it is less frequently represented than mitral stenosis. All these facts point to one conclusion, viz. that mitral incompetence is not a deadly form of heart disease; I consider it to be less serious than aortic stenosis. It is not merely that in a large number of cases the actual damage to the valve and the consequent functional imperfection is only slight, but there is ample provision for compensatory adjustments, and very extensive change, if it is stationary, may be survived twenty or thirty years, and not prevent the patient reaching old age in comfort.

## Mitral Incompetence without Damage to Valves.

In the large group of cases of mitral regurgitation now to be considered, the cause of the reflux is not actual damage to the mitral valves, but stretching of the orifice or imperfect closure of the valves, due to dilatation of the left ventricle.

Such dilatation may be secondary to aortic disease, or the result of prolonged high arterial tension; but mitral regurgitation due to these causes need not be considered here, as its prognosis and treatment are those of the primary affection, and have been discussed elsewhere.

The chief causes of mitral incompetence in the group to be considered, are: anæmia, acute febrile disorders, and conditions associated with advancing age.

The so-called hæmic mitral murmurs which have sometimes been supposed to have some other significance than actual reflux, as they disappear with improving health, are not unfrequently met with in anæmia, especially in young women, or at times after acute febrile diseases, such as acute rheumatism, typhoid fever, or measles; the systolic mitral murmurs so commonly present in chorea sometimes belong to the same class, and mitral regurgitation, coming on late in life, not unfrequently has a similar causation, although it may not be removed by treatment.

It is to all this class of cases that McAlister's* explanation of mitral reflux without disease of the valves or enlargement of the orifice, already referred to, applies. It had been forgotten or overlooked, notwithstanding ocular demonstration on the living heart, and preparations

* *British Medical Journal*, August, 1882.

showing the heart in systole and diastole by Sibson, notwithstanding also measurement of the circumference of the heart in the contracted and relaxed condition and the fact that the opening was only the upper end of the ventricular cavity, that contraction of the orifice contributed in an important degree to its perfect closure by the valves. When regurgitation occurred, which was not explained by changes in the valves, it was accounted for by irregular action of the papillary muscles, or by the supposition that the papillary muscles, and with them the tendinous cords, were carried by dilatation of the ventricle to such a distance from the base of the valves that the margins, being dragged down by the chordæ tendineæ, could not meet. It was demonstrated in McAlister's paper, that all that is required in order that the reflux in question may occur, is that from languid contraction of the cardiac muscular fibres, or from resistance in the peripheral circulation, the due constriction of the orifice should not take place; the valvular mechanism will then be deranged and the apposition of the flaps be incomplete. It must be added, however, that if the contraction of the orifice is imperfect, so will be the ventricular systole as a whole, so that the position of the papillary muscles may contribute to the derangement.

The mitral murmur of anæmia, though only a particular case of regurgitation from dilatation, is worthy of separate consideration. It is met with in only a small proportion of cases of anæmia, and may be absent when the bloodlessness is extreme. It does not, therefore, mark a certain degree of impoverishment of the blood, and may indeed be found when this is by no means advanced. The remarks apply equally to chlorotic anæmia, to anæmia from loss of blood, and to pernicious anæmia. The fact that a mitral murmur is so often absent in fatal pernicious anæmia is perhaps the most remarkable. It seems probable that while the poverty of the blood and the consequent innutrition of the heart are the predisposing influences, the proximate cause is some overstrain, which may be sufficient even in the absence of anæmia.

As an instance of this, may be quoted the case of a young lady whom I saw from time to time during a period of four years. She was well nourished, with well-developed muscles, as well as a fair amount of adipose tissue, and the lips and face were a good colour. When first seen she had a pronounced mitral murmur, and the apex beat was displaced to the left of the nipple line. There were no murmurs in the neck or over the pulmonic area or aorta; the catamenia were excessive.

This was her condition in July; in October the murmur had disappeared and the apex had receded. In the following January, after the death of a relation by drowning, which she witnessed, the murmur and dilatation had returned. A month later the murmur could not be heard, but the apex was still outside its normal situation. On examination in July, September, and December of that year, the apex beat was normal and the murmur absent, although the menses were suspended for long periods, and she had lost flesh. No further relapse had occurred when I last saw her. The influences which appeared to determine the occurrence of the regurgitation were the relaxing climate in which her home was placed; the frequent necessity, from the situation of the house, of walking uphill when tired; and, probably more than all, domestic worry.

There is, however, in anæmia, a cause of dilatation of the weakened left ventricle independent of external and accidental circumstances; this is high arterial tension, which, as has been elsewhere pointed out, nearly always attends this state of the blood. Undue arterial tension implies increased resistance to the emptying of the ventricle, and this gradually distends it. When regurgitation is not produced, there are still very frequently the signs of dilatation in displacement outwards and downwards of the apex, and a diffuse character of its beat. The operation of this cause perhaps throws light on the production of permanent valvular disease by anæmia, which Goodhart has shown to be probable. The peripheral resistance throws extra stress upon the mitral valves, the action of the heart is liable to be excited and violent in anæmic subjects, which will intensify the effects of the strain, and so valvulitis may be set up.

## Differential Diagnosis.

It may sometimes be difficult to decide whether a mitral murmur is due to conditions such as have just been described, or to actual changes in the valves. Where there are obvious compensatory changes in the left or right ventricle, there can be no doubt, and in many cases the state of health of the patient with the history will be a sufficient guide; but difficulties may arise, for example, when there is marked anæmia in a woman who has had acute rheumatism, or when a murmur is present, without anæmia adequate to account for it, in a patient who is not known to have suffered from rheumatism. In such doubtful cases, the character of the murmur may afford useful information. If the murmur is soft and blowing, and a murmur is heard not only at the apex, but at the pulmonic and aortic areas, the probability is that it is due to anæmia, and not to actual valvular change.

Hæmic murmurs are usually soft and blowing in character, not harsh or musical, and they do not replace or extinguish the first sound. Generally speaking, they are not conducted to the axilla or heard over the back, and are not accompanied by much displacement of the apex beat. While this is the rule, I have known several cases in which it was departed from, the apex being displaced, and the murmur heard towards the axilla or over the back.

Furthermore, it is the hæmic murmur which is most frequently late-systolic in time, that is, it follows the first sound at an appreciable interval instead of commencing synchronously with it.

These indications, together with the history of the case and the physical signs present, will as a rule be sufficient to clear up the diagnosis in doubtful cases.

**Regurgitation in Acute Febrile Diseases.**—Regurgitation of similar character resulting from acute disease lasts for a short time only, and is chiefly interesting from the fact that it is not uncommon after acute rheumatism, the great cause of true valvular lesions. It is often impossible to say whether a soft mitral murmur heard towards the close of an attack of rheumatic fever, indicates the beginning of actual disease, or is the result of temporary functional imperfection. If it occurs after the commencement of systole, and especially if a pulmonic systolic murmur is also present, it may be that the regurgitation is due to dilatation from anæmia or loss of tone of the muscular fibres, the result of myocarditis; but time alone will decide with certainty.

**Chorea.**—The mitral murmur associated with chorea frequently persists after the chorea is cured, and may be the result of endocarditis which has damaged the valves during acute or sub-acute rheumatism, which is so frequently an antecedent or accompaniment of chorea. It may, however, be due to temporary dilatation of the heart, and disappear as the chorea subsides and the patient improves in general health.

The cases considered constitute the mitral incompetence of early life. But the mitral incompetence may be established during the decline of life, from other causes, and this class of cases must now be considered.

**The Mitral Regurgitation of Middle and Old Age.**—It is astonishing how frequently this is met with, and how imperceptibly it is established. In some cases there is no obvious organic valvular, or structural alteration; commonly, however, there is considerable dilatation of the auriculo-ventricular opening, and no definite diagnosis can be made between this condition and degenerative changes, such as thickening and calcification, slowly taking place in the valves.

**Mitral Incompetence and High Arterial Tension.**—The mitral orifice may be greatly stretched so as to admit three or four fingers. Sometimes, from the condition of rigor mortis in the muscle, the valves seem to be apparently capable of closing it more or less perfectly when tested by water after death, though during life regurgitation was permitted as a result of imperfect coaptation. Dilatation of the ventricle and stretching of the auriculo-ventricular opening usually take place together, but by no means to a corresponding extent; either orifice or ventricle may be disproportionately enlarged. The regurgitation may be said to be only an incident of dilatation. Undue arterial tension will have a most important place among its causes, and I have watched in many cases the gradual supervention of a murmur upon sounds which have had the loud and sharp character produced by excessive peripheral resistance; but I have also found a mitral murmur when there has been no arterial tension, the pulse being large, soft, short, and compressible. In chronic disease of the kidneys, which can scarcely escape mention when the effects upon the heart of protracted high tension in the arteries are under consideration, mitral regurgitation is less frequent than might perhaps have been expected, and when it occurs, there is usually actual lesion of the valves. This is probably due to the fact that the hypertrophy, which is associated with the dilatation, and is usually the predominant change, renders the ventricular systole efficient in constricting the orifice.

## TREATMENT.

Mitral incompetence is met with in such varied degree and has such varied causation, that it is necessary in discussing the treatment to differentiate between the most important varieties.

1. When there is no valvular lesion, and the regurgitation is due to imperfect systolic narrowing of the orifice as in anæmia, and occasionally after acute disease, the principal treatment will be that of the condition which has given rise to the atony of the cardiac muscle. When the heart is dilated after acute disease, a period of absolute rest may occasionally be necessary. Violent or sustained exertion in such cases and in anæmia, must be avoided, as acute dilatation may be produced, or a pre-existing dilatation may be increased by a comparatively slight cause. Gentle regular exercise will be of great importance, and may be gradually increased in duration and vigour, as the heart regains its tone.

A daily period of repose in the recumbent position should be enjoined, and a complete rest for a certain time before and after meals should be insisted on.

Climate has an extraordinary influence in this condition of heart, and the Œrtel system of graduated exercise at a moderate elevation is often of great service.

Iron, quinine and strychnine may be given for the anæmia and general weakness, and small doses of digitalis will often make a great difference in the results obtained.

The systolic apex murmur may be confidently expected to disappear in time, as a result of suitable treatment.

2. In the case of a systolic apex murmur with extremely little regurgitation, common after middle age, when not due to dilatation of the left ventricle, little treatment is required.

In most cases, instead of restriction in exercise being necessary, regular exercise will have to be ordered, and a sedentary, self-indulgent mode of life modified, as these patients often plead a weak heart as an excuse for avoiding fresh air and exercise, which they dislike.

When the incompetence is real, and has required compensatory changes to neutralize its effects, it is still desirable that the patient should take regular exercise, the duration and vigour of which must be determined by his strength and breath. So long as respiratory distress is not induced, outdoor exercise will do good and not harm. Standing about indoors is much more likely to be injurious.

The one contingency to be specially guarded against is bronchitis, or any acute affection of the lungs. The pulmonary circulation is already carried on under difficulties, and superadded obstruction may intercept the compensatory high pressure maintained in the left auricle by the right ventricle; the result being that there is less opposition to the mitral regurgitant stream, the left ventricle is imperfectly filled, and the systemic blood supply is impaired: further, the right ventricle, unable to contend with the double obstacle to the transmission of blood through the lungs, becomes over-distended and crippled, so that tricuspid regurgitation and venous stasis result. The dreaded ulterior effects of mitral regurgitation are thus anticipated, and, besides this, recovery from the bronchitis is retarded by the congestion in the pulmonary capillaries.

**High Arterial Tension.**—Precautions must also be taken against high arterial tension, which may be due to renal disease or gout, or may be produced by too nitrogenized a system of diet, or by habitual consumption of beer or strong wines, or by constipation. With high arterial tension there will be increase in peripheral resistance, and thus increase in the amount and force of the mitral reflux, causing an additional continuous strain on the compensatory mechanism. Suitable dieting and the habitual use of a mild mercurial purge once or twice a week, will tend to keep down high arterial tension when it is present.

3. When serious symptoms set in, and especially if any exciting cause can be traced, there is more chance of making head against them, and of improvement under treatment, than in other forms of valvular disease. The result of mitral regurgitation is always backward pressure, taking effect first on the lungs, then on the right ventricle, and finally giving rise to obstruction to the systemic venous return, when the right ventricle breaks down. Tricuspid regurgitation does not appear to add appreciably to the obstruction in the great veins, and, indeed, is thought by some to prevent paralysis of the right ventricle from over-distension. The two problems in the treatment are the relief of the venous stagnation and the strengthening and restoration of tone and vigour to the right ventricle, so that it can again perform its work efficiently. There is no constricting barrier opposing a fixed mechanical obstruction to the blood current as in mitral stenosis; the task is therefore easier.

For the **Relief of the Venous Obstruction**, purgatives, of which mercury in some form is a constituent, will usually be sufficient, repeated according to their effect, and according to the condition and strength of the patient every second or third day. The application of leeches over the liver, if it is enlarged and tender, will often be of great service, and almost invariably affords relief. Dry cupping may be useful. Venesection is not often absolutely required, though probably it might more frequently be resorted to with advantage than is the case.

Concurrently digitalis should be given, and it is in the treatment of dropsy and advanced conditions of mitral incompetence, that it may be administered with the greatest confidence and least apprehension of its so-called cumulative effects. It increases, it is true, the peripheral resistance, but as long as the structures of the heart are sound, it appears to increase the vigour of its contraction in greater proportion; this is especially the case with the right ventricle, and the improvement in the transit of blood through the lungs is perhaps the most important element in its beneficial results. It may be given with satisfactory results for any length of time, as there is no barrier in the shape of a stenosed orifice, against which the increased energy expended by the heart will be exhausted: the only reason for discontinuing it will be nausea or loss of appetite, to which it sometimes gives rise, or marked diminution in the amount of urine excreted.

# CHAPTER XII.

## MITRAL STENOSIS.

ETIOLOGY—PREDOMINANCE IN THE FEMALE SEX—MORBID ANATOMY—PHYSIOLOGY OF THE CHANGES IN THE HEART—BROWN INDURATION OF LUNGS—NUTMEG LIVER—THE PHYSICAL SIGNS—THE PULSE—THE CHANGES IN THE HEART—THE CARDIAC MURMURS—THREE STAGES IN THE PROGRESS OF THE DISEASE AS DEFINED BY AUSCULTATORY SIGNS—THE CHARACTERISTICS OF THESE THREE STAGES—SYMPTOMS—DIAGNOSIS—PROGNOSIS—TREATMENT.

CONSTRICTION of the mitral orifice is on many grounds the most interesting of the valvular affections of the heart. It is a common, and at the same time a serious form of valvular disease, and its clinical history presents peculiarities, some of which have long been recognized, while others have not received adequate notice. It was the last of the valvular diseases to be associated with distinctive physical signs, and to Gairdner the credit of this discovery is due. It also presents greater difficulties in diagnosis than any other of the valvular affections.

### ETIOLOGY.

Acute endocarditis is the commonest cause of mitral stenosis, but a certain interval must elapse before constriction of the mitral orifice results, as this is mainly due to cicatricial contraction of the fibrous tissue formed in the process of repair of the damaged valves after inflammation.

A remarkable fact is the relative frequency of its occurrence in women, whether the basis of the estimate is post-mortem or clinical. Of fifty-three patients dying in St. Mary's Hospital and examined after death, thirty-eight were females and only fifteen males — seventy-two and twenty-eight per cent. respectively. Of eighty-one cases collected by Hayden fifty-four were females and twenty-seven males—66·6 and 33·3 per cent. Dyce Duckworth, in eighty cases, found no fewer than sixty-three women—78·75 per cent. It cannot be said that any satisfactory explanation of this great disproportion of women affected by mitral stenosis has been given. It is true that rheumatism is more common in girls than in boys, but were this the only reason, there ought only to be a general predominance of valvular disease in women, and not of this particular condition. Possibly the greater liability of girls to anæmia at the period of puberty may have some bearing on the greater incidence of mitral stenosis in the female sex, especially when it is borne in mind that anæmia is frequently attended with augmented arterial tension which, by increasing the stress on the mitral valves, is a cause of insidious damage. These two factors may tend to keep going the chronic inflammatory process, which results in adhesion of the cusps of the mitral valve, and in further constriction of its orifice by cicatricial contraction of the fibrous tissue thrown out around it.

## MORBID ANATOMY.

**The Heart.**—As a rule the heart is not very large. Weights of ten and twelve ounces are common, and fourteen or fifteen will represent about the average. The left ventricle is usually not increased in size, the left auricle is dilated and hypertrophied, and the right ventricle much enlarged and its walls greatly thickened. The left ventricle, however, may be enlarged and its walls thickened if mitral incompetence preceded the mitral stenosis, and there may therefore be great differences in the weight of the heart and dimensions of its cavities in different cases.

**The Mitral Orifice.**—The condition of the mitral orifice may vary greatly, and an extreme degree of stenosis does not seem to be incompatible with life. The orifice may be so constricted that it will scarcely admit a penholder, and very commonly it will only admit the tip of the little finger. To such conditions the term "button-hole" has been applied, but it is scarcely applicable, as the margins of the orifice are usually rigid and unyielding. In other cases the aperture may be funnel-shaped. Frequently there is no trace of the mitral valves remaining as such, as they are adherent at the margins, contracted down to form a rough irregular lining to what is left of the original mitral orifice.

The characteristic physiological effect of the lesion upon the heart is dilatation of the left auricle with more or less thickening of its wall, and great hypertrophy with some dilatation of the right ventricle. The left ventricle is not correspondingly enlarged, and may retain its normal size, while the right ventricle, by its growth, may displace it backwards, so that no part of it appears on the anterior aspect of the heart, and its apex is no longer in contact with the chest wall.

When the mitral orifice is narrowed, it is the left auricle and right ventricle only which are called upon to exert increased force, since there is no obvious cause of increased resistance in the systemic circulation. The same may be said when the valvular lesion is mitral incompetence with regurgitation; but here another element of change comes in, which makes a difference between obstruction and incompetence. The high pressure in the pulmonary veins and left auricle, which is a result of the damming back of the blood and of the increased force of the right ventricle, causes a forcible inrush into the left ventricle during diastole; and this, so long as the orifice remains of the natural size, must distend, and in the long run dilate its cavity, taking effect, as it does, during the unresisting period of the ventricular rhythm. But an increase in the capacity of the cavity multiplies by so much the force required to expel its contents, and this constitutes a demand for hypertrophy. We have, then, as a result of mitral incompetence, dilatation, and more or less hypertrophy of the left ventricle; but the hypertrophy here is required as compensation for the dilatation, and not to overcome any direct effect of the impairment of the valvular apparatus. In stenosis of the mitral orifice, the pressure which thus affects the left ventricle is intercepted by the narrowed orifice. There is scarcely time for it to be adequately filled during diastole, still less for any distending effect to be produced. We see, then, how it is that the left ventricle usually remains of normal size and does not increase *pari passu* with the right. Frequently, however, the left ventricle is dilated and more or less thickened, and here our reasoning appears to be at fault. But the difficulty disappears on reflection. Not uncommonly the change in the valves, which eventually glues them together and narrows the orifice, only interferes at first with their apposition and permits of regurgitation, which may, indeed, be for a long time the predominant result; and, in point of fact, incompetence often precedes the establishment of obstruction. We have here abundant cause for differences in the condition of the walls and cavities of the heart found after death, and, it must be added, for variations in the clinical history, and especially for diversity of physical signs.

**The Lungs. Passive Hyperæmia. Brown Induration. Œdema.**—As a result of prolonged obstruction to the flow of blood from the lungs to the left auricle in mitral incompetence and stenosis, there is passive hyperæmia of the lungs. To a certain extent this is overcome by the increased driving power of the hypertrophied right ventricle. But the high pressure thus induced in the pulmonary circulation gives rise to certain pathological changes in the lungs.

The capillaries in the walls of the alveoli are overdistended, and become tortuous, projecting into the alveoli. Exudation of white and red blood cells into the alveoli takes place and occasionally capillaries rupture, giving rise to slight hæmoptysis, which is frequently met with in mitral stenosis even in the early stages. Some of the extravasated blood may be thus expectorated, some is taken up by the alveolar cells and lymphatics, and the walls and lymphatics of the alveoli are often loaded with granules of pigment derived from the disentegrated hæmoglobin.

As a result of the irritation, proliferative changes take place in the alveolar walls, which become thickened, lose their elasticity, and tend to shrink and collapse, so that the surface available for aëration of the blood is seriously impaired and diminished. It may be still further diminished by patches of catarrhal inflammation.

This condition of lung, from its tough, inelastic feel, resulting from the diffuse fibrosis, and the brownish colour due to the deposit of blood pigment, is known as "Brown Induration."

As will be readily understood, this condition is most likely to arise in cases of mitral stenosis, where the hypertrophied right ventricle has to keep up sufficient pressure in the pulmonary circulation to force the blood through the narrowed mitral orifice which constitutes, in severe cases, an almost impenetrable barrier to the on-flow of the blood. In mitral incompetence the back pressure is more variable and is usually not so severe, and we are more likely to meet with a condition of congestion varying in degree from time to time. When the stagnation of the circulation in the lungs becomes more intense, œdema of the bases of the lungs may supervene, the alveoli becoming filled with serum exuded from the congested vessels.

**Infarction.**—In the later and final stages of mitral stenosis, or of mitral stenosis and incompetence combined, infarction of the lungs is very liable to occur.

As the lung is freely supplied with blood vessels, infarction does not occur from embolism of a small artery in a normal lung, as is the case in the spleen or kidney, since collateral circulation is readily established. This has been proved experimentally by Welch in dogs, and has also been verified at post-mortems by the finding of occluded vessels without any resulting infarct. When, however, there is extreme congestion of the lungs and the circulation is obstructed and stagnant, embolism will give rise to an infarct, as collateral circulation cannot be established. It has been supposed that, in mitral stenosis, embolism occurs from clots forming in the right auricle during life and portions becoming detached and carried to the lungs. I have never seen any foundation in fact for this theory, and it is scarcely conceivable that clotting should take place in the heart during life if its walls are healthy.

It is probable that the infarction which is common in the later stages of mitral stenosis is the result of thrombosis. There is intense congestion and stagnation in the capillaries and small arteries, and the limit at which the circulation can be maintained is reached at last. Stasis and gradual thrombosis occur in one or more of the smaller arteries, and the result is the same as in embolism. The blood-supply to the area supplied by the artery is cut off, and temporarily it becomes anæmic. But blood soon flows from the adjoining capillaries into the empty vessels, the walls of which, deprived of their nutrition, give way or allow the blood to pass through them into the alveoli, by actual rhexis, or diapedesis, so that we get a large hæmorrhagic infarct. The name "pulmonary apoplexy" has been applied by some authors to this condition, but it scarcely seems a suitable term, as it is not the rupture of a vessel which is primarily responsible for the lesion.

The infarcted areas are usually of considerable size, and more or less wedge-shaped with their base at the pleura, and may measure from half-inch to three or four inches across at their widest part. They are often multiple, and are usually among the incidents of the closing scenes in the disease.

**The Liver.**—As the pressure in the pulmonary circulation is greatly increased, it stands to reason that the pressure in the right ventricle in systole must be raised in proportion. If the ventricle is unequal to the task of maintaining the high-pressure circulation it may dilate, giving rise to incompotence of the tricuspid valve, or may incompletely empty itself during systole, which tends, in either case, to dam back the blood in the right auricle. This will cause obstruction to the return of blood to the auricle from the great veins. The blood in the inferior vena cava, and consequently that in the hepatic veins being dammed back, will give rise to congestion of the liver. The intra-lobular veins and the capillaries entering them in the centre of the liver lobules, become distended and engorged with blood. The pressure on the adjoining cells in the centre of the lobule, and impairment of their nutrition results in atrophy of these cells, while fatty degeneration is prone to occur in the cells in the periphery of the lobule. The liver is engorged with blood, and greatly increased in size; and on making a section of the liver post-mortem, we see, naked eye, the congested capillaries and vein in the centre of the lobules as small red areas surrounded by yellowish, opaque rings of cells in a state of fatty degeneration, a condition which is known as a "Nutmeg Liver" from its appearance. A certain amount of secondary fibrosis may occur in chronic cases of long duration, especially in mitral stenosis.

**The Kidneys.**—As a result of chronic congestion prevalent throughout the venous system, the kidneys become congested. The stellate veins are especially prominent, and the capillaries of the malpighian tufts are swollen and distended with blood. The organ is often of a bluish colour, when seen at the post-mortem, and is hard, rounded, and very firm on section from secondary diffuse fibrosis chiefly marked round the congested vessels. This condition is known as "Cyanotic Induration."

## PHYSICAL SIGNS.

**The Pulse.**—The pulse of mitral stenosis is interesting. It is almost always regular until the heart is obviously failing, unless the obstruction be complicated by regurgitation or by valvular affection of the right side of the heart.

The artery at the wrist is small, and is full between the beats, presenting the characters of moderately high tension —that is, it can be rolled under the finger and is not very easily compressed. In my experience this modified high tension pulse is almost constant, and it points to resistance in the capillaries; but the cause of such resistance is not readily perceived. It may be due to contraction of the arterioles, either reflex or by direct stimulation, consequent on the blood being charged with impurities from imperfect elimination, or possibly be caused by backward pressure in the veins, which makes itself felt through the capillary network. More probably, however, it is simply an effect of the contracting down of the entire arterial system owing to the diminished supply of blood from the imperfectly filled left ventricle.

When irregularity comes on, it is usually at first inequality in the force of the beats, without marked disturbance of the rhythm. Then some of the beats of the heart fail to reach the wrist—no doubt from inadequate filling of the ventricle; the action of the heart may thus continue to be regular when the pulse is irregular. In some rare instances, there is only one beat of the pulse for every two beats of the heart, the contraction of the left ventricle at every alternate systole being inadequate to raise the aortic valves; and, on listening to the heart, there will be no aortic second sound with the alternate systoles, the rhythm as expressed by the sounds being one—two—*one*, one—two—*one*, with an accent on the third sound heard. The heart-beats follow each other in couples, and the accentuated first sound, unaccompanied by an aortic second sound, is mainly produced by the abrupt contraction of the right ventricle.

**The Heart.**—The cardiac sounds and murmurs are varied, and sometimes perplexing; but it has appeared to me that they afford a means of estimating approximately the degree of constriction which the mitral orifice has undergone. The contraction does not take place all at once, but increases by slow degrees through many months or years, and it is to be expected that corresponding change in the physical signs will accompany this change of mechanical conditions. The physical signs are not the same in a given case from beginning to end, and by following the modifications of the sounds and murmurs which gradually supervene, I have been led to recognize three stages of the disease.

The heart is not usually greatly enlarged; the apex is displaced to the left and sometimes also downwards, but it is found, as a rule, not far from the normal situation.

The dilatation of the left auricle gives rise to an extension of dulness outwards, along the fourth and third left intercostal spaces, and the dilatation of the right auricle causes dulness beyond the right border of the sternum.

The apex beat is not well defined, and in advanced cases a sharp and distinct shock is felt on palpation, which has not the deliberate thrusting character of hypertrophy, but is more like a tap. A thrill, presystolic in time, may usually be felt at the apex or just internal to it. The impulse of the right ventricle is powerful, lifting the lower end of the sternum and adjacent costal cartilages, and making itself seen and felt in the epigastrium.

Changes in the dimensions of the heart, however, have not the same direct relation to the degree of valvular mischief in mitral stenosis as in other valvular diseases, and it is by means of auscultatory signs that the division into stages is effected.

The pathognomonic sign of mitral stenosis is usually given as a presystolic murmur heard over a limited area at and to the inner side of the apex beat, between it and the left border of the sternum. It is not a smooth, blowing murmur, but has a rough, vibratory character, and is often accompanied by a thrill perceptible to the hand at the same spot. A further distinctive feature is the way in which it runs up to and suddenly ends in the first sound, which tends to become short and sharp, and is itself highly characteristic.

Sometimes in children after an attack of pericarditis, possibly as a result of pericardial adhesions, or in association with a mitral systolic murmur, a kind of rumbling presystolic murmur is audible, when no constriction of the mitral orifice exists. This murmur has not, however, the vibratory character of the true murmur of mitral stenosis ; nor does it terminate abruptly in the first sound; nor is the first sound modified in the manner described above. Reduplication of the first sound should not be mistaken for a presystolic murmur.

The pulmonic second sound is accentuated, as a result of the backward pressure in the pulmonary circulation, and very frequently there is reduplication of the second sound, from want of synchronism in the closure of the pulmonic and aortic valves.

## Characteristics of the Three Stages in the Progress of the Disease, as defined by Auscultatory Signs.

In the first stage a second sound, as well as a presystolic murmur and first sound, will be audible at and to the left of the apex. It is the persistence of the second sound at the apex which is the chief distinctive feature of this stage. The second sound may be reduplicated.

Under these conditions I have never known serious symptoms to arise from the condition of the heart, and I have seen illnesses of different kinds, even serious attacks of bronchitis, passed through without the intervention of embarrassment of the circulation. It is very rarely that patients are admitted into hospital presenting simply the signs above enumerated, but they are frequently met with in out-patient practice and in consulting-rooms.

**The Second Stage.**—This is marked by the disappearance of the second sound at the apex, and by the short, sharp character of the first sound, which also usually becomes very loud; the first sound, in effect, comes to resemble a second sound. Mistakes in diagnosis may now be easily made. In mitral stenosis, at this stage, and in mitral incompetence there is alike heard at the apex a murmur followed by a short, sharp sound; but in the former the murmur is presystolic in time, and the sound is the modified first sound, while in the latter the murmur is systolic and the sound is the second sound. Very slight attention would, in most cases, suffice to prevent any confusion between the two, but an apex murmur is liable to be set down as the familiar systolic murmur of regurgitation without further investigation, and thus mitral stenosis, the most serious of the diseases of the valves, at a period, too, when symptoms may be impending, is taken for incompetence, which is attended with less danger than any other of the valvular affections. To bear this source of error in mind is to avoid it; but cases are sometimes met with in which, from absence of cardiac impulse and from the similarity between the sounds, it is not easy to follow the rhythm of the heart and time the murmurs and sounds. Flexible stethoscopes are here at a disadvantage as compared with the rigid wooden instrument, which communicates to the ear and head, not only sound, but a sense of shock which at once indicates the moment of the systole, and this when there is no impulse perceptible to the hand. To attempt to time the first sound by the radial pulse is, of course, fallacious. The carotid pulse is a safer guide, but it is not always easy to co-ordinate tactile and auditory impressions.

The most trustworthy method of determining the relation of sounds to the cardiac rhythm is to find a spot in the region of the base where the first and second sounds are unmistakably recognized, and then from this point to follow the sounds, step by step, toward the apex, when it will be found which of them it is that disappears, or which maintains some distinguishing peculiarity.

The presystolic murmur itself usually undergoes a modification in this stage. As commonly heard, it occupies the end of the diastolic interval, running up to the first sound, and corresponding therefore with the auricular systole. But it may be a long or a short murmur, and may indeed occupy the entire diastolic interval, when it will correspond, not only with the auricular systole, but also with the active diastolic rebound of the ventricle from contraction; that is, the murmur is produced by the current of blood sucked into the ventricle as it dilates, as well as by that driven into it by the systole of the auricle. This murmur, occupying the whole of the diastolic interval, is most frequent in bad cases. But it may further be cut in two, and, instead of being a continuous rumble from the second sound up to the first, may subside as the active dilatation of the ventricle ends, and before the auricular systole begins; or the proper presystolic part of the murmur may be lost while the diastolic part remains audible, so that the only murmur heard is diastolic, *i.e.* a diastolic mitral murmur, strictly speaking. These varieties

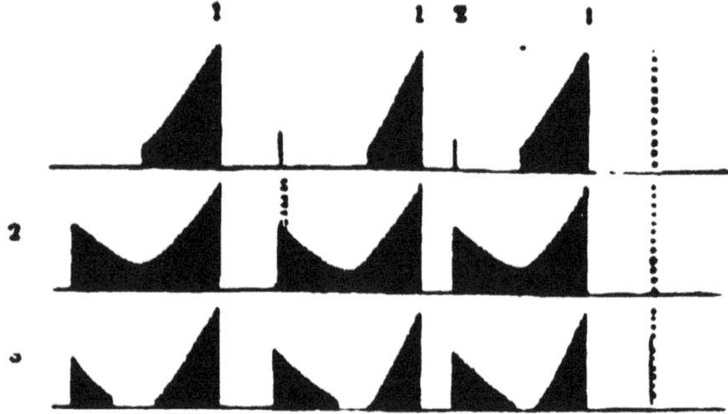

FIG. 19.—1. PRESYSTOLIC MURMUR CORRESPONDING WITH AURICULAR SYSTOLE. 2. MURMUR OCCUPYING WHOLE DIASTOLIC INTERVAL. 3 MURMUR DIVIDED INTO DIASTOLIC AND PRESYSTOLIC PORTIONS.

of murmur may be represented diagrammatically as shown in Fig. 19.

The disappearance of the second sound at the left of the apex, which, with the short, sharp character of the first sound, marks the second stage of mitral stenosis, is probably explained by the following considerations. In the normal heart, a second sound is always audible at and to the left of the apex; and repeated careful examinations have convinced me that it is the aortic second sound which is here heard, and not the pulmonic, even when this is accentuated and unduly loud. In mitral stenosis, there are two influences tending to prevent the aortic second sound from reaching the surface of the chest. First, the left ventricle, not undergoing dilatation and hypertrophy, while the right enlarges greatly, is overlapped by the latter, which usurps the position of the apex, and thus the left ventricle cannot conduct the aortic sound to the chest wall. Again, the aortic second sound will be weak, because the diminished amount of blood entering the ventricle, in consequence of the narrowed mitral orifice, will not distend the aorta, and will, therefore, fail to produce a powerful recoil such as is necessary for the production of a loud second sound.

The modification of the first sound in mitral stenosis is remarkable, and in searching for an explanation of this, one is struck by the analogy of the sharp, sudden, and tapping character of the apex beat to the shortness and sharpness of the first sound, which would seem to imply that some common cause has been instrumental in the production of these peculiarities in both instances. If this be the case, it is clear that the ventricular wall must be one of the factors, and the following explanation may be suggested. Owing to the narrowing of the mitral orifice there is not time in the diastolic interval for a sufficient amount of blood to flow into the left ventricle to completely fill it. At the commencement of systole, therefore, the ventricular cavity is not fully distended with blood, so that the muscular walls at the first moment of their contraction meet with no resistance; then, closing down rapidly, they are suddenly brought up and made tense as they encounter the contained blood. It seems plausible that this sudden tension of the muscular walls and the abbreviated systole of the left ventricle, would account both for the sharp and tapping apex beat and for the short first sound.

In severe palpitation and tachycardia the first sound is also extremely short and sharp, and probably a similar explanation holds good here, namely, that the brief diastolic interval which is the rule in such cases does not afford sufficient time for the complete filling and distending of the ventricle with blood.

The third stage is characterized by the disappearance of the presystolic murmur, so that, the second sound being already lost, the only sound at and outside the apex is the short sharp first sound described. This is not unlike the first sound heard in dilatation with thinning of the left ventricle; but the absence of the second sound to the left of the apex constitutes a diagnostic difference, since this is distinct in dilatation.

No careful observer who has devoted much attention to the study of mitral stenosis has failed to notice that the presystolic murmur is sometimes absent in cases in which an advanced stage of this condition is met with after death. The principal justification, however, for taking the disappearance of the presystolic murmur as a distinct stage in the clinical history of mitral stenosis is that, very commonly when pulmonary complications set in, or other serious symptoms arise, the presystolic murmur is lost, and that it again becomes audible when these subside and the patient improves.

It is a matter of repeated and familiar experience for cases to be admitted into hospital on account of serious symptoms with only the short sharp first sound audible at the apex, and to leave after recovery with a presystolic murmur. The third stage, however, is not necessarily attended with serious symptoms, though this is the rule.

The probable cause of the disappearance of the murmur is the establishment of tricuspid incompetence. The giving way of the tricuspid valve and the occurrence of considerable reflux into the right auricle, make it impossible for the right ventricle to sustain the same high pressure in the pulmonary circulation and left auricle as was present previously. There is not, therefore, sufficient pressure to force the blood through the mitral orifice rapidly enough to generate a murmur.

## Symptoms.

The patient, up to a somewhat advanced stage, has not the look of heart disease, is neither pallid, nor dusky, nor anxious-looking, but often has a bright colour and cheerful expression. There is some breathlessness on exertion, but not infrequently, up to the moment when, from some cause or other, serious symptoms set in, he or she is unconscious of serious embarrassment of the circulation, and capable of ordinary work. The capillaries over the cheek bones are frequently congested, giving a ruddy colour which might be taken for a sign of good health, were it not contradicted by the dusky cyanotic tinge of the lips. The cyanosis tends to become more marked and permanent and the dyspnœa more severe in the later stages, from the diminution in the aërating capacity of the lungs, which supervenes as their condition approximates that known as "Brown Induration." Such patients are liable to cough and hæmoptysis from the constant high pressure in the pulmonic circulation. In the early stages the hæmoptysis is slight, being due to rupture of capillaries, and consists of mucus streaked with blood. In the advanced and terminal stages it is often very profuse and repeated, being due to infarction. Cough is often a troublesome symptom, from the bronchial catarrh to which the patient is especially liable. Attacks of tachycardia or palpitation are common and may cause great distress. Another condition more frequently met with as a consequence of mitral stenosis, than in other valvular affections, is great enlargement of the liver, with true pulsation of this organ, which often feels hard and firm on examination; it is not uncommon to find fluid in the peritoneal cavity before there is œdema of the feet and legs, or the œdema will disappear with rest in bed, while ascites persists, whereas dropsy, in cardiac failure, due to mitral incompetence, as a rule, begins in the connective tissue of the most dependent parts, and ascites is not common. A reference to the section on morbid anatomy will make clear the causation of most of the symptoms.

## Diagnosis.

In the first stage, where the vibratory presystolic murmur ending in the short sharp first sound, and the second sound are present, there will be little difficulty in arriving at a diagnosis. The short, rumbling, presystolic murmur often met with during or shortly after an attack of peri- or endo-carditis, more especially in children, may, however, lead to some confusion. This murmur, however, is not of the loud vibratory character of the typical presystolic murmur, but is usually short and rumbling; it does not indicate the presence of mitral stenosis, at any rate, in the sense of an established organic lesion. A further distinctive feature in diagnosis will be the absence of the typical modification of the first sound, which, instead of being short and sharp, will be dull, low-pitched, and possibly reduplicated.

In the second stage, when the second sound is lost at the apex and only the presystolic murmur and first sound are present; these may possibly be taken for a systolic murmur and second sound which the first sound has come to resemble in character; the case would then be mistaken for one of mitral incompetence in which the prognosis is much less serious. Due care and accurate timing of the sounds will prevent this. Confusion is, however, liable to occur when mitral regurgitation is present as a complication, which is of very common occurrence. It is then possible to mistake the presystolic and systolic murmurs together for a prolonged systolic murmur, the short sharp first sound being taken for an accentuated second sound. But attention to the character and time of the murmurs will obviate such a mistake. The systolic murmur of mitral regurgitation is blowing or musical, and begins with an accent, whereas the presystolic murmur is vibratory and ends with an accent. Accurate observation of the time at which the short sharp sound is heard will also prevent the mistake, but this will not perhaps be so easily distinguished as the character of the murmurs.

They may be represented diagrammatically as follows:—

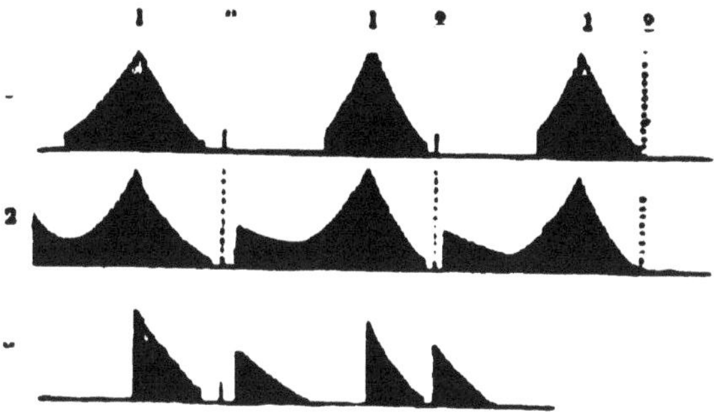

FIG. 20 (Dark shading = presystolic murmur; light shading = systolic murmur).

1. ORDINARY PRESYSTOLIC WITH SYSTOLIC MURMUR. 2. PRESYSTOLIC MURMUR OCCUPYING THE WHOLE OF DIASTOLE, WITH SYSTOLIC MURMUR. 3. DIASTOLIC PORTION ONLY OF PRESYSTOLIC MURMUR WITH SYSTOLIC MURMUR.

In the third stage, complicated by mitral regurgitation, recognition of mitral stenosis will often present great difficulties. There will be no presystolic murmur, and only a first sound with a systolic murmur will be audible at the apex. The absence of the second sound will be of great value in identifying the stenosis. If, however, the mitral regurgitation has preceded the onset of stenosis, it may have given rise to a degree of hypertrophy and dilatation of the left ventricle, such that the apex-beat, which comes into contact with the chest wall, is still that of the left ventricle and not of the right, so that the aortic second sound is still conducted to the chest wall. In such cases the modification of the first sound is an important aid to diagnosis; regurgitation tends to destroy the first sound, stenosis to shorten and intensify it, so that the presence of a short sharp first sound with a systolic murmur, in a case where there is obviously serious cardiac mischief, should at once suggest the probability of the presence of mitral stenosis.

When, however, compensation has broken down in a case of combined stenosis and regurgitation, extraordinary fluctuations in the physical signs may be present; at one time a systolic, at another a presystolic murmur, at another time both may be heard, or perhaps only a short sharp sound alternating with murmurs, which it is impossible to time. At the same time the action of the heart will be rapid and markedly irregular. In such cases the extraordinary fluctuations must themselves give the chief clue to the diagnosis, though it will be impossible to estimate the extent of either lesion.

It would appear that when the high pressure in the left auricle is well sustained it generates a presystolic murmur, and prevents regurgitation, so that no systolic murmur is generated, and there is no reflux, even though the typical "buttonhole" mitral orifice is present, in which closure of the orifice is absolutely impossible, as no valves in fact remain as such. When, on the other hand, the pressure in the left auricle and pulmonary circulation falls below a certain point, either from break-down of the right ventricle or from the onset of tricuspid regurgitation, mitral reflux takes place during systole, and there is not sufficient pressure in the left auricle during diastole to generate a presystolic murmur. We may thus explain these extreme and confusing varieties in the physical signs of the third stage of mitral obstruction complicated by regurgitation, and account for the absence of a systolic murmur in many cases where, from the condition of the mitral orifice post-mortem, we should have expected mitral regurgitation to have been present during life.

In aortic incompetence a presystolic murmur is sometimes present in addition to the diastolic murmur, which does not necessarily imply the existence of mitral stenosis. The probable significance of this murmur and the explanation of its presence have already been discussed in the chapter on Aortic Incompetence.

## PROGNOSIS.

Mitral stenosis stands next to aortic regurgitation among valvular affections in the order of gravity. The average age at death, as deduced from 53 cases abstracted from the post-mortem records at St. Mary's Hospital, was found to be 33 for males and 37 or 38 for females, which is higher than one would expect.

A suggestive inquiry is, why mitral stenosis should be so serious, and especially why it should be attended with greater danger to life than mitral incompetence. One reason is, that the effects of obstruction here are not so easily neutralized as are the effects of regurgitation. The high pressure maintained in the pulmonary circulation and in the left auricle, by hypertrophy of the right ventricle, will antagonize incompetence of the valve in two ways—by resisting the reflux during systole, and by more rapid filling of the ventricle during diastole. In stenosis this high pressure can only be of service by increasing the rapidity of the passage of blood through the narrowed orifice during diastole; and, as diastole only lasts for a certain time, if the contraction be extreme, the ventricle cannot be properly filled before the systole is again due. When such is the case, the compensation is inadequate. On the other hand, since the constriction may reach a degree which, in the absence of experience, would seem quite incompatible with life, and since the subjects of such extensive change must have lived through all the intermediate degrees, it can scarcely be simply that obstruction, as such, is specially dangerous. Probably the explanation of the greater danger of obstruction, as compared with regurgitation, lies in the fact that, when once adhesion between the flaps of the valves has set in, it tends to go on, the friction and strain keeping up chronic inflammation, which gives rise to further adhesion of the valves and contraction of the orifice.

When mitral stenosis is established in childhood or early adolescence, the prognosis is more serious than when it occurs in later life. This is partly owing to the progressive tendency of the constriction of the orifice, which is more marked in early life, and partly to the fact that the stenosed orifice does not increase in size while the growth of the heart continues, so that even though no further actual narrowing takes place, the relative disproportions between the mitral orifice and the cavities of the heart will increase as the heart attains its full development.

The important point in prognosis, however, is the comparative prospect of life in individual cases, and it is in the estimation of this that the recognition of the different stages is of service. The extent of the hypertrophy and dilatation of the walls and cavities of the heart does not afford very great assistance, as we have seen that mitral stenosis does not give rise to any marked change in the left ventricle; a certain amount of information, however, as to the amount of obstruction may be gathered from the degree of hypertrophy and dilatation of the right ventricle, on which has fallen the work of overcoming the obstruction. A careful study of the sounds and murmurs will give more precise information, so that the three stages in the disease, as described above, must be borne in mind in attempting to form a prognosis. So long as the second sound is heard at and beyond the apex, there is little or no liability to the occurrence of symptoms, and there is no immediate danger. It must, however, be borne in mind that, owing to the tendency of the stenosis to increase, the prognosis as to prolonged life in the future is not favourable in the majority of cases.

When the second sound is lost at the apex, that is, when the second stage is reached, there may still be immunity from symptoms under ordinary conditions of life; but there is no capacity for the adjustment of the circulation to deviations from these, so that any imprudence or slight over-exertion, or even mental worry, on the part of the patient is liable to bring about a break-down of compensation. One must not, therefore, be thrown off one's guard by absence of complaints, or by the apparent good health of the patient. With suitable precautions and care, however, the condition of the patient may remain the same for years, though any tendency to increasing shortness of breath or any fresh attack of rheumatism will be reasons for apprehension, as indicating that the constriction is increasing.

When the third stage is reached and serious symptoms, such as dyspnœa, dropsy, pulmonary infarction, and other effects of venous congestion and over-distension of the right side of the heart, are present, the first element in the mental calculation will be the severity of the symptoms. But recoveries are witnessed in conditions apparently so desperate that if it is the first time the patient has suffered from a similar complete break-down of compensation, the case must not be pronounced absolutely hopeless. The number of times severe symptoms have arisen and the readiness with which they have been provoked become the most important considerations. If the patient has had similar attacks previously, and if a very slight cause has been sufficient to induce them, the danger is very great, and the chance of even temporary recovery is a poor one.

## TREATMENT.

The first stage of mitral stenosis is attended with few symptoms, and rarely calls for treatment. So long as the narrowing of the orifice is only moderate, compensation appears to be easily effected, and the patient suffers little or no inconvenience. The fear is that once the flaps of the valve have begun to adhere, the adhesion will extend and gradually narrow the fissure between them. If this could be prevented by any means, the treatment effecting it would be of extreme value. We have no power, however, of directly influencing the process of adhesion, and can only endeavour to obviate causes tending to keep up or excite inflammation of the valves. Every possible precaution should be taken against rheumatism, which is extremely prone to attack the damaged valves; and slight rheumatism, which might be neglected in a sound individual, should receive attention in a patient suffering from mitràl stenosis of however small degree. Unduly high pressure in the arterial circulation will react on the valves by giving rise to high intra-cardiac pressure, and stress upon them will tend to keep up or revive irritation. Over-eating and drinking, again, and constipation, giving rise to accumulation of impurities in the blood, will have a like tendency. Precautions based on this knowledge should therefore be inculcated upon the patient.

Bronchitis and other affections of the lungs will increase the resistance in the pulmonary circulation and the strain on the right ventricle, and should be specially guarded against.

As the narrowing of the orifice progresses, or when the affection is found on examination to have reached the second stage, and when symptoms such as breathlessness and cardiac pain or oppression or weight are readily induced, or are more or less constantly present, or when hæmoptysis has occurred, the precautions suggested above should be urged more emphatically. Mercurial purgatives will then be of service, and rest in the recumbent position, and, if necessary, confinement to bed for a time should be ordered. Strychnia and iron, with nitroglycerine or nitrites and stimulants, may be prescribed, but digitalis should not be given unless there are symptoms of right ventricle failure, and not then until after free purgation; on no account should it be given for a long period.

The rules for exercise will be the same as in other forms of valvular disease. Sufferers from mitral stenosis of slight or moderate degree are perhaps more liable to do themselves harm by imprudent exertion than the subjects of mitral incompetence, as they are often not checked by breathlessness, but persist in overtaxing their strength till severe pain in the heart, or perhaps an attack of hæmoptysis is induced. At an advanced stage of the disease exertion may prove suddenly fatal, but never while the patient is free from serious symptoms; more commonly it is by overthrowing the compensatory balance already inclined to the wrong side, and so aggravating the existing venous stasis, or by detaching a thrombus, which gives rise to embolism, that effort or excitement proves injurious and ultimately fatal. Hæmoptysis is rarely considerable, and seldom requires any other treatment than rest and aperients.

When from neglect of precautions, or from overtaxing of strength by unavoidable duties, or from depressing emotions, or from the advance of the disease, decided symptoms of right-ventricle failure have supervened, such as great weakness, cough, dyspnœa, with evidences of venous stasis in swollen jugulars and enlarged liver, and dropsy, then energetic measures will be required. These will be mainly such as will relieve the venous engorgement and the overloaded right ventricle and auricle, smart purgation by calomel or blue pill and colocynth, followed, if necessary, by salines.

When the symptoms are very urgent, venesection may be of striking service, and in certain cases there is no other treatment that will take its place and avail to avert a speedy fatal termination.

The indications will be, not a full bounding pulse, but the opposite—a small, weak, irregular pulse, many of the beats being scarcely perceptible; the heart, on the other hand, more especially the right ventricle, will be beating violently, epigastric pulsation being very marked, while the apex beat is scarcely perceptible. The liver will be enlarged, and perhaps pulsating, and the jugulars will be full and pulsating. The contrast between the powerful right ventricle impulse and the small, weak, irregular pulse is very striking, and is one of the most important indications for venesection. The sufferer will be in a state of dyspnœa, though not always of an agonizing kind, and not always compelling him to sit up; the face may be dusky and the lips blue, but it may also be pale with a red patch of injected capillaries on the cheeks.

The narrowed mitral orifice constitutes a fixed obstacle, which keeps up an unremitting backward pressure in the pulmonary circulation, and makes it difficult or impossible for the right ventricle to overcome the paralyzing over-distension to which it is subjected. Venesection lessens the amount of blood arriving by the veins, and gives the right ventricle a chance of recovery, so that it can again contract down more or less efficiently on its contents.

Venesection does not, however, dispense with the necessity for relieving the portal circulation by purgation. Stimulants which without these measures afford no relief, and may indeed do harm, will then be of the greatest service, and digitalis and like remedies will find their opportunity.

When the symptoms are less urgent or venesection is objected to, seven or eight leeches applied over the liver may be of service, and in hospital patients, where rest and care and proper nourishment make such an enormous difference in the influences acting on the patient, leeches will usually be sufficient.

The administration of digitalis in the early stages of the disease is seldom if ever called for; it is only when there are symptoms of right ventricle failure, and then only after free purgation and, if necessary, venesection have been employed, that it should be prescribed. Up to a certain point in such cases its influence is often most beneficial, but sometimes it fails to relieve, and even appears to aggravate the symptoms. If continued too long in cases where it has been of signal service, unfavourable effects may supervene, marked by slowing of the pulse, a sense of præcordial oppression, and by coupled heart-beats, the first of which alone reaches the wrist, the second being unaccompanied by an aortic second sound.

In many cases the coupled heart-beats with two beats of the heart to one beat of the pulse at the wrist can be induced at will by the administration of digitalis.

Digitalis, therefore, must be employed with caution in mitral stenosis, and its effects should be carefully watched. Under no circumstances should it be prescribed unless the patient is under observation, and it should rarely be given for a long period of time.

Nitro-glycerine and other vasodilators may sometimes be given with good effect for many weeks or even months in conjunction with general tonics, such as iron, quinine, and nux vomica.

# CHAPTER XIII.

## VALVULAR DISEASE OF THE RIGHT SIDE OF THE HEART.

TRICUSPID INCOMPETENCE AND STENOSIS—PULMONIC INCOMPETENCE AND STENOSIS—SYSTOLIC PULMONIC MURMURS WHICH DO NOT INDICATE STENOSIS.

PRIMARY tricuspid valvular disease is rare, and for the most part is congenital.

Tricuspid regurgitation is so common when the right ventricle is overdistended by violent exertion (the so-called safety-valve action) that it may be looked on as physiological; it is not usually attended with a murmur. Tricuspid incompetence, again, with or without a murmur, is an early and almost constant effect of back pressure through the lungs when there is serious valvular disease of the left ventricle. In both instances the cause of the regurgitation is dilatation of the right ventricle, temporary or permanent, as the case may be.

The tricuspid valve may, however, be damaged during intra-uterine life, or more rarely in childhood or adolescence by endocarditis of rheumatic origin, or, where serious valvular disease of the left ventricle exists, may undergo thickening and contraction from chronic inflammation set up by the irritation and undue strain caused by protracted high pressure in the pulmonary circulation.

The murmur attending tricuspid regurgitation is systolic

in time and is usually blowing in character, having its maximum intensity about one-third of the distance between the left edge of the sternum and the vertical nipple line. It is usually audible outwards towards the apex, and sometimes at the apex itself, where it may be mistaken for a mitral murmur. Such a murmur, when constant and not occasional only, may be looked on as indicative of definite tricuspid insufficiency, with probably actual change in the valvular flaps and chordæ tendineæ. A musical tricuspid systolic murmur may sometimes be heard over a limited area, but it seldom has any important significance.

It is not, however, from the character of the murmur, or from its presence, that conclusions as to the degree of tricuspid incompetence are to be drawn. More important information is gained from the condition of the veins of the neck and from enlargement of the liver. The veins of the neck are more or less distended according to the degree of regurgitation, and the external jugulars may attain even the size of the little finger. Frequently they will fill from below when emptied by pressure.

Pulsation is usually present when there is much regurgitation, and is often very conspicuous. It is sometimes seen to be double, the contraction, first of the auricle, then of the ventricle, sending a reflux wave along the jugulars. At times the pulsation in the internal jugular vein is so marked, and extends so high, that at first sight it may be taken for the carotid throb of aortic regurgitation; but it is of course easily extinguished by light pressure.

The effect of tricuspid incompetence, causing damming back of the blood in the inferior vena cava, is felt by the liver, which gradually becomes much congested and enlarged, and eventually may pulsate as the reflux becomes considerable.

## TRICUSPID STENOSIS.

Tricuspid stenosis is of rare occurrence, and is usually associated with mitral stenosis. It seldom, if ever, occurs as an isolated valvular lesion. It is in most cases the result of an attack of endocarditis affecting mitral and tricuspid valves simultaneously, and is rarely a congenital affection.

The most characteristic physical sign, when it can be recognized, is a presystolic murmur, audible in the tricuspid area, but it is not always present, and when present is not easily distinguished from a concurrent mitral presystolic murmur. In many cases in which tricuspid stenosis has been diagnosed from the symptoms during life and found on post-mortem examination, and when consequently the presystolic murmur has been carefully and perseveringly sought for over a long period, it has been impossible to recognize and distinguish it. There can be no doubt, however, that the murmur has been frequently heard and recognized. Another important physical sign of tricuspid obstruction is distension of the jugular veins with little or no pulsation. Mackenzie* of Burnley has obtained graphic records of jugular pulsation, and describes an auricular and ventricular type: when the right side of the heart is distended, the double jugular pulsation—the first wave auricular and the second ventricular—is frequently very distinct. But if the tricuspid valves are contracted and rigid and the orifice narrowed, the ventricular wave is cut off, while the auricular may be present. If, however, the auricle is paralyzed by over-distension, the auricular wave may also be missing.

When any considerable degree of tricuspid stenosis exists, the symptoms of embarrassment of the circulation and of venous back pressure are present in a marked degree. When it supervenes on mitral stenosis it is

* *Edin. Hosp. Reports*, 1894, vol. ii.

possible that it has a beneficial effect in postponing the supervention of and limiting the degree of tricuspid regurgitation, but this is doubtful. The symptoms are usually severe. Cyanosis and dyspnœa are prominent features, and œdema of the legs is commonly present.

## The Pulmonic Valves.

Disease of the pulmonic semilunar valves is rare, and of the two conditions, insufficiency and stenosis, the former is the more uncommon.

**Pulmonic insufficiency** gives rise to a diastolic murmur, best heard in the left third intercostal space, and conducted downwards. It must, however, be borne in mind that the murmur of aortic regurgitation is also frequently heard at this spot, so that before venturing on a diagnosis of pulmonic regurgitation, it must be ascertained, not only that the pulmonic second sound is impaired, but also that the carotid throb and collapsing pulse are absent, and that the aortic second sound is unimpaired. No special train of symptoms can be attributed to pulmonic regurgitation.

**Pulmonic stenosis** is nearly always a congenital defect, and as it is fully discussed in the chapter on Congenital Malformations, little need be said here. The murmur to which it gives rise is systolic in time and usually loud and rough, varying in intensity. It is most distinct in the third left space, about three-quarters of an inch from the margin of the sternum, but it is conducted along the branches of the pulmonary artery and is often audible over the whole cardiac area and far beyond, sometimes over the entire chest, front and back. Pulmonic stenosis is often associated with some other congenital defect, such as a perforate interventricular septum or patent foramen ovale. When the last-named condition exists cyanosis is, in the majority of cases, present in a more or less pronounced degree, or is easily induced by exertion.

Systolic pulmonic murmurs are very common without change in the orifice or valves.

A pulmonic murmur may be present in a patient suffering from anæmia and disappear as the blood regains its normal character; it is then properly termed "hæmic."

Again, a murmur in this situation may be induced by severe or protracted exertion, and last for some hours or days. There will probably be at the same time indications of dilatation of the right ventricle, though it is not easy to explain how this could give rise to the pulmonic murmur.

A third variety of systolic murmur in the pulmonic area, which may be loud and rough, and often varies greatly in the same subject and without obvious cause, or especially on change of position, is not unfrequently met with in adolescents of both sexes, which cannot be attributed to anæmia or to dilatation of the right ventricle. It is not indicative of temporary weakness or organic unsoundness of heart, nor is it incompatible with capacity for vigorous and sustained exertion, as boys and men in whom it is present can play football and train for races with impunity. Its presence may be made a pretext for rejecting candidates for the army on medical grounds, but I have known many men in whom such a murmur was present go through arduous campaigns without breaking down. I have never known such a murmur develop into actual heart disease; on the contrary, it usually disappears in adult life, except now and then in women.

The causation of such a murmur is apparently as follows. Usually the conus arteriosus of the pulmonary artery is covered by the thin edge of the overlapping left lung. In the cases under consideration the covering by lung is incomplete, and a part of the conus comes into contact with the chest wall, and during systole is flattened more or less against the chest wall. An eddy is thus formed in the current of blood rushing into the pulmonary artery, which gives rise to a murmur. Evidence in support of this explanation is afforded by the fact that the murmur usually disappears when the patient is told to take a deep breath and hold it, as a cushion of lung is then brought over the conus arteriosus between it and the chest wall. The result is the more striking if the murmur happens to be loud and vibratory.

## CHAPTER XIV.

## CONGENITAL MALFORMATIONS.

VARIETIES OF CONGENITAL MALFORMATIONS—RELATIVE FREQUENCY OF OCCURRENCE—OF SINGLE AND COMBINED DEFECTS—PHYSICAL SIGNS—SYMPTOMS—CYANOSIS—CAUSE OF CYANOSIS—DIAGNOSIS—PROGNOSIS.

SOME of the most important varieties of congenital malformations of the heart and great vessels are—

1. The heart consisting of two or three cavities, the interventricular or interauricular septum, or both, being absent. This is of rare occurrence.

2. Incomplete interventricular septum, usually taking the form of a perforation in the upper third of the septum.

3. Patent foramen ovale.

4. Persistence of patent ductus arteriosus.

5. Stenosis of the pulmonary orifice due to constriction of the trunk of the vessel itself, or of the infundibular portion of the right ventricle, or to the adhesion or malformation of the valves.

6. Transposition of pulmonary artery and aorta.

7. The aorta and pulmonary artery may both arise from the same ventricle.

8. Malformations of the aortic, tricuspid, or mitral valves are not of common occurrence. In most cases, where the tricuspid valve is found to be affected at birth, the probabilities will be that it has been damaged by endocarditis occurring during fœtal life.

**Pulmonic Stenosis.**—Of these varieties by far the most common is stenosis of the pulmonary orifice. Of 181 cases of congenital malformation collected by Peacock, in 90 more or less contraction of the pulmonary orifice was present, and in 29 others the orifice or trunk of the vessel was obliterated.*

The narrowing may be due to constriction of the conus arteriosus above the valves, or to adhesion between the cusps of the valves. The artery may be very small and ill developed and the valves present but impervious.

The most common varieties of congenital heart disease, after pulmonic stenosis, are deficiency of the interventricular septum and patency of the foramen ovale.

**Deficiency of the interventricular septum** usually takes the form of a perforation in the upper third of the septum, in the undefended or membranous space, so called because normally the septum here only consists of two layers of endocardium. It is rare as an isolated lesion, but is not uncommon in association with other malformations which give rise to unequal pressure in the two ventricles. For instance, it is frequently found coexisting with pulmonic stenosis, in which the pressure in the right ventricle is in excess of that in the left. Not unfrequently in such cases the right ventricle is greatly hypertrophied and the septum is deviated to the left, and in some cases the aorta arises wholly or in part from the right ventricle.

**Patency of the foramen ovale** may occur in connection with pulmonic stenosis; but this cannot be always attributed to excess of pressure in the right auricle, as it is sometimes found as an isolated lesion; and also cases are recorded in which the foramen was found closed, though excess of pressure must have existed in the right auricle.

The **ductus arteriosus** may remain patent in consequence of some obstruction to the passage of blood through the

* Peacock, "Malformations of the Human Heart," p. 193.

lungs or systemic vessels; not infrequently a patent ductus arteriosus occurs in association with a patent foramen ovale, the patency of both being due to similar causes; hence the two may be found together with, and as a direct result of, pulmonic stenosis.

In a case recently under my care at St. Mary's Hospital, patency of the ductus arteriosus existed as an isolated lesion.

**Transposition of Pulmonary Artery and Aorta.**—The aorta may arise from the right ventricle, and the pulmonary artery from the left. The ductus arteriosus will usually remain patent. The aorta and pulmonary artery may both arise from the same ventricle. In a specimen in the St. Mary's Hospital Museum, both aorta and pulmonary artery arise from the right ventricle. The interventricular septum is absent in the upper third, so that there is free communication between the two ventricles. The right ventricle is greatly dilated and hypertrophied and the left very small. The pulmonary artery is very small and ill developed, and its lumen is only about 2 mm. in diameter.

In spite of this the child from which the specimen was taken lived to the age of three months, though cyanosed and dyspnœic from birth, and very poorly developed.

## Physical Signs.

In pulmonic stenosis a loud, rough, systolic murmur is usually to be heard over the præcordial region with its maximum intensity at the level of the nipple, midway between the nipple and the sternum. It will be conducted along the branches of the pulmonary artery so that it will be heard over a large area on both sides of the chest; but it will be heard more distinctly on the left side of the chest between the base of the heart and the clavicle than over the aorta. In association with this the right ventricle will usually be hypertrophied.

**Deficiency of the interventricular septum** may give rise to a systolic murmur whose seat of maximum intensity is, according to Roger and Potain, in the fourth left space half an inch above the nipple; but as this defect commonly coexists with pulmonic stenosis, such a murmur would probably be masked by that due to the pulmonic lesion. A murmur that may occur in cases of deficient interventricular septum, and which I look upon as diagnostic, is one quite different in character to any that occur in the usual forms of valvular disease. It is harsh and loud, but its great peculiarity is that it never ceases, becoming suddenly louder and higher pitched with the systole, and subsiding into a continuous rumble during diastole, reminding one of the kind of noise of varying intensity made by a knife-grinder's wheel when a knife is being sharpened.

**Patent foramen ovale.**—There is no known auscultatory or other physical sign by which a patent foramen ovale can be diagnosed. Peacock quotes one case of patent foramen ovale without other defect, in which the patient, a girl, lived to the age of sixteen, when she died of pulmonary tuberculosis. There was no cyanosis, and till she began to suffer from tuberculosis there were no symptoms other than those of general debility. In a case under my care the patient was a man, who died at the age of thirty from bronchitis. There was no marked cyanosis during infancy, there were no special symptoms of morbus cordis, and no cardiac murmurs; the patient was, however, dull and of sluggish intellect, but could take long walks without seeming distressed in any way, or appearing the worse for it. During the fatal attack of bronchitis cyanosis developed, attended with torpor. A noteworthy point was that the cyanosis deepened during sleep, and there was no spontaneous waking up, and the patient was roused with difficulty. Eventually the torpor had under my care a case, already referred to, in which patency of the ductus arteriosus existed as an isolated lesion The only physical sign was a soft blowing systolic murmur of moderate intensity audible over most of the cardiac area, most marked in the third left intercostal space; it diminished in intensity towards the clavicle and towards the aortic area, but was very distinct at the apex. There was no cyanosis, and there were no symptoms directly attributable to the condition, but the child died of diarrhœa and vomiting. It was 7 months old.

## Symptoms.

The child suffering from a serious congenital affection of the heart is usually irritable and fretful, and may be subject to fits. The fingers and toes are clubbed, and the extremities cold. He may be always cyanosed to a varying degree, or only become cyanosed on exertion. There will usually be constant shortness of breath, and paroxysms of dyspnœa may occur, in which cyanosis becomes so intense that the extremities become almost black. He will remain stunted in growth and backward in development, intellectually as well as physically. The symptoms will of course vary, according to the nature of the lesion. They will be most marked in a case of severe pulmonary stenosis, and may, as has already been seen, be entirely absent in a case of uncomplicated patent foramen ovale.

**Cyanosis.**—In many instances of congenital malformation of the heart, the most marked and striking feature is the cyanosis of the patient; hence the various forms of congenital heart disease have been grouped together under the names morbus cœruleus, or blue disease, by English, and cyanose, or maladie bleue, by French authors.

The explanation of the cause of this peculiar discoloration is still a matter of dispute. Sénac, Corvisart, Gintrac, and others attribute it to the mixture of arterial and venous blood in the heart or great vessels, owing to defective septa or patent ductus arteriosus. Cruveilhier attributed it to venous congestion. It has been proved, however, that cyanosis may exist without the intermixture of currents of blood, also that complete intermixture may take place without the occurrence of cyanosis.

It is obvious, therefore, that neither of these explanations are sufficient. Stillé, with a view to determining the cause of cyanosis, collected 77 cases of congenital morbus cordis in which cyanosis was present. In 53 instances the pulmonary artery was constricted or impervious, or its orifice was obstructed in some way. He came to the conclusion, therefore, that cyanosis was due to venous congestion usually dependent on obstruction at the orifice of the pulmonary artery, or on some other cause giving rise to obstruction to the venous return. This is clearly not a complete explanation, as there is often no cyanosis in cases of morbus cordis in adults where the venous congestion is extreme. Peacock makes another important suggestion, that deficient aeration of the blood is a contributory cause of cyanosis; he says, "where only a small proportion of the blood is submitted at one time to aeration in the lungs, the whole mass must be of a dark colour, consequently the hue of the surface will be proportionately dark." This is especially the case in pulmonic stenosis, and Stillé's statistics, which show that pulmonic stenosis is the commonest cause of cyanosis, afford strong support to this view, that aeration of a small proportion only of the blood is the essential cause of cyanosis.

## Diagnosis.

Though in severe cases it is usually easy to arrive at a diagnosis of congenital heart disease from a history of cyanosis and dyspnœa since birth, with the clubbing of the fingers and toes, it is difficult and in many instances impossible to be certain of the exact nature of the malformation.

Where with a history of cyanosis and paroxysms of dyspnœa since birth we find a loud, rough, systolic murmur, with its maximum intensity on the left side at the level of the nipple, midway between the nipple and sternum, together with a hypertrophied right ventricle, we may be fairly certain that pulmonary stenosis is the main lesion; but whether a patent foramen ovale or perforate interventricular septum, or patent ductus arteriosus, is present as well, it will often be impossible to decide.

## Prognosis.

The lesion is in this case stationary, and not progressive, but the malformations being widely different, the effect they have on the duration of life will vary considerably.

1. In cases of moderate constriction of the pulmonary artery without other malformation, for which hypertrophy of the right ventricle is sufficient to compensate, there will be no cyanosis, and the patient may live many years without serious inconvenience, except on violent exertion.

2. In cases where the foramen ovale is open the pulmonary stenosis is usually greater, and hence the duration of life will probably be less; but out of 20 cases which Peacock collected, 11 lived to the age of 15 years and over, 1 living to the age of 57.

3. Where with pulmonary stenosis the interventricular

septum is also deficient, the prognosis is much less favourable, for not only must the pulmonary constriction be considerable to have given rise to this deficiency, but, further, in such case the aorta usually arises in part from the right ventricle. Of 64 such cases collected by Peacock, only 14 survived the age of 15. If, however, the degree of pulmonic stenosis is slight and the perforation in the septum small, life may be prolonged, and two patients are now living, at the age of 30 or upwards, in which I believe this condition to exist; one has borne a child.

4. Where the pulmonary artery is impervious, the duration of life rarely exceeds a few months, though of 28 such cases of Peacock's, 3 lived to the age of 9 or 10, and 1 to 12 years.

In a case under the care of Dr. Cheadle in St. Mary's Hospital in 1902, a child lived to the age of 14 months with an impervious pulmonary artery and a heart consisting of only two cavities, an auricle and ventricle. It was cyanosed and dyspnœic from birth.

5. Transposition of the main arteries, or arrest of development, so that the heart consists of two or three cavities only, is usually incompatible with life for any long period after birth, but 4 cases are recorded by Peacock where with one ventricle only and two auricles persons lived to the ages of 11, 16, 23, and 24 years respectively.

6. Patency of the foramen ovale uncomplicated by any other defect may not of itself give rise to any serious symptoms; doubtless in most instances where the opening is valve-like it will become closed before adolescence is reached. Where it persists or allows of extensive leakage, any lung affection, such as bronchitis, which tends to increase the pressure in the right side of the heart and cause a flow of non-aerated blood from the right to the left auricle, will be especially dangerous and liable to prove fatal.

# CHAPTER XV.

## PROGNOSIS IN VALVULAR DISEASE (GENERAL).

THE NATURE OF THE LESION: THE RELATIVE DANGER ATTACHING TO EACH PARTICULAR LESION—SUDDEN DEATH: THE VALVULAR DISEASES IN WHICH IT IS LIABLE TO OCCUR—THE EXTENT OF THE LESION—THE STATIONARY OR PROGRESSIVE CHARACTER OF THE LESION AS INFLUENCING PROGNOSIS.

In cases of heart disease, prognosis is of special importance, since a patient who knows that he is suffering from some affection of the heart immediately dreads the worst. It is always necessary to allay his fears as far as possible, as these in themselves tend to aggravate the danger attending the disease. In some cases this may be done with absolute confidence; in others, the apprehensions may be only too well founded; in others, again, the issue may be uncertain and may be dependent on other conditions than the state of the heart. It will be most important in all instances that the medical attendant should form a definite idea of the probable effect the heart disease will have in shortening life, so that he may guide the patient and his friends in making arrangements on which the welfare of the family may depend.

The following are the points which should specially be considered in regard to prognosis:—

1. The valve affected and the relative danger attaching to the particular lesion.

2. The extent of the lesion.
3. The stationary or progressive character of the lesion.
4. The degree of soundness and vigour, functional and nutritional, of the muscular substance of the heart, of the arterial walls, and of the tissues generally.
5. The age of the patient.
6. The family history, especially in regard to whether there is any hereditary tendency to heart disease.
7. The habits and mode of life of the patient.
8. The presence or absence of other diseases—such as anæmia, bronchitis, renal affections—as complications.

## The Relative Danger attaching to the Different Valvular Lesions.

According to Walshe, the valvular affections stand in the order of relative gravity as follows: tricuspid regurgitation, mitral regurgitation, mitral constriction, aortic regurgitation, pulmonary constriction, aortic constriction. Tricuspid regurgitation, however, as has already been said, is rarely primary, but usually occurs as a result of obstruction to the transit of blood through the lungs either from disease in these organs, or from valvular disease in the left side of the heart. It is therefore an effect of serious valvular lesions of the left side of the heart, and can scarcely be regarded as a cause of the fatal termination.

My own experience would lead me to modify Walshe's arrangement somewhat, and to give this order of relative danger: aortic incompetence, mitral stenosis, aortic stenosis, mitral incompetence. Aortic incompetence is most rapidly fatal when it comes on late in life at a period when compensatory hypertrophy is established with difficulty, more especially when due to degenerative change in the valves. In childhood and early adolescence, mitral stenosis is often more serious than aortic incompetence, owing to the progressive nature of the lesion and to imperfect development of the left ventricle. It is, however, difficult to estimate with any accuracy the relative danger of different valvular lesions, as so many other factors must be taken into consideration in prognosis.

## SUDDEN DEATH.

One of the first questions to be discussed is the liability to sudden death in heart disease. In the mind of the general public, disease of the heart and sudden death are so closely associated that the mention of the one immediately suggests the other, and in a nervous patient, a pain or a sense of weight or oppression in the cardiac region, easily exaggerated by the concentration of his attention upon the heart, will make him think the end is near.

It is therefore of the greatest importance that we should know with certainty, in what form of heart disease sudden death is liable to occur, and be able in cases where no such danger exists to say so with confidence. It must be understood that the sudden death under consideration is such as is meant by the familiar phrase "dropping down dead," with little or no warning, the individual having been up to the moment in apparent health, or so far well as to be able to go about his duties, or at any rate not suffering from dropsy or other serious symptoms of cardiac embarrassment.

In all forms of heart disease, when the effects on the circulation have become very decided, and such symptoms as engorgement of the lungs, with dyspnœa, dropsy, effusion into the pleural cavities, albuminuria, have set in, the final struggle may come on abruptly and end speedily. This, however, is not the mode of death which is the special dread attending heart disease.

Walshe, in speaking of the different forms of valvular lesions, says that only one causes sudden death, namely, aortic incompetence.

In a paper read before the Harveian Society in 1866, I gave as the conclusion at which I had arrived that "sudden death is a contingency which may almost be left out of consideration in valvular disease, except in aortic regurgitation." This would still express very nearly my individual experience. As will be shown in the part of this book on the structural changes in the wall of the heart, there are other conditions more likely to give rise to sudden death than aortic regurgitation. Here, however, we are considering only the valvular lesions.

As individual experience is not altogether a trustworthy guide, some years ago Sidney Phillips, at my request, went through the post-mortem records of St. Mary's Hospital of four hundred cases in which the heart had undergone marked change, in order to see what light they threw on the question of heart disease and sudden death. Of these, 151 were cases of valvular disease, 204 examples of changes in the wall of the heart. Of aortic regurgitation there were thirty-eight cases. Three were brought to the hospital dead, a fourth died in the hospital suddenly during convalescence from acute rheumatism. In six more the final symptoms came on abruptly and were rapidly fatal, one dying within twenty-four hours of his admission to the hospital, another within two days. There were eleven examples of aortic stenosis without one sudden death in the sense of the patient being overtaken by death while in apparent health or free from symptoms arising from heart disease.

Of mitral stenosis there were fifty-three instances. One patient only was brought in dead, a young girl who was picked up in the street. From the condition of the lungs there was no doubt that she must have been suffering severely from symptoms due to the heart affection.

Of mitral insufficiency there were forty-nine cases. Of these, two may be said to have died suddenly, but both had serious symptoms and were under treatment in hospital, and in both the pericardium also was universally adherent.

In three more a final attack of dyspnœa set in abruptly and proved rapidly fatal.

These numbers are not given as representing with anything like accuracy the proportion of sudden deaths in the different forms of valvular disease, but they afford confirmation of the opinion formed from personal experience that aortic insufficiency is the only form of valvular disease attended with danger of sudden death.

## The Extent of the Lesion.

In a previous chapter the indications by means of which the extent of the lesion may be estimated, have been discussed. A certain limited amount of information on this head is obtained from the character of the murmur. Further help is derived from the pulse, and still more from the amount of hypertrophy and dilatation which the heart has undergone in consequence of the lesion. A valvular murmur, accompanied by dilatation or hypertrophy or both, is attended with greater danger than a similar murmur not so accompanied; not, however, because the hypertrophy and dilatation add new elements of danger, but because the valvular change causing the murmur has given rise also to mechanical difficulty when these changes are present, whereas their absence shows that it has given rise to no serious obstacle to the circulation.

It must be understood, however, that when hypertrophy and dilatation are taken as a measure of the valvular lesion it is in the absence of any evidence of functional inefficiency. Where, in addition to the disease of the valves, there is degeneration of the muscular substance of the heart, this will give rise to further dilatation. Still, however, the amount of dilatation may be taken as expressing the relation between the mechanical difficulty and the power of the heart to cope with it. Naturally the more extensive the lesion, as estimated by the changes in the heart, the more serious the prognosis, because the compensatory balance has been established with difficulty and is more easily upset.

## The Stationary or Progressive Character of the Lesion as influencing Prognosis.

A given state of valve existing—a certain degree of obstruction or incompetence—it will be obvious that the future of the patient will be very greatly influenced by the question whether the morbid process which has damaged the valve is still in progress, or has come to a standstill. In the one case, where the change has reached its maximum, we know what we have to deal with—the hypertrophy and dilatation give an approximate idea of the functional imperfection; they compensate it or they do not, and the prognosis varies accordingly: in the other there can be but one course and issue, a gradual or swift aggravation of symptoms, unless indeed sudden death interferes.

Such a difference exists arising out of the character of the pathological process by which the valve is affected. Speaking generally, the question is whether the valvular change has had its origin in an acute inflammatory attack or is the result of a chronic degenerative process. Fortunately the distinction is for the most part easy.

In the chapter on the ætiology of valvular disease the various causes of lesions of the valves and orifices have been enumerated and briefly discussed. They are, acute endocarditis, chronic endocarditis, and degenerative changes in the valves, rupture of valve, dilatation of the orifice.

**Acute Endocarditis.**—When the valvular lesion can be

traced definitely to an attack of acute endocarditis, there is this favourable element in the prognosis, that the lesion once established is not progressive. If the lesion was slight it remains slight, and does not increase in severity after the endocarditis has subsided; consequently the dilatation and hypertrophy of the heart will be small, if indeed they are appreciable; if the lesion is extensive, the dilatation and hypertrophy which will follow are proportionate. Hence we are able to arrive at a definite conclusion as to the extent of the lesion, and give an approximate idea as to the probable effect it will have in shortening life, and say how far exercise and exertion can be allowed. The only exception to be made will be in cases of mitral stenosis, where the orifice may become gradually further narrowed after the initial damage has been done, owing to cicatricial contraction of the inflammatory products.

**Chronic Endocarditis.**—The fatal feature about this chronic inflammatory or degenerative change in the valves is, that once begun it is inevitably progressive. The heart and system may have accommodated themselves to a degree of obstruction or regurgitation, but this does not remain the same; slowly or rapidly the valvular lesion will increase, and with it the obstacle to the due transmission of the blood through the heart. This takes place at an age when the heart is little able to adapt itself to change or to meet the increasing difficulty, and is, moreover, itself liable to structural decay; further, the cause which has worn out the valves, the excessive resistance in the peripheral circulation giving rise to unduly high tension in the arterial system, is probably still in operation.

Before, however, we take so serious a view of any given case in which a valvular murmur has been developed late in life, and accept it as necessarily indicative of progressive disease, we ought to make sure that it is due to degenerative changes, and not to mere roughening of the valve. To prove the former we ought to have evidence of actual damage to the valve, either in the shape of symptoms traceable to functional inefficiency or of modifications of the physical signs. It is common in elderly people to find a mitral or aortic systolic murmur develop, which persists for years without any symptoms of heart disease, due to a slight roughness or rigidity in the case of the aortic valve which sets up vibrations; or, in the case of the mitral valve, to a little thickening or want of pliability which prevents an accurate apposition of the flaps of the valve, but does not allow of any appreciable regurgitation.

**Rupture of Valve.**—Rupture of a valve is of rare occurrence and is always a serious lesion. The valve affected is usually the aortic, and the sudden and severe strain on the heart, which has no time to accommodate itself to the altered conditions of the circulation, leads to dilatation of the left ventricle and the consequent onset of severe symptoms when the rupture of a cusp is complete. The accident is usually accompanied by sudden pain in the chest, and the patient may be seized by a syncopal attack, which will at once prove fatal. The early symptoms may, however, not be very severe. The patient may appear to progress favourably for a time, but dyspnœa and other symptoms of cardiac embarrassment will soon set in, for the accident usually takes place at a time in life when degenerative changes are already beginning to take place in the walls of the heart, and it is incapable of undergoing sufficient hypertrophy to compensate for the valvular lesion. Hence the ultimate cause of death, if the patient survives, is a gradual stasis of the circulation, the premonitory indications being a rapid increase in the size of the liver, with dilatation of the right ventricle following on that of the left, and later the onset of œdema of the extremities. It may be some weeks or months after the accident before the fatal termination ensues.

**Dilatation of the Orifice.**—(*a*) *The Aortic Orifice.*—The aortic orifice is less liable to dilatation than the mitral, owing to the strong fibrous ring surrounding it. When dilatation does occur, it usually takes place comparatively late in life as a part of a general dilatation of the aorta due to degenerative changes in the walls of the vessel or its orifice: it is therefore progressive in character and the prognosis is unfavourable, more especially as these same degenerative changes may lead to the production of aneurysm.

Syphilitic disease of the aorta, invading the orifice and valves and giving rise to incompetence, carries with it a grave prognosis.

(*b*) *The Mitral Orifice.*—Speaking generally, mitral regurgitation, established by means of dilatation of the left ventricle, in the young, or as a result of acute febrile conditions or anæmia, is, under favourable conditions, curable. When it is secondary to aortic disease, the prognosis necessarily merges in that of the primary lesion. When it occurs as a result of protracted high tension or a kidney disease, it may be temporarily curable by suitable treatment, but will be liable to recur.

In later life and old age it may be gradually and imperceptibly established without any obvious cause for it, and it is difficult to diagnose between dilatation of the orifice and changes such as gradual thickening and contraction of the valves. It is in such cases, however, very slowly progressive, as a rule.

# CHAPTER XVI.

PROGNOSIS CONTINUED—AGE, SEX, HEREDITY—EFFECTS OF HIGH ARTERIAL TENSION—HABITS AND MODE OF LIFE OF THE PATIENT—ANÆMIA—THE CIRCUMSTANCES UNDER WHICH PROGNOSIS MAY HAVE TO BE MADE: (1) IMMEDIATELY AFTER ACUTE ENDOCARDITIS; (2) WHEN THE VALVULAR LESION IS SLIGHT AND HAS GIVEN RISE TO NO STRUCTURAL CHANGES IN THE HEART; (3) WHEN COMPENSATORY CHANGES HAVE TAKEN PLACE BUT NO SYMPTOMS OF EMBARRASSMENT OF THE CIRCULATION ARE PRESENT; (4) WHEN SYMPTOMS OF FAILURE OF COMPENSATION HAVE SET IN; (5) IN ADVANCED VALVULAR DISEASE WHEN SEVERE SYMPTOMS OF CARDIAC FAILURE HAVE SUPERVENED.

**Age.**—Little need be said with regard to age as affecting the prognosis of heart disease. Late in life, degenerative processes are almost invariably in operation, and the hypertrophy which is needed, in order that the effects of valvular affections may be neutralized, is established with difficulty; moreover, compensatory hypertrophy, which has served its purpose for twenty or thirty years, may at the end of this time be undermined by fatty or fibroid degeneration of the cardiac walls.

**Childhood.**—In early childhood, the outbreak of rheumatic endocarditis is always a matter of grave prognostic significance: firstly, because it is so frequently accompanied by pericarditis, which may prove fatal at the time of the attack or leave the heart permanently hampered and disabled by pericardial adhesions; secondly, because, even though the heart escapes serious damage from the first attack of either peri- or endocarditis, both are extremely liable to recur. Further, it would appear that when a valvular lesion of some severity is established, the heart cannot both answer the demand for hypertrophy and keep pace with the active growth of this period of life, so that the child is liable to remain small and stunted, with clubbing of the fingers and toes, and to be generally backward in development.

**Sex.**—It is a remarkable fact that mitral stenosis is very much more common in women than in men. The post-mortem statistics previously referred to, show that out of 53 cases of mitral stenosis, 38 were in females, and only 15 in males, which is approximately a proportion in accord with the experience of most observers. No satisfactory explanation of this predominance has yet been given.

On the other hand, aortic insufficiency is more frequently met with in men, which again is borne out by the same statistics, as out of 36 cases, 30 were males, and only 6 females. This appears to be explained by the occupation and mode of life of men; in my own experience, however, aortic regurgitation has been much more common in boys than in girls at a period of life long before the influence of occupation would begin to operate.

When valvular disease has been established in childhood, girls are, according to my experience, more likely to break down at the trying period of puberty than boys, and, speaking generally, the compensatory changes in the heart walls are less perfectly effected in the female than in the male.

**Hereditary Tendencies.**—In no class of cases is it more necessary to inquire into the family history than in diseases of the heart. It is more particularly in affections of the muscular walls that a family tendency to heart disease is seen, which may take the form of fatty degeneration, or of fibroid change secondary to high arterial tension. I have known a family in which three out of four brothers died suddenly before reaching the age of fifty-five from disease of the heart or aorta, and other examples almost equally striking; similar histories must be known to most medical men of large experience. It is not, however, only a special liability to structural degeneration of the heart at a certain age which is important. In any valvular affection, and at any stage, the constitution of the patient is an element in the prognosis which must be kept in view. We have to take into account, not simply the cardiac lesion and the functional derangement of the circulation caused thereby, but also the behaviour of the system under this disturbing influence and its power of endurance, and in a short-lived family we cannot have the same confidence in the tissues as in a family noted for longevity. More than once in my own experience, a prognosis based upon the state of the heart has been falsified through failure of general constitutional power.

**Effects of High Tension in the Circulation.**—High tension in the arterial system, frequently a hereditary condition, may in itself be a cause of chronic valvular disease in later life, as has been already stated in discussing the causes of chronic endocarditis. It increases the shock of every closure of the aortic valves, and renders necessary more powerful contraction of the left ventricle to drive on the blood, and thus increases the stress on the mitral valve and its tendinous cords. The unremitting strain thus imposed on both aortic and mitral valves is more injurious than the occasional strain due to violent muscular efforts. Hence, when there is high arterial tension in addition to valvular disease, it will greatly tend to aggravate the mischief already effected, and will contribute a grave addition to the unfavourable elements of prognosis, unless carefully watched and relieved by diet and treatment.

**Habits and Mode of Life of the Patient.**—These have a very important bearing on the prognosis. Violent efforts or sustained exertion impose a great strain on the valves of the heart; vicissitudes of temperature tax its power of accommodation to different conditions of circulation, while unfavourable hygienic influences tend to malnutrition and degeneration. The man, therefore, who must labour with his hands, who is exposed to all weathers, whose food is of inferior quality and sometimes insufficient in quantity, who breathes impure air and indulges perhaps in strong drink, who seeks advice only when he can no longer toil, and abandons all precautions as soon as he leaves the hospital, has far less chance of long life than the man who can seek advice early and has adequate means to carry it out. There can be little probability of existing compensation being maintained, or of reparative hypertrophy being established under such circumstances. The first condition of recovery from the effects of disease, the removal of the cause which gives rise to these effects, is wanting. Conversely, protection from adverse influences which have precipitated the access of symptoms, together with rest, warmth, good food, and care, may reverse an apparently hopeless forecast, as is not unfrequently seen in the all but miraculous recoveries which take place in hospitals. In the same way, persistence in habits of eating and drinking, which may lead to valvular disease, directly, by overloading the blood with impurities, which give rise to high arterial tension, or indirectly, through gouty inflammation, will affect the prognosis unfavourably, while obedience to rules of diet carefully laid down and supervised as to their effect will incline the balance to the opposite side.

**Anæmia.**—Anæmia, as is well known, is very common at the period of adolescence, and especially in girls; and its effects may be most prejudicial. About middle age, essential or pernicious anæmia may complicate heart disease, and in at least two instances which have come under my observation, has been the real cause of death which was attributed to the state of the heart.

But, in addition to primary anæmia, a deterioration of the blood is a common and almost inevitable result of heart disease when this reaches a point at which it begins to affect the circulation. The slow movement of the blood through the systemic capillaries and through the lungs, whether due to deficient *vis a tergo*, as in aortic disease, or to venous stasis in mitral disease, prevents those active changes from taking place by means of which the blood is constantly purified and renewed. Absorption of food, again, will be more or less hindered by the languid movement of the blood in the gastro-intestinal mucous membrane, and by the congestion of the liver, which result from obstruction to the return of blood to the heart.

Anæmia, therefore, existing at a time when prognosis is called for, and especially a tendency to recurring anæmia, is a serious element in the forecast.

Anæmia, however induced, has always a detrimental influence on the heart. It may of itself, aided by the high arterial tension which often accompanies it, give rise to dilatation of the left ventricle and leakage of the mitral valve; it will, therefore, tend to aggravate such dilatation as has already been produced by valvular disease, while it will retard compensatory hypertrophy by impairing the quality of the nutritive material supplied. It is also often attended with palpitation of the heart, and will add to the liability of the valvular disease to this distressing and sometimes dangerous symptom.

Anæmia, again, may of itself give rise to œdema, and it will precipitate the occurrence of dropsy when a tendency thereto exists from the nature of the cardiac lesion.

## The Circumstances and Conditions under which a Prognosis may have to be made.

1. We are frequently asked, during convalescence after acute endocarditis—sometimes, indeed, before the attack has subsided—how far the heart is likely to be ultimately affected. This is a question to which no prudent man will give a definite reply. It is impossible at this time to appeal to the changes in the walls and cavities of the heart for guidance, as there has been no time for their development. The cardiac murmurs are not trustworthy guides, as a systolic apex murmur, or sometimes an aortic murmur, which has developed in the course of acute rheumatism, may disappear afterwards. If, however, aortic regurgitation is actually established, the prognosis is serious, although no definite opinion can be formed as to the probable rate of progress.

2. When the lesion is one of old standing we may have an individual in apparent health and vigour, scarcely conscious of any inconvenience arising from derangement of the circulation even on exertion, but in whom the discovery of a valvular murmur has been made. There is no modification of the pulse, the murmur accompanies and does not replace the sound with which it is associated, and there is no marked hypertrophy or dilatation of the heart. In such a case the valvular change is slight and unimportant, and of present danger there is none.

With regard to the future of such a patient, everything depends on the question whether the existing state of the valves is an old-standing, permanent condition traceable to a long past attack of rheumatic endocarditis, or is just the beginning of mischief, such as chronic valvulitis, or atheroma, which will go on increasing. In the former case the patient may live to old age and weather all storms of illness and hardship; in the latter, if we take as an illustration the most serious form of disease, aortic regurgitation, he will probably not live more than four or five years, though a definite judgment as to the course and duration of the affection can only be formed after repeated and careful examination at long intervals.

3. In another case, while no symptoms are present, there is hypertrophy or dilatation of the heart, or both. Here the presence of structural changes testifies to the existence of mechanical difficulty due to obstruction or regurgitation, and shows that the valvular lesion is real: there will almost certainly be some corresponding modification of the pulse, and although compensation has been established, the equilibrium may be disturbed by causes, which would have no effect on the normal heart, and once overthrown will not be very easily restored. While, therefore, under favourable circumstances, the health may remain unaffected for many years, an illness of any kind, and especially an attack of bronchitis, may be attended with dangerous disturbance of the circulation.

In such a case, again, it is of the utmost consequence whether the valvular disease is stationary or progressive: should it be progressive, the prognosis will necessarily be grave, though much will depend on the seat and character of the valvular lesion. The age, sex, general constitutional vigour, and family history must be taken into account, as also the position in life and habits of the patient.

4. In another patient, symptoms of embarrassment of the pulmonary or systemic circulation are present, habitual shortness of breath on slight exertion, violent or irregular action of the heart on slight provocation, which does not readily subside, pain or a feeling of oppression in the præcordial area, incipient œdema about the ankles and perhaps albuminuria with a thick deposit of pink or high-coloured urates in the urine; further evidences of imperfect compensation are also found in the pulse, in the

enlargement of the liver and fulness or pulsation of the veins of the neck.

Here danger is never far off and may be imminent, though by suitable precautions it may be guarded against and warded off for years. Speaking generally, there is less probability of prolonged life and comfort after such symptoms have set in, in aortic than in mitral disease. There are more chances of obviating the effects of obstruction by compensatory changes than of making up for failure of *vis a tergo.* As a rule, the earlier in the course of valvular disease symptoms supervene, the more serious is their significance.

5. In another case we are called upon to give a prognosis when grave consequences of a valvular disease have already been developed. The occurrence of these serious symptoms may have taken place in spite of compensatory changes in the shape of hypertrophy of the right or left ventricle or both, as the case may be, or for the want of them; we must therefore consider whether by opportunity for the restoration or establishment of compensation and by suitable treatment a working equilibrium can be attained. The most important question will be whether the symptoms have been brought on by any temporary or removable cause, such as over-exertion, exposure, anxiety, recent acute illness, pulmonary disease such as bronchitis, anæmia, or debility or the like, or whether there is no recognizable cause for their appearance. In the latter case, the prognosis is far more serious, as some degenerative change in the cardiac walls or organic weakness of the heart or system generally, or possibly some further complication in the shape of adherent pericardium, is to be apprehended. A working man admitted into hospital will almost certainly recover, only however to break down again when he resumes his occupation, and is again exposed to the injurious influences which brought on the symptoms of compensatory

failure. A patient in easy circumstances may by care maintain for a long time the *statum quo*, but he will not easily retrace downward steps taken in spite of all favouring conditions. The character of the valvular change loses none of its importance, the only hope of prolonged immunity from further consequences of failing or obstructed circulation will be the absence of any tendency to aggravation of the lesion in the valve. Subject to this the soundness of the patient's organs and tissues and the tenacity of life exhibited by the family history will be elements of great consequence.

6. When we are called upon to form an opinion of the chances of recovery of a patient who is suffering from advanced dropsy, with severe pulmonary congestion and extreme dyspnœa, then indeed the stationary or progressive character of the lesion has no longer any bearing on the immediate issue of the case. If the symptoms have been gradually increasing in severity without any apparent cause, and the dropsy has crept on from the legs and invaded the trunk, and the dyspnœa is extreme even while the patient is at rest in bed, then there is little hope of recovery. If, on the other hand, the access of severe symptoms is traceable to over-exertion or a chill or intercurrent pulmonary trouble, such as bronchitis, then there is a hope that suitable treatment may for a time restore the compensatory balance, provided that there is evidence of a certain degree of vigour and force in the cardiac impulse, more especially in that of the right ventricle. If it is a second attack of this kind, there will be less chance of recovery, and any complication, such as kidney disease, will diminish materially this chance. The occurrence of a pulmonary apoplexy at this stage, or of thrombosis of the veins of the leg, will be of very serious import, rendering the prognosis as regards the prolongation of life, even for a short period, almost hopeless.

## CHAPTER XVII.

## TREATMENT (GENERAL).

TREATMENT OF VALVULAR DISEASE IN GENERAL—PROPHYLACTIC MEASURES—GENERAL RULES, IN CASES WHERE LESION IS NOT OF SERIOUS EXTENT, AS TO EXERCISE, ŒRTEL AND SCHOTT TREATMENTS, CLIMATE, CHOICE OF RESIDENCE, DIET, STIMULANTS—TREATMENT WHERE LESION IS OF MORE SERIOUS NATURE AND HAS GIVEN RISE TO MARKED HYPERTROPHY AND DILATATION OF THE HEART—PRECAUTIONS TO BE TAKEN—SELECTION OF WINTER RESORT—REST IN BED—DIET—STIMULANTS—EMPLOYMENT OF DRUGS—TREATMENT OF VENOUS CONGESTION—VENESECTION—TREATMENT IN AORTIC DISEASE.

THE treatment of valvular disease of the heart has been foreshadowed in the consideration of its prognosis. Whatever influences have been seen to affect unfavourably the condition of the circulation and of the patient, such must be averted or counteracted, and injurious tendencies arising out of the particular lesions of the valves must be combated. The order also in which the therapeutic methods and resources employed for the above ends must be discussed is dictated by the arrangement adopted in the consideration of the prognosis.

One of the most important prophylactic measures is the prevention, as far as possible, of the ill effects on the heart of a recently established valvular lesion. When an attack of endocarditis has subsided, leaving behind it some valvular lesion, the exercise of caution and care will prevent undue cardiac dilatation, which might prove rapidly fatal or cripple the heart seriously in the future.

The patient should be kept in bed, or confined to his room for some weeks, or perhaps even months, according to the degree of severity of the lesion, cases of aortic incompetence requiring the longest period of rest. The object of protracted rest is to allow time for the necessary compensatory hypertrophy of the cardiac walls to take place. In many cases, more especially when pericarditis accompanies the endocarditis, as it frequently does in children, the heart is left dilated and weakened after the subsidence of the attack, so that the risk from premature exertion will be doubly serious, and the period of rest required afterwards will be proportionately longer.

In children, in whom the joint manifestations of rheumatism are usually slight, while the heart is frequently attacked, the heart should be examined from time to time if there is the slightest suspicion of rheumatism, such as fugitive pains in the joints or limbs, with rise of temperature, still more if there are obvious manifestations such as rheumatic nodules; for the onset of pericarditis or endocarditis is often very insidious, and serious mischief may result before it is detected, if the child is allowed to go about as usual.

When the lesion is established, and sufficient rest after the attack of endocarditis has been allowed, the next question to be settled will be, how far the patient may live his ordinary life, or what rules must be laid down for his future conduct, and what precautions should be taken. Everything will of course depend on the nature and the degree of severity of the lesion, and in discussing the treatment the less severe class of cases will be first considered, in which there is no evidence in the shape of marked cardiac dilatation or hypertrophy that the lesion is considerable.

**Exercise.**—Almost the first question will be as to the

rules to be laid down with regard to exercise and exposure to changes of temperature. These will necessarily vary according to the character and seat of the lesion, but not so only—the constitution, strength, habits, and disposition of the patient will also have to be considered. One man is timid and apprehensive; he will scarcely move out of doors lest he should overtax his heart, or eat a sufficient meal for fear of palpitation, or go away for change of air lest he should die away from home. He must be encouraged or even compelled to take exercise. Another is only too ready to ignore the state of his heart, and will run or row or swim or take part in violent games; he must be warned against imprudence, and it may be necessary to forbid such forms of exertion as are liable to be indulged in to excess. In another, an eager temperament and impetuous disposition may reside in a weakly frame, and ordinary duties and an average amount of work may be done with injurious energy and haste. It is not possible, therefore, to draw up definite regulations applicable to all cases. To make the restrictions imposed too severe will in one person directly injure the sufferer's health; in another, will make him unnecessarily depressed and miserable; in a third, will provoke revolt and lead to rash and dangerous violation of all rules. The principle on which recommendations must be based will be to interfere as little as possible with the avocation, habits, and mode of life of the patient, as long as these are not injurious, and especially to allow a maximum of exercise in fresh air compatible with safety.

Nothing can be worse than to debar all patients who are found to have valvular disease from games and vigorous exercise, and to forbid them to go upstairs or to walk uphill, and on no cases do I look back with greater satisfaction than on those, and they have not been few, in which I have liberated boys and girls from such orders. In the class of cases under consideration, supposing a sufficient time to have elapsed after the acute attack in which the valvular affection was established for the necessary compensatory changes to take place, a girl may be allowed to take long walks, to play lawn tennis, to ride, cycle, swim, and dance, and a boy to play cricket and racquets, to hunt, box, and fence, provided that these exercises are not attended with undue breathlessness and distress, and that they are entered upon gradually and practised with moderation and discretion. On the other hand, football, paper-chases, long house-runs, training for races of any kind, are scarcely permissible.

While discussing the question of exercise the Œrtel and Schott methods may be described.

The **Œrtel Treatment** consists in systematic, graduated muscular exercise carried out at a certain elevation, about two thousand feet above sea-level. The patient is required to walk a certain distance up a gentle ascent each day, the distance and pace being gradually increased. At the same time the diet is carefully regulated, and the amount of fluids ingested is strictly limited. The object of the treatment is: firstly, to stimulate the heart by muscular exercise, carefully adjusted to the capacity of the patient, so as to bring about hypertrophy of its walls; secondly, to diminish the volume of blood in circulation by restricting the amount of water consumed, and increasing the amount eliminated. Œrtel claims that this treatment is successful in cases of fatty heart uncomplicated by disease of the coronary arteries, in cardiac dilatation, and in valvular disease, even when compensation has broken down, and dropsy with other evidence of venous congestion is present.

In cases of valvular disease, in which compensation has completely given way, this treatment is certainly not advisable, nor in many instances would it be possible; but where compensation has been established after a recent valvular lesion, or has been restored by rest and suitable treatment, or where it is maintained with some difficulty, gentle climbing exercise in fresh and pure and somewhat rarefied air will certainly do more to develop further compensatory hypertrophy of the heart, than mere walking on the level, which has not the same beneficial effect on the circulation, and where the air is not so pure or invigorating.

It is more especially in cases of fatty infiltration of the heart without fatty degeneration of the cardiac muscle, arising from overeating and drinking and insufficient exercise, that this treatment by dieting and systematic muscular exercise may be of real service. At the commencement of the treatment, great caution should be observed as to the nature and amount of exercise. The patient should only be allowed to walk a certain distance up a gentle slope, and each day the distance may be gradually increased. By this means, and by the limitation of the fluids ingested, the superfluous adipose tissue is gradually got rid of, and the tone of the heart muscle is restored. Not infrequently this treatment is employed as a sequel to the Nauheim methods.

**The Schott Treatment.**—The treatment by baths and exercises by the method of Schott, of Nauheim, may be of service in suitable cases. The waters of Nauheim are remarkably rich in free carbonic acid gas, as well as in mineral constituents, the chief of which are chloride of sodium, and chloride of calcium, and carbonate of iron. At the beginning of the treatment the baths should contain about 1 per cent. of chloride of sodium, and 1 per 1000 of calcium chloride, and should be free from carbonic acid gas. The bath at first should last from six to eight minutes, and should be of the temperature of 92° to 95° Fahr. As time goes on the proportion of solids in the bath should be increased, also the duration of the bath, while the temperature is gradually lowered. Eventually, baths containing free carbonic acid gas, and about 3 per cent. of sodium chloride and 3 per 1000 of calcium chloride, may be taken. Baths can be artificially prepared in imitation of those at Nauheim, the essential ingredients being the chlorides of sodium and calcium and the free carbonic acid gas.

The exercises consist of a series of simple movements of each limb and of the trunk made against slight resistance, so that every muscle of the body, as far as possible, is in turn brought into play. The movements should be made slowly and systematically, and a short interval of rest should be interposed between each; they should be stopped if the patient experiences any distress in breathing or discomfort, but may be proceeded with again as soon as he is rested. The movements consist of flexions, extensions, adductions, abductions, and rotations of each limb in turn, and of flexion, extension, and rotation of the trunk.

The effects produced on the circulation and the heart, whether by the baths or exercises, are similar; the pulse frequency is diminished, its volume and force are increased, and the area of cardiac dulness in cases of cardiac dilatation is diminished, while the apex beat recedes and comes nearer to the normal position.

Such are the immediate results which appear to indicate an improvement in the contractile power of the heart and a reduction of its dilatation; but these are not permanent.

Similar temporary results may, indeed, be obtained in a normal individual as the immediate effect of a simple hot or cold bath without any saline constituents.

Too much importance is attached by advocates of the Schott treatment to the percussing out of the area of cardiac dulness and to the diminution it is said to undergo after each bath, more especially when the so-called auscultatory method is employed. This method lends itself very much to the imagination, and is absolutely untrustworthy. A shifting inwards of the apex beat is of importance, but in cases of dilatation from over-exertion a similar inward movement of the apex may sometimes be effected by making the patient walk rapidly two or three times across the room. It is also probable that the diminution of percussion dulness is due, not so much to fluctuations in the size of the heart as to encroachment by the lungs on the cardiac area, due to deeper respirations taken while the patient is in the bath. **It does not therefore follow that, because the area of cardiac dulness diminishes after a bath, the heart was previously dilated.** Moreover, accurate delineation of the outline of the heart by percussion is in many cases impossible, and even in the mere percussing out of the area of superficial cardiac dulness there may be many difficulties and sources of error in the adult, from the solid nature of the chest walls and the thickness of their coverings, from an emphysematous condition of the lungs, or from pleuro-pericardial adhesions. It is difficult, therefore, to attach any real value to the remarkable diagrams of the cardiac dulness "before" and "after" the bath, published in quantity by the enthusiastic advocates of this treatment, and one is compelled to question their accuracy if not their honesty. Even if they approximate the truth, they are worth nothing if there is not other evidence of improvement in the general condition of the patient and in the symptoms and physical signs of the affection from which he is suffering. The treatment cannot, of course, cure a valvular lesion, but it may give beneficial results in suitable cases. But it is rather in cases of cardiac dilatation from loss of tone after influenza, or some depressing disease, and in cases of functional and neurotic heart disease, than in actual valvular disease, that it is satisfactory. The change of air and scene, the sedative effect of the baths, the enjoined rest after each bath, the quiet, uneventful life, the early hours and regular meals, together with freedom from excitement and worry, and the satisfaction engendered by "taking a cure," will be among the most important factors which contribute to its success in this class of cases.

**Exposure to Change of Temperature.**—As regards exposure to vicissitudes of temperature and to changes of weather, we have to bear in mind that the subjects of valvular disease have, in most cases, already manifested a susceptibility to the effects of cold and wet, or an inherited predisposition to rheumatism. One of the things, therefore, most to be feared and guarded against, is another attack of rheumatism. Flannel or woollen underclothing of some kind should be worn next to the skin winter and summer, and standing or sitting with wet feet or in damp clothes, or lying down on the grass after games, involving the risk of getting chilled after perspiration, must be forbidden. But we must not go to the other extreme and cultivate an undue susceptibility to cold by excessive care. The patient need not be kept indoors by rain or cold, or forbidden to get into a perspiration. Excessive precautions defeat the object for which they were enjoined, and it is easy to reduce the power of resistance to changes of temperature until the slightest exposure is attended with risk. While, however, the primary aim ought to be to maintain and confirm such hardihood as the constitution possesses or is capable of, there are cases in which safety consists in flight from too severe a climate, or from a situation or soil conducive to rheumatism. There is full opportunity for the exercise of judgment in deciding how much may be dared and how soon the patient must yield.

**Climate.**—Climate may do much to influence the course of heart disease. On *a priori* grounds, we should say that a mild, dry, bracing and equable climate, in which the patient could have a maximum of exercise in the open air, would be the best; but, independently of the question where these desiderata are to be found, all such general statements have to be qualified to meet the idiosyncrasies of individuals; the great majority of our patients, moreover, are tied down by circumstances to a particular spot, and the most important practical problem usually is how to make the best of a given neighbourhood.

**Choice of Residence.**—If the choice of a residence is open we should direct the patient to seek a gravelly or sandy soil at a moderate elevation, where the rainfall is below and the sunshine above the average, and the water not hard; conditions best realized—in England—in Kent, Surrey, and Sussex. The exposure of the house should be to the south, and there should be protection from the north and east. The immediately surrounding country should not be too hilly, and especially the house itself should not be on the top of a steep hill, making every walk necessarily end in an ascent. There would be danger, some day or other, of dilatation or other ill effect from the exertion after a longer or more tiring walk than usual or when out of sorts. It must always be borne in mind that the good results obtainable from the best climate may be neutralized by faults of detail in the placing or construction of a house.

**Diet.**—About food little need be said. Excess should be avoided, but, subject to this condition, the diet may be liberal and varied. It is important, however, that there should be a due proportion of farinaceous and vegetable articles of diet; when the food is highly nitrogenized, as when it consists largely of meat, imperfectly oxidized waste accumulates in the blood, and this is a great cause of resistance in the capillary circulation, which constitutes a serious addition to the work imposed upon the heart, and puts a continued strain upon the compensation by which it adjusts itself to the imperfect state of the valves. This recommendation is specially important in the case of constitutions disposed to gout, since the valves may be further damaged by gouty inflammation. Habitual excess of food beyond the requirements of the system will have the same effect.

The food, again, should be divided into three fairly equal meals, and not taken in excessive quantity at dinner, or at breakfast and dinner. If the nourishment for the twenty-four hours is consumed at one huge repast, the blood, in the long interval, is drawn upon for the nutrition of the tissues and for the supply of the secretions and its volume being reduced, the vessels are depleted; the products of digestion are then rapidly absorbed, the amount of blood is increased, and the vascular system is rapidly filled and perhaps overcharged. Wide variations in the volume and pressure of the blood are thus liable to result, and are harmful to the patient.

When its valvular apparatus is unsound, or its structure is impaired, the heart does not easily adjust itself to such extremes, and, if it so far effects this that no particular discomfort is experienced, the increased work thrown upon a weak organ cannot fail to be injurious in the long run. A very large meal, again, must distend the stomach, and the diaphragm may be pushed up and hindered in its action so as to embarrass the heart directly by pressure, and indirectly by interference with respiration. A dilated stomach by upward pressure may so embarrass a heart which is diseased as to give rise to irregularity of rhythm, anginoid pains, and even syncopal attacks, one of which may prove fatal.

**Stimulants.**—Strict moderation must be observed in the matter of alcoholic drinks; in comparatively few cases are they necessary, and if taken they should be taken only as part of a substantial meal. Their effects as excitants of the heart may, to some extent, be neutralized by the relaxation of the peripheral vessels which they induce, but their general tendency is to interfere with due metabolism and elimination, and to bring about degeneration of structure.

Unduly high arterial tension, from whatever cause, must be combated. Its injurious effects have been already pointed out. The regulations as to diet and drink have for one of their objects the prevention of high blood-pressure. When this condition exists from inherited tendency, or from gout or renal disease, it must be kept down within safe limits by suitable eliminants.

**Regulation of Bowels.**—It is always important to take measures against constipation. Accumulation of fæcal matters in the large intestine, with the associated flatulent distension, will more or less embarrass the heart, both by direct pressure upwards of the diaphragm and indirectly by interference with respiratory movements. Palpitation, again, is a frequent result of constipation, and both the effort required to unload the bowel and the different pressure on the abdominal veins before and after a large evacuation put stress upon the heart. A further ill-result is the retention of toxic matters in the blood, which provoke resistance in the capillaries and tend to the production of high tension.

**Anæmia.**—While everything is done to maintain the general health, special precautions must be taken to guard against anæmia. We have seen that it may itself give rise to dilatation of the left ventricle, which is a most serious aggravation of valvular disease. Valvular disease, moreover, tends to deteriorate the blood in so far as it interferes with its free movement through the glands and tissues generally, and to produce anæmia. It does not follow that we are to be always giving iron or other reconstituent tonics, but it is a valid reason for careful choice of residence and for frequent change of air, and for attention to and treatment of the earliest indications of anæmia.

## Treatment in Cases of Severe Valvular Lesion.

When the presence of dilatation and hypertrophy indicate that the damage to the valve has been such as to interfere perceptibly with transmission of the blood through the heart, while the principles with regard to exercise remain the same, some modification in their application will be necessitated. Each form of valvular disease gives rise to a certain kind and degree of interference with the efficient pumping of the blood through the heart, lungs, and system, which tends to the production of results injurious to health, and in the long run dangerous to life. We must not wait for the recognition of such tendencies till they are forced upon our attention by the appearance of symptoms; they can always be foreseen, and they may often be prevented. Again, it must be borne in mind that when valvular disease of any importance, as indicated by changes in the walls and cavities, exists, the heart has to some extent lost the power of responding to sudden calls for variations in the rate or force of the circulation; more than this, its power of recovering itself after disturbance is impaired. The compensation effected by hypertrophy is efficient only for ordinary purposes, or within certain limits more or less restricted. When the muscular pressure on the veins all over the body, which attends vigorous exercise, brings the blood in increased quantity to the right cavities of the heart, it cannot be sent on against the resistance in the pulmonary circulation, which results, as we have seen, from most forms of valvular disease. Even in health there is a period of breathlessness before the right ventricle succeeds in driving the blood through the lungs as fast as it arrives from the system, when we begin to run, and in disease, this breathlessness is more readily provoked and is easily exaggerated to painful dyspnœa; the distended condition of the right ventricle and auricle, which is induced by exertion in health, and which acts as a reservoir for the blood till it can be delivered to the lungs by the increased action of the heart, may already exist in disease, so that the provision for the emergency is already exhausted, and there is no margin left for severe exertion.

While, therefore, we avoid unnecessary and injurious restrictions on exercise, sudden and violent exertions must be forbidden, and it must be understood that anything which gives rise to painful breathlessness is injurious. A patient, however, will often, by beginning gradually, arrive at a rate of walking which attempted at first would have been impossible, and may eventually, by the exercise of similar caution, mount with ease an incline which would otherwise have brought him to a standstill. So long as the equilibrium of the circulation is not disturbed, there is no particular danger in going uphill. The danger arises from the fact that on coming to an ascent, the tendency is to maintain the same pace as on level ground until we are checked by shortness of breath. The sufferer from heart disease cannot afford to do this. What would be a mere fugitive inconvenience to a man in health may be a risk and injury to him. If, however, he will exercise a little foresight and slacken his pace immediately on coming to an incline, he may afterwards gradually increase it again within certain limits and so climb hills. The same conclusions apply to stairs. So long as the subject of a valvular affection can go upstairs quite comfortably, there is no objection to his doing so; and if by ascending them quietly he avoids breathlessness, this need not be forbidden even when symptoms are already manifest. Sometimes he can go up backwards without distress, when to take them step by step in the ordinary way is difficult. But there comes a time when stairs must be avoided as far as possible, and when the patient must be carried up or must live on one floor. This will especially be the case when not mere breathlessness but faintness is produced by slight exertion, and the patient feels giddy or has dimness or temporary loss of vision, or weakness and trembling of the knees after going uphill or upstairs. It is in aortic disease that such symptoms are most likely to be experienced, but they may occur whenever the left ventricle is greatly dilated or is weak from any cause.

**Age.**—In applying any rules for the management of valvular disease of the heart, a great difference will be made between the young and those who have reached or passed middle age. After a certain period of life, varying greatly according to constitution and habits, there is a liability to dilatation of the heart on exertion, and this condition, attended at once by symptoms and leading to a speedy fatal issue, is often brought about by an imprudent effort independently of any pre-existing affection of the valves. The risk of such an event is indefinitely increased when dilatation, attendant on valvular lesion, is already present; or when the tendency thereto has only been neutralized by compensatory hypertrophy. The ventricle is tried by chronic overwork, and the nutrition of the increased amount of muscular tissue in the walls is maintained with difficulty, the heart is consequently more ready to break down under stress. We may, therefore, allow a boy to play cricket, or the young of either sex to play lawn tennis, to boat, or even swim in moderation, provided always that no distress of breathing or tendency to syncope is induced, while a corresponding amount of exertion would be altogether forbidden at middle age.

Under no circumstances, and at no age, must fatigue be carried to the point of exhaustion. There is less chance of recovery from the effects of overtaxed endurance than from those of a brief violent effort.

**Selection of Wintering or Holiday Place.**—In deciding upon a place for temporary change of air for a patient suffering from valvular disease, we must be guided very much by the previous experience of the patient. In some cases a trip by sea will be of the greatest service, but this could be recommended only to good sailors. A winter in Egypt, Algiers, or Rome may be good in others, or, if this is not practicable, a few months on the south coast of England, at places where exercise can be taken without much up and downhill. In summer the seaside is most generally useful; but some people tell us it does not suit them, that it makes them bilious. This is often a mere temporary effect, which quickly passes off, or it may be a result of the constipation, which is common. In all cases constipation must be provided against.

When change of air is recommended, great caution must be exercised in sending patients suffering from heart disease to any considerable height, such as 5000 or 6000 feet. The effects of the reduction of atmospheric pressure cannot be foreseen; palpitation is often set up which is absolutely intractable without removal to a lower level, and this is sometimes difficult. One reason for this may possibly be the expansion of the gases in the stomach and intestines, permitted by the diminution in the atmospheric pressure at high altitudes. Every year people arrive in the Engadine with unsuspected heart disease, which is revealed or perhaps developed by palpitation and dyspnœa, rendering a hasty retreat imperative. On the other hand, in a case in which the absence of dilatation and hypertrophy shows the valvular lesion to be slight and the patient is capable of all ordinary forms of exercise without suffering, high altitudes will usually give rise to no inconvenience or danger.

Moderate heights, say 2000 or 3000 feet, are usually well borne, even when there is decided valvular disease, and graduated exercise at such elevations is systematically employed as a means of improving the tone and vigour of the muscular walls of the heart, and of removing fatty deposit which may have taken place upon its surface and in its substance.

**Complete Rest in Bed.**—Rest is, in many cases, an important part of the treatment, and when the state of the patient demands it, rest in bed is of the greatest service; but one of the questions calling for the greatest exercise of judgment is to decide when absolute rest is necessary. There are circumstances in which a month or six weeks in bed will prolong life for as many years. On the other hand, the disturbance of compensation and the supervention of symptoms often date from some slight injury which has confined the patient to his couch or to the house for a month or two. Even when severe symptoms are present, to insist upon confinement indoors is sometimes to add to the suffering of the last few months of life without adding to its duration. When the onset or exacerbation of symptoms is distinctly attributable to work persisted in from necessity, as in the case of most hospital patients, or from courage and defiance of pain, as we sometimes see; or when the aggravation is due to imprudent exertion or exposure, or to some intercurrent pulmonary complication or other illness, there can be no hesitation in ordering rest. The doubt arises in cases in which the effects of valvular disease are gradually creeping on, and the increasing breathlessness and evening œdema are the direct result of the obstruction to the circulation and of failing compensation. Under such circumstances it is difficult to decide when to interfere. The patient will say he is worse in bed than up, that he cannot lie down, but has to be propped up by pillows; that he cannot and dare not sleep, and that if he drop off into a dose he wakes up in indescribable fright and distress. His attendants, it is true, may tell us that he has had more sleep than he supposes, but all the same the nights are long and miserable, and it is no light matter to condemn a sufferer, who has looked and longed for morning, to a couch which, in his experience, is associated with his worst moments. Not uncommonly, however, after sleepless tossing till early morning, with inability to lie down, quiet sleep may come, and the sufferer may slip down into a comfortable position in which he gets real repose, and sometimes after twenty-four or forty-eight hours in bed, relief is experienced, which reconciles the patient to the confinement. We must be guided by results and by our knowledge of the patient.

A similar difficulty frequently confronts us in advanced stages of heart disease, especially when attended with dropsy. The patient implores us to be allowed to sit up, and in paroxysms of dyspnœa he is compelled to do so and to throw his legs out of bed and let them hang down. It is an unequivocal dictate of experience, not easily accounted for by theory, that the heart in disease is often relieved by an upright posture of the body and a dependent position of the legs. Such is the case, not merely because in dropsy the swollen abdomen and thighs make it impossible to sit well forward in bed when the legs are raised, but because in some way the position facilitates the action of the heart, it may be by taking off the pressure of the abdominal viscera from the diaphragm, or by allowing blood to gravitate from the right auricle into the vena cava inferior and abdominal veins, or it may be in consequence of a physiological diminution of the arterial tension which, according to Dr. Oliver, attends the erect position. There are few medical men of large experience who have not seen instances in which the sufferer has not gone to bed for months, but has slept all this time in an armchair with some support contrived for the head. On the other hand, our results are better when the patient can be kept in bed; there is a better chance of removal of dropsical effusion and of recovery generally in the recumbent position. While, therefore, we do not carry too far our resistance to a patient's entreaties to be allowed to sit up in a chair for a part or the whole of a day, recognizing, also, that a few days or weeks of life may be dearly purchased if it is at the expense of increased suffering, it is our duty sometimes, and especially when there is a chance of recovery from the existing complications, to exercise firmness in keeping the patient in bed in spite of great temporary distress.

There is less uncertainty with regard to exposure to cold, though in an advanced stage the patient often complains of subjective heat, and throws off his coverings, or insists on the window being opened on the coldest day to satisfy his want of air. External cold contracts the arterioles of the surface, and increases the resistance in the systemic circulation, and it should be prevented from reaching the sufferer. The open window, however, may be permitted, on condition that the patient is efficiently protected. The play of cool, fresh air on the face, and a deep draught of it into the lungs, are indescribably refreshing. The cold and livid lower limbs in aggravated dropsy appear to be almost insensible to changes of temperature, but they should none the less be carefully covered.

**Diet.**—Little need be said about nourishment. The patient may have whatever he can eat and digest, but his appetite will leave deficiencies, which must be supplied partly by liquid food of different kinds, and partly of preparations of pounded meat, fish, or chicken.

When **dropsy** is present the use of common salt and of chlorides in general should be restricted as far as possible, for the reasons given in the chapter on dilatation, page 308.

**Stimulants.**—Alcoholic stimulants afford valuable help, and will be required more or less in every case of severity. At first a small quantity of any wine which suits the patient may be taken with food, and frequently a little spirit in hot water at night will help to procure sleep. Ultimately stimulants, especially spirits, may have to be given freely; but great caution must be exercised in the early periods, since the struggle against the encroachments of the malady is often very long and trying, and if the good effects of alcohol are exhausted by abuse of it, the patient is left without resource when the time of greatest need arrives. As to the actual amount required, I should consider about six ounces of brandy per diem the maximum likely to be useful in the most urgent cases. This should be reached very gradually from two or three ounces, and whenever an emergency has led to an increase of the allowance, it should be reduced when the occasion has passed. We must, above all, be careful not to be misled by the patient's demands. He is conscious of relief from the stimulant, and not unnaturally asks for it whenever the oppression or depression becomes severe; but it is easy to pass the limits of usefulness, and to produce a feeling of depression which is only reaction from an excess of alcohol.

In larger quantities than six ounces the effects become uncertain, and I have often seen improvement from diminution of a dose which seemed to be imperatively required.

**Drugs.**—When symptoms have arisen requiring the employment of medicinal treatment, the first question to be considered is whether the heart can be relieved, in any degree, of work to which it is no longer equal. It is very rarely that this is not the case, and not uncommonly a lessening of stress upon the heart is sufficient of itself to restore the circulatory equilibrium. A diminution in the volume of the blood by eliminants of various kinds, removal of portal congestion and of distension of the abdominal veins by purgatives, which will relieve the right side of the heart and lower the arterial tension, are among the measures most generally useful and most commonly required.

The fatal result is reached through various secondary

consequences, the prevention or removal of which postpones the final issue, and not only does this, but also relieves suffering. These consequences, therefore, must be studied, and it will be necessary to revert to the modes of death from valvular disease of the heart and to consider the tendencies thereto which we have to counteract. Leaving out of consideration thrombosis, whether systemic or pulmonary, which will best be averted by the prevention of stagnation of blood in the heart, heart disease tends to the arrest of the circulation in two different ways—by failure of propulsion through the arteries and by damming back in the veins. It is not to be understood that one or other of these tendencies is alone in operation in any given case; the rule is that both are present, as has been already seen. While, however, in most cases of valvular disease which have proceeded so far as to give rise to serious symptoms, the double effect on the circulation—the damming back in the veins and the imperfect propulsion through the arteries —is recognizable, one or other will be a primary tendency, and will predominate, and the treatment must be directed to the rectification of the tendency which is most concerned in placing life in danger. By far the more common is venous stasis, since it not only follows directly from both forms of mitral disease, but may also be a secondary result of aortic disease, and it gives rise to a characteristic train of phenomena. Inadequate arterial supply is of itself more likely to cause sudden death than to produce symptoms.

With venous obstruction the liver will be enlarged and greatly congested, perhaps pulsating, and one of the first objects of treatment is the relief of this engorgement of the liver. Thereby relief will also be afforded to the nausea and sickness dependent on the congested state of the gastro-intestinal mucous membrane, and also to the over-distended right side of the heart, which is constantly receiving from the liver, which acts as a kind of reservoir, more blood than the right ventricle can transmit through the lungs. The means to be employed for the purpose are chiefly aperients, and all purgatives will have the desired effect in a greater or less degree; but it is not a matter of indifference what drugs we employ. The best results are undoubtedly to be obtained, according to my experience, from purgatives, in which calomel or other mercurial preparation is a constituent, such as calomel and compound jalap powder, calomel, blue pill, or grey powder, with colocynth and hyoscyamus, followed or not by salines. Hydragogue cathartics of greater violence may be necessary in some cases, but the effect on the liver and heart is not proportional to the degree of purgation, and the relief of dropsy is not due simply to the amount of liquid carried off by the intestinal surface, but is frequently the effect rather of the diuresis which follows improvement in the circulation. Digitalis is often useless, and appears only to add to the embarrassment of the heart and to produce sickness, until the way has been cleared for its operation by a mercurial purge, and where its good effects on the heart seem to be expended, a fresh start will often follow a calomel and colocynth pill.

A troublesome, watery diarrhœa, which is not unfrequently present, is no contra-indication for purgatives, but, on the other hand, constitutes a distinct call for a decided aperient. It is due to the passive congestion of the gastro-intestinal mucous membrane which results from the obstruction in the portal system, and is relieved by free secretion from the mucous surface and from the liver.

**Venesection.**—But the venous obstruction may reach a point which it is out of the power of purgatives to affect. The lower edge of the liver is at or near the level of the umbilicus (or this organ may be prevented from swelling by cirrhosis), the right cavities of the heart are almost paralyzed by over-distension, which, with regurgitation through the tricuspid orifice, reduces the transmission of blood through the lungs to a minimum, and the left ventricle receiving little blood has little to forward into the arterial system. The pulse is weak, small, irregular, both from the irregular action of the heart usually present, and from some of its beats not reaching the wrist. Unless the circulation is to come to a standstill the right side of the heart must be promptly relieved of the over-distension which is the immediate cause of the threatened arrest, and this can be most quickly and effectually done by venesection. The withdrawal of a few ounces of blood (8-16) so far reduces the pressure in the right auricle and ventricle when the latter is checked at the very beginning of its systole by resistance which it is unable to overcome, that it regains command over its contents, and is once more able to drive the blood through the lungs. Nothing can be more striking or satisfactory than the effect of bleeding from the arm under such conditions. The face may be livid and bedewed with cold sweat, the extremities blue and cold, but as the blood flows warmth and colour will return, the dyspnœa will be relieved, and the pulse will improve. The condition of the right ventricle is of critical importance when venesection appears to be required. If it is weak and degenerated, and unable to take advantage of the relief afforded by the withdrawal of blood, the desired result does not follow. We ought, therefore, for bleeding to be successful, to have a powerful right ventricle impulse heaving the left costal cartilages, and perhaps the lower end of the sternum itself, and felt below the costal margin.

In some cases, where the circulation is so nearly at a standstill that blood will not flow from the vein when opened, a hypodermic injection of ether or strychnia in the præcordial region may cause the blood to start flowing, and save the patient from impending death.

Very frequently, especially in hospital patients, the

Digitalis may sometimes be of great service, but its ffects are not constant, and may be unfavourable, or may ecome so after a period of marked benefit. The reasons r the apparently uncertain and inconstant results of igitalis in aortic incompetence will be discussed in the xt chapter.

desired relief may be obtained by leeches, and I have usually selected the region of the liver for their application, not of course with the idea of taking blood from this organ, but because there is, as a rule, local pain here which is relieved: six or eight may be applied at a time. The abstraction of blood will be followed up by a mercurial purge and digitalis. Brandy and other stimulants may be given at the same time; there is nothing inconsistent in helping the oppressed organ at the same time that it is being relieved from the special difficulty with which it has to contend.

When, as in aortic incompetence, a spasmodic and imperfect supply of blood is the cause likely to lead to arrest of the circulation, there is no such conspicuous train of symptoms. There may be præcordial pain, dyspnœa, syncopal attacks, etc.; but since a momentary failure of the circulation in the vital nerve centres is fatal, sudden death may occur before the warnings of danger have arrested attention. Such warnings are sudden attacks of faintness and dimness of vision, giddiness, anginoid pains, sudden weakness and trembling of the knees.

In this condition, measures suitable for the relief of venous stagnation would be fatal. We cannot resort to bleeding; purgation must be employed with caution. The treatment must rather be directed to stimulation of the failing heart, by drugs such as strychnine, ammonia, and ether, together with good, easily digested, nourishing food, and alcohol regularly administered in small quantities. Vascular dilators, such as nitro-glycerine and nitrite of amyl and sodium nitrite, or perhaps erythrol, or mannitol nitrate, the effects of which are more lasting according to Bradbury, may be of great service in cases in which the incompetence is due to degenerative change and not to endocarditis, especially where anginoid pains are a prominent symptom.

Digitalis may sometimes be of great service, but its effects are not constant, and may be unfavourable, or may become so after a period of marked benefit. The reasons for the apparently uncertain and inconstant results of digitalis in aortic incompetence will be discussed in the next chapter.

# CHAPTER XVIII.

## TREATMENT BY DRUGS.

USE AND ABUSE OF DIGITALIS—SUBSTITUTES FOR DIGITALIS—THE GROUP OF CARDIAC TONICS OF THE DIGITALIS TYPE—THEIR PHYSIOLOGICAL ACTION: THERAPEUTIC EFFECTS—USE OF DIGITALIS IN AORTIC STENOSIS, IN MITRAL INCOMPETENCE, IN MITRAL STENOSIS.

### USE OF DIGITALIS.

IT is too commonly taken for granted that the existence of valvular disease constitutes an immediate indication for the administration of digitalis. But to make the discovery of a murmur the signal for giving digitalis is fatal to anything like precision in treatment, and may deprive the sufferer of the advantage to be derived from this remedy when it is really needed. The special indications for its use are frequency, weakness, and irregularity of pulse, and œdema of the extremities, with scanty, turbid, concentrated urine. When these are absent, it is rarely of service; but even when these symptoms begin to show themselves gradually or occasionally on slight provocation, it will be well to combat them at first with strychnine, iron, quinine, and general tonics, rather than resort at once to digitalis, the salts of potash and any suitable vegetable diuretic being employed to promote secretion of urine. When the use of digitalis is called for, the most trustworthy evidence of its beneficial effects will be increase in the amount of urine secreted, with an improvement in the tone and vigour of the pulse, as well as a more regular and less hurried action of the heart. When there is no response in the form of diuresis, the pulse and general symptoms must be carefully watched lest harmful effects should arise.

Digitalis may be given in combination with nux vomica or strychnia, or with caffein, or with ammonia or ether, or various other drugs, according to circumstances, which cannot be minutely laid down. In most cases it will be advisable to give a mercurial purge before its administration, and to repeat this from time to time.

In cases where there is high arterial tension, the exhibition of a mercurial purgative from time to time is especially important, and it may be well to give with the digitalis some vaso-dilator such as spiritus ætheris nitrosi, liq. trinitrin, erythrol tetranitrate, etc., to counteract the tonic effects of the digitalis on the arterioles and capillaries. As alternatives to digitalis, strophanthus, convallaria, caffein, spartein, cactein have been advocated.

*Convallaria* has been extensively tried, but either its effect or its preparation is uncertain, and it does not appear to be of great service.

*Strophanthus* may be a most useful alternative when digitalis produces sickness, and may even succeed where digitalis has failed. It is claimed for strophanthus that its tonic action is mainly confined to the heart, and that it does not cause contraction of the arterioles and thus increase the peripheral resistance in the same way as digitalis.

*Caffein* is said to increase the solids in the urine, which would make it a useful complement to digitalis, which promotes a flow of water. It is also a cardiac stimulant. In my hands it has often been a most useful accessory to digitalis, diuresis and general improvement setting in promptly on the administration of 5 gr. doses of citrate of caffein three times a day in addition to digitalis, which had failed to produce any decided effect without it. I have not, however, found that caffein alone is an efficient substitute for digitalis.

*Theobromine and diuretin*, the latter of which is a sodio-salicylic compound of theobromine, are powerful diuretics, and have a similar stimulant action on the heart to caffein; they may be used with advantage in cases of cardiac dropsy, and sometimes succeed where caffein fails.

Digitalis and its congeners, which contribute the most important group of cardiac tonics, possess special interest, and merit a separate discussion, since they not only render important service in the treatment of disease, but furnish one of the best illustrations of the relation between physiological and therapeutic action. Digitalis, the best known and longest employed, as well as the most important of them, will be taken as the general representative of the class. Their physiological action will first be briefly mentioned.

## Their Physiological Action.

The physiological action is a stimulation of the muscular fibres of the entire cardio-vascular system, giving rise, on the one hand, to more deliberate and powerful action of the heart, and on the other to tonic contraction of the arterioles and capillaries. After death from the poisonous effect of digitalis, the arterioles are narrowed to an impervious thread, and the ventricles of the heart are found firmly contracted upon themselves, and empty. The drug appears to act directly upon the muscular structures, and not through an intermediate influence upon nerves; we have not, therefore, in considering the effects upon the heart, to discuss the question whether they are produced by inhibition of the sympathetic or stimulation of the vagus.

## Their Therapeutic Action.

There are various ways in which the physiological action thus briefly sketched may come to the aid of the circulation when the transit of blood through the heart is hampered by valvular or other disease. Besides the more complete expulsion of their contents by the energetic contraction of the ventricles, which will help to fill the arterial side of the circulatory system, there will be improved suction action during diastole, which will tend to withdraw from the veins the blood which has been dammed back and remains stagnating in the liver and abdominal venous plexuses. Another effect is that not only are the force and effectiveness of the systole increased, but the general vigour of the heart is renewed, through the increased physiological rest resulting from the relative prolongation of the diastolic period, which gives opportunity for nutritive repair of the cardiac muscular fibres, and for the reaccumulation of energy expended in the systole.

The primary effect of the tonic contraction of the arterioles will be to increase the resistance in the peripheral circulation, thus throwing more work upon the heart; and it is conceivable that the arterio-capillary contraction may, under certain conditions, more than neutralize the increased force of the ventricular systole, as, for example, when the cardiac muscular fibres have undergone serious degeneration, and, as a matter of observation, this is found sometimes to be the case. For the most part, however, the disease, and especially valvular disease, which has given rise to the necessity for cardiac tonics, will have brought about considerable hypertrophy of the muscular walls of the heart without any corresponding hypertrophy of the muscular walls of the vessels. The balance of advantage, therefore, when the contractile energy of both heart and vessels is increased, is largely on the side of the heart, its muscular fibres having greatly increased in number and size.

It might seem, again, that the contraction of the arterioles would more or less intercept the *vis a tergo* in the veins which is already lacking, as is often manifested by the presence of œdema. If, however, we bear in mind that the contraction affects not only the arterioles but the capillaries also, it will be evident that the narrowing of these channels will give rise to increased rapidity of the current of blood within them which will carry to the venules the propulsive force communicated by the heart better than a sluggish and irregular movement through a network of flaccid, dilated and bulging capillaries. This more rapid onward flow of the blood will again favour the taking up of fluid effused into the inter-cellular spaces.

It would seem that the effects just enumerated ought to be of equal service in all forms of heart disease, excepting structural degeneration of the walls, and certainly in all forms of valvular disease. As a matter of observation, however, such is not found to be the case. In one valvular disease, mitral incompetence, all observers agree that digitalis is of the greatest possible service; in another, mitral stenosis, there is almost equal concurrence of opinion that this remedy is not of the same benefit, and, indeed, that it is capable of doing harm and of aggravating the bad effects of the disease. In aortic incompetence opinions are divided, some maintaining that the cardiac tonics in general and digitalis in particular are injurious, others that they are helpful. The same may be said of aortic stenosis.

It appears to me that an explanation of this difference, if it can be arrived at, will make our comprehension of the beneficial effect more clear, and render our employment of these remedies more precise.

The question of the effects of digitalis is often argued

on theoretical grounds; but it must be pointed out that it is upon experience and not upon theoretical considerations that the conclusion just stated as to the difference in its remedial influence is based. Long before the physiological action of digitalis was ascertained, it had been noted that this remedy was not always beneficial in its action, and was sometimes obviously injurious, and much was said by old writers as to intolerance of the drug and especially as to its cumulative effects. When mitral stenosis was not distinguished from incompetence of this valve, the varying effects of digitalis must have been most perplexing, and, indeed, incomprehensible.

**In aortic regurgitation** failure of compensation is manifested in two distinct ways, and there are two different modes of death. In one, the effect is defective propulsion of blood into the arterial system, manifested by faintness, giddiness, and sudden weakness of the legs, sometimes by anginoid pain; death is by syncope; in the other, there is obstructive backworking through the lungs and right heart, giving rise to venous obstruction and dropsy, exactly as in mitral insufficiency. There are, in effect, aortic physical signs with mitral symptoms.

We have in this, it appears to me, an explanation of the different views as to the influence of digitalis in aortic insufficiency. When the tendency indicated by the symptoms is defective propulsion with failure of arterial blood supply to the brain, the effects are uncertain and even doubtful. While sometimes apparently beneficial for a while, a frequent result is the production of irregularity of the pulse with aggravation of the symptoms, and occasionally of vomiting attended with rapidly increasing weakness of the heart's action. Cases are met with, indeed, in which there is grave reason to suspect that it has precipitated a sudden fatal termination.

When, on the other hand, the symptoms are due to

secondary dilatation of the left ventricle not adequately neutralized by hypertrophy, with or without mitral regurgitation, and to the effects of this upon the pulmonary circulation and right ventricle, we have exactly the same opportunity for the beneficial influence of digitalis in reinforcing the right side of the heart, and the same favourable results as in mitral regurgitation. The effects, indeed, are sometimes much more striking, and the removal of dropsical effusion more rapid. I have observed, however, that not uncommonly patients suffering from serious aortic insufficiency, after recovering from the mitral symptoms, die suddenly from failure of the left ventricle, and this whether the digitalis has been continued or left off, and sometimes before the patient has begun to get up and move about.

Aortic stenosis, like aortic incompetence, leads up to a fatal termination in two ways—directly, by limiting the supply of arterial blood, and indirectly, by giving rise to back pressure in the pulmonic and venous circulation, through secondary mitral incompetence. It is only when symptoms arise from the latter that digitalis is useful. In the earlier stages the left ventricle may be injured if stimulated to drive its contents through a narrowed orifice. More relief is often obtained by relaxing the arterioles by means of nitroglycerine, deducting thus the arterio-capillary resistance from the total work with which the heart has to contend.

### Mode of Action of Digitalis in Mitral Regurgitation.

Mitral regurgitation, being the disease in which the action of the cardiac tonics is almost always beneficial, a study of the conditions presented may enable us to arrive at some comprehension of the way in which the good effects are brought about.

What takes place in mitral regurgitation is as follows: The regurgitation into the left auricle dilates this cavity (there may be some hypertrophy of its muscular walls, but no compensatory influence of any consequence is gained thereby) and at the same time drives back the blood which is flowing to the left auricle and ventricle by the pulmonary veins. The obstruction in the pulmonary veins necessarily gives rise to resistance to the onward flow through the capillaries, to overcome which increased pressure is required in the pulmonary artery, and therefore greater driving power on the part of the right ventricle. From this results hypertrophy of the right ventricle, which is the great compensating agency by which the leakage of the mitral valve is more or less perfectly neutralized. If the blood pressure in the pulmonary veins could be maintained at such a point as to be greater than the pressure in the aorta, there would be no reflux into the auricle during the contraction of the ventricle, even were the mitral valve completely destroyed; but, however powerful the action of the right ventricle, this can never be absolutely the case. The walls of the pulmonary capillaries and veins and of the left auricle, are too weak to resist such a distending force, and moreover the suction action of the left ventricle during diastole will always temporarily reduce the pressure in the left auricle.

Another change in the heart resulting from mitral regurgitation must be noticed. This is, a dilatation of the left ventricle, produced by distension of this cavity during the defenceless diastolic period, by the high pressure in the pulmonary veins and left auricle. It involves some consecutive hypertrophy of the ventricular walls.

These familiar and elementary explanations are enumerated in order once more to emphasize the fact that the work of compensation for mitral regurgitation falls upon the right ventricle, and that, when systemic venous stasis and other late effects of mitral regurgitation show themselves, it is because the right ventricle is beaten by the resistance in the pulmonary circuit and can no longer keep up adequate pressure in the left auricle.

Applying now our knowledge of the physiological effects of digitalis, we shall see that the favourable results of its administration are due almost entirely to reinforcement of the right ventricle. On the left side of the heart and in the systemic circulation there will be produced a certain degree of arterio-capillary contraction, with slight increase in the peripheral resistance and in the intermediate arterial tension, and a more deliberate and energetic action of the left ventricle in systole, which makes room for a large volume of blood in diastole, while the elastic rebound at the end of systole exercises a better suction action on the contents of the distended left auricle. The hypertrophy of the ventricular walls, which will more than neutralize the increase of resistance in the peripheral circulation, and the greater capacity of the cavity would, in the absence of regurgitation into the auricle, result in the projection of a larger charge into the arteries at each systole. The effect of this is undoubtedly good, but the regurgitation into the left auricle is a set-off against it, and this will be increased with the increase of resistance in the arterial system. So far, however, as these good effects on the left ventricle and systemic circulation are concerned, they would be much more conspicuous in aortic regurgitation than in mitral regurgitation, since the ventricle is stronger and its capacity larger, and yet we do not find that digitalis is more useful in this affection, but very often the contrary.

Looking now at the effects upon the right side of the heart and the pulmonary circuit, there may or may not be contraction of the arterioles and capillaries in the lungs with increase of resistance. This could, however, in any case only be slight, while the ventricular walls being greatly hypertrophied, increase of vigour in their contraction will at once raise the blood pressure in the entire pulmonary circulation and in the left auricle. Improved pressure in the left auricle, as has been seen, will fill the left ventricle better during diastole, will resist reflux through the mitral orifice in the systole, and so will increase the amount of blood thrown into the aorta.

It is here that the beneficial influence of digitalis really comes in. As has been before stated, the neutralization of the effects of mitral regurgitation is almost entirely the work of the right ventricle, and it is by increasing the efficiency of its compensatory action that digitalis is of service. Additional evidence of this is, on the one hand, the fact that relief of over-distension of the right side of the heart by venesection or leeches and purgation is an important corroborative measure, in many cases absolutely essential to the result, and, on the other hand, that digitalis fails when the right ventricle is seriously degenerated or hampered by pericardial adhesions.

Among the conspicuous favourable results of the administration of digitalis is diminished irregularity of the pulse. This is entirely due to the higher blood pressure in the left auricle, and the more regular supply of blood to the ventricle. Mitral incompetence is the one among the valvular affections which is specially liable to give rise to irregularity of the pulse. This will be understood from the following considerations. The left auricle is exposed to the respiratory variations of pressure which its thin walls resist only imperfectly. When, therefore, these variations are exaggerated, as when the breath is held or when there is dyspnœa from bronchitis or asthma, the amount of blood carried on into the left ventricle will vary, and the pulse will be more or less irregular. During inspiration the negative pressure will tend to keep the auricle dilated, and to prevent it from contracting properly, so that the ventricle will not have a full charge of blood, and its systole will be brief and abortive. During forced expiration the auricle will be compressed, and its contained blood will be forced on into the ventricle, with opposite consequences. In mitral regurgitation a further effect will be that the negative pressure of inspiration will encourage the reflux into the auricle, while the positive pressure of expiration will oppose it. In this way—the ventricle sometimes being imperfectly, at other times perfectly, filled, sometimes sending back more, sometimes less, of its contents into the auricle—we have ample explanation of irregularity of the pulse. Now, the lower the internal blood-pressure in the auricle and pulmonary veins, the greater will be the effect of variations of external pressure, and the higher the pressure within the auricle, the more independent it will be of pressure from without. It will be seen, therefore, how digitalis steadies the action of the heart and renders the pulse more regular.

### Effects of Digitalis in Mitral Stenosis.

If we examine the effects of digitalis in mitral stenosis, we may perhaps see why they are less certainly favourable, and sometimes clearly unfavourable. In an uncomplicated case the left ventricle is neither dilated nor hypertrophied, and the arteries generally are already small and contracted. No obvious advantage can be seen in further contraction of the arterioles, and, in point of fact, the symptoms are somewhat relieved by causing them to dilate. No great improvement in the output of blood, again, is to be gained by more vigorous contraction of the walls of the left ventricle, as they are not specially strong, and the cavity is small. But it would seem that increased vigour in the contraction of the right ventricle should have the same good effect here as in mitral regurgitation, and marked beneficial influence is indeed very commonly observed if it is judiciously administered when the right ventricle is beginning to give way. The conditions, however, are different, and if given in the early stages of mitral stenosis it may do actual harm. In mitral regurgitation the increased amount of blood driven by the right ventricle into the pulmonary artery, by raising the pressure in the pulmonary circulation, antagonizes the reflux into the auricle, so that more blood finds its way into the left ventricle, whereas in mitral stenosis the blood cannot be forced through the constricted mitral orifice beyond a certain rate of speed, and if the right ventricle is stimulated to contract more than is required for this, it encounters an insuperable obstruction, and becomes embarrassed in its action, its energy being uselessly expended. A common result is irregularity in the beats, accompanied by a sense of precordial oppression, and not infrequently the heart-beats are in couples, the first of which alone reaches the wrist, the second having no aortic second sound.

In many cases of advanced mitral stenosis, in which there is fair compensation, the coupled beats can be produced at will by giving digitalis. The second of the two beats is evidently a supplementary systole of the right ventricle: there is a right ventricle impulse felt over the lower left costal cartilages, while the apex beat is scarcely, or not at all, perceptible. At the second of the coupled beats both right ventricle sounds are heard, while the aortic second sound is absent, and if there is a systolic mitral murmur as well as the presystolic, it is audible only with the first of the two beats. When compensation has broken down and there are pulsation of the veins in the neck, œdema of the extremities, and other evidence of secondary tricuspid regurgitation, digitalis may be given, oftentimes with marked benefit, but its effects should be carefully watched, and it should not be persevered with too long if good results do not follow.

# CHAPTER XIX.

## STRUCTURAL CHANGE IN THE HEART.

HYPERTROPHY—CAUSES OF HYPERTROPHY OF THE LEFT VENTRICLE, OF THE RIGHT VENTRICLE—PHYSICAL SIGNS—SYMPTOMS—PROGNOSIS—TREATMENT.

THE muscular walls of the heart are liable to changes of various kinds, some of which constitute diseases which shorten life and give rise to much suffering. Of these structural alterations, some are common—**hypertrophy**, dilatation, fatty degeneration, fibrosis; others rare—cancer, syphilitic gumma, abscess, aneurysm. We shall concern ourselves mainly with those which are comparatively frequent; the others, obscure as well as uncommon, are very seldom recognized during life, and a diagnosis is only made when an exceptionally clear case comes under the notice of an exceptionally acute observer.

Even when the common and familiar affections—hypertrophy, dilatation, and degeneration—only are taken into consideration, we find ourselves on much less secure ground than when dealing with lesions of the valves. The latter we can localize with great confidence; and knowing, partly by experience, partly by the application of mechanical principles, their effects and tendencies, we can, by making out how far such effects are manifest, form an opinion as to the probable course of the symptoms and as to the future of the patient. On examination after death, again, we can understand the connection between the lesion and the symptoms, and can follow the sequence of secondary changes in the heart and vessels which are set up by the original valvular defect. In the case of structural changes, on the contrary, the diagnosis cannot be made with the same precision, and we are often left in some degree in the dark even by a post-mortem examination. In one patient fatty degeneration has apparently proved fatal at so early a stage that the naked-eye characters of the condition are scarcely perceptible, and it is only by the microscope that its existence is definitely established; in another the change has proceeded so far that the fingers sink into the pale greasy walls, and the muscular fibres have almost disappeared, so that it is scarcely conceivable how the heart has been able to impress any movement whatever on the blood, or how life has been sustained through the intermediate stages of disintegration. So with regard to dilatation, there is no fixed relation between the degree of enlargement of the cavities and thinning of the walls found after death and the interference with the circulation observed during life. One man will live for years with a heart which has reached the extreme limits of dilatation, while another succumbs when it is but moderately advanced. If, therefore, we could make out with great exactness the dimensions of the heart, the size of its separate chambers, and the thickness of their respective walls, which is no easy task, we could not on these grounds alone compare one case with another, and decide upon the relative danger.

Many other considerations of extreme importance will come into the estimate—the functional vigour of the muscular walls as well as their thickness, the liability to palpitation, the state of the great and small vessels, the degree of peripheral resistance, the presence or absence of reflex irritation of the heart from gastric or other derangement. The question of prognosis thus becomes extremely complicated, and is beset with uncertainty. An element of chance or luck even comes in—the subject of advanced disease is at the mercy of the slightest accident; many a patient lives for years with a dilated or fatty heart who would be killed by an attack of influenza, or by a powerful emotion, or by tripping over a stone or a mat. A serious obstacle to the attainment of the minute and definite knowledge which alone is of real use in arriving at a sure prognosis in structural disease of the heart, is the fact that a large proportion of the cases occur in private and consulting practice, and comparatively few come under observation in hospital. It is difficult, therefore, to keep such cases in sight and to watch their progress, and seldom possible to obtain a post-mortem examination to confirm the diagnosis.

While, however, the great difficulty of prognosis and diagnosis in structural diseases of the heart is acknowledged, it is of the utmost consequence that such approximation to a forecast of the prospects of life as is possible should be an object of serious endeavour. The cases are numerous, far more numerous at and after middle age than those of valvular disease, and everything which has been said as to the importance of prognosis in general applies here. An early recognition of these changes, indeed, is often of greater service to the subject of them than in the case of valvular affections, since it reveals also the tendencies which are in operation, and often at a time when they can be successfully combated by treatment.

Too commonly, however, no attempt is made to recognize the existence and extent of degeneration or dilatation. The symptoms due to derangement of the circulation force themselves upon the attention of the medical man, but no murmur being detected, the only diagnosis ventured upon is that of "weak heart," a vague term which covers the entire ground, from temporary functional debility to disease inevitably and imminently fatal. Such a diagnosis reacts unfavourably upon the mind of the observer who rests upon it, and makes him less exact and trustworthy, while it may be full of danger to the patient.

These considerations alone would justify an attempt to render the prognosis of structural diseases of the heart more definite, but a study of these affections from the point of view of prognosis also leads to closer observation, and to the recognition of the importance of details which do not force themselves upon the attention so long as diagnosis in the ordinary and limited sense of the word only is the object.

A further justification of the prominence given to prognosis is that the grasp of all the facts of the disease and of the individual case, which is necessary to the formation of a just forecast of the result, is the best guide for treatment, whether this may demand chiefly patience and caution, or must be energetic and prompt. Prognosis is not merely a well-instructed conjecture as to the ultimate issue, it is a deliberate judgment as to the processes and tendencies of the disease, and as to the constitutional soundness and strength of the patient. The foresight relates to the dangers which attend the attack, to the course it will run, and to the influences and contingencies which make for or against the sufferer. To this there has only to be added a knowledge of the therapeutic measures by which the tendency to death or structural injury can be antagonized, and by which the patient can be guided and helped, together with skill, courage, and promptitude in applying it, and we have all the requisites for successful treatment.

Treatment, therefore, will form a natural sequel and corollary to prognosis.

## HYPERTROPHY.

This condition of the heart will not detain us long. The prognosis of cardiac hypertrophy, like the symptoms, is that of its cause, and the character and degree of hypertrophy are important, not so much in themselves or on account of danger likely to arise out of them, but as indicating the existence of some condition which has given rise to the increase in thickness and contractile power of the muscular walls of the heart, and which is serious, possibly, in proportion to the hypertrophy which it has provoked.

### Causes of Hypertrophy of the Left Ventricle.

The causes which give rise to hypertrophy must be enumerated. The left or right ventricle may be affected alone or predominantly, or both may have undergone change. The causes which bring about hypertrophy of the left ventricle are, in the first place, valvular diseases, stenosis, or insufficiency of the aortic valve, or mitral insufficiency. With these we are not now concerned, as they have been fully discussed in the chapters on the respective valvular lesions. Next in frequency will be protracted high arterial tension. When high pressure in the systemic arteries is recognized, and especially when there are evidences of its having been habitual for some time, such as large, thickened, tortuous, radial and temporal arteries, or a dilated ascending aorta, the underlying condition to which it is due must be identified. The causes of high arterial tension and the mechanism of its production have been dealt with in Chapter II., so they will only be briefly enumerated here. They are renal disease, gout, diabetes, lead poisoning, excessive nitrogenous diet, constipation, alcohol, tobacco, and, above all, a hereditary predisposition.

Left ventricle hypertrophy, again, may in rare instances

have no other assignable origin than adherent pericardium, a condition which is difficult to diagnose, and with regard to which prognosis is, as a rule, unfavourable if the heart is much enlarged.

If hypertrophy is at any time produced by a mode of life entailing sustained muscular exertion, it is physiological and not pathological, and has no claims on our attention; unless, indeed, the initial change has been dilatation caused by violent and sustained effort, such as racing, the hypertrophy being secondary to this; but even here it is the dilatation and not the compensatory process which has to be considered.

### Causes of Hypertrophy of the Right Ventricle.

Hypertrophy of the right ventricle, as of the left, has its most common cause in valvular disease—in this instance chiefly mitral stenosis or insufficiency;—and after valvular disease, in conditions which give rise to obstruction in the pulmonary circulation.

Emphysema and bronchitis are the lung affections which most frequently give rise to hypertrophy of the right ventricle, but the hypertrophy is rarely dissociated from dilatation, which is the primary effect of the obstruction in the pulmonary capillaries. Collapse of a portion of the lungs, contraction of a lung from pleural adhesions, fibroid phthisis, or any condition which throws a considerable area of lung surface out of gear, will to a certain degree give rise to overwork and consequent hypertrophy of the right ventricle.

### Hypertrophy of the Left Ventricle. Physical Signs.

**The Pulse.**—The pulse will be that of the condition which has given rise to the hypertrophy. When this has been high arterial tension due to renal disease, gout, lead poisoning, pregnancy, etc., the character of the pulse will be as follows: The artery will be full between the beats, will not be easily flattened under the fingers, and can be followed some distance up the forearm like a cord. The pulse wave will not have a violent ictus, but will rise gradually and subside slowly, and as it makes little impression on the fingers it is sometimes described as weak, but when the attempt is made to arrest the wave very firm pressure is required. When the cause of the hypertrophy has been valvular disease, the character of the pulse will be as described in the chapters on the particular lesion.

**The Heart.**—On inspection, there may or may not be recognizable bulging over the cardiac area; the impulse is not extensive or violent in uncomplicated cases; the apex beat, if visible, is seen below the normal point, frequently in the sixth, sometimes even in the seventh, space, and is probably also displaced somewhat outwards; it is a circumscribed gentle heave. Occasionally one or more of the intercostal spaces above and to the inner side of the apex line may be seen to be retracted, but this is very rare, and is never so well marked in hypertrophy without valvular disease as it may be seen in aortic regurgitation.

By palpation, which is always an extremely important part of the physical examination of the heart, the apex beat is further defined, and is felt as a powerful but deliberate thrust in the space, sometimes distinctly lifting the adjacent ribs. The more the fingers are pressed into the space, the more distinctly is the thrust recognized. When the flat of the hand is laid over the cardiac region, a general heaving impulse can usually be felt, but when the left ventricle is alone or mainly affected, it is not very conspicuous. As a rule, no impulse is felt to the right of the sternum except when the aorta is dilated, in which case pulsation may be felt when the fingers are thrust into the second and third spaces near the sternum. It must be added that sometimes neither apex beat nor impulse can be seen or felt when the hypertrophy is considerable. Mostly this is in deep-chested individuals with large, overlapping lungs, but occasionally hypertrophic enlargement takes a direction which carries the heart away from the chest wall.

**Percussion** maps out more or less accurately the enlargement of the heart downwards and to the left. This demarcation should be done with extreme care, but it must not be taken for granted that the outline drawn on the surface corresponds exactly with that of the organ, or gives a trustworthy idea of its size. To say nothing of the difficulty of defining deep dulness, the heart may enlarge backwards instead of laterally. The results of percussion must be correlated with all the other evidence as to the size of the heart.

**Auscultation**, besides teaching the character and intensity of the sounds, must be made to contribute to the information on this point by careful noting of the seat of maximum intensity of the sounds in the apex region.

The left ventricle first sound as heard at the apex is longer and of lower pitch than in a normal state of the heart; either the mass of muscle enters into contraction more slowly, and the muscular tension being less sudden yields a duller sound, or the thickness of the walls masks the sound produced by the sudden tension of the valves and tendinous cords. The aortic second sound, heard at the apex, is usually louder than normal, and is often heard at or near the apex more distinctly even than in the right second space.

The systole is usually somewhat prolonged. The first sound may be reduplicated, due to the two first sounds, produced by the right and left ventricles respectively, not coinciding. This indicates that the left ventricle is no longer quite equal to the extra work imposed upon it, and marks the supervention of a tendency to dilatation.

At the base of the heart the left ventricle first sound is less distinct than at the apex, and is frequently inaudible, while the accentuation of the second sound is rendered more evident by the absence of the first. When this sound is not only accentuated but low-pitched and ringing, it indicates that the root of the aorta is more or less dilated, and the sound will be heard for some distance to the right of the edge of the sternum.

The sounds of the right ventricle undergo no modification of sufficient importance to require notice.

## Symptoms.

Various symptoms are described as resulting from hypertrophy of the heart—discomfort from the violence of the impulse, or actual pain in the region of the heart, tenderness on pressure in the neighbourhood of the apex, throbbing sensations in the head and neck, pulsatile noises in the ears, or audible pulsation in the carotid and other arteries. The action of the heart may be unduly frequent, or too easily excited, or abrupt and irritable, or irregular with falterings and bounds, which are very disturbing to the subject, and the heart may be prone to palpitation. There may be a sense of respiratory oppression, with sighing and desire to fill the chest with air.

Some of the symptoms are simply the result of the size of the heart and of the vehemence of its beat; others are due, not to the hypertrophy itself, but to its cause, whether in the valves or in the vessels, or to external influences which have given rise to it; others, again, are common to various affections of the heart, functional or organic, besides hypertrophy. They have no such direct or definite bearing on prognosis as would warrant a discussion of their significance, though a sustained frequency of the pulse is an unfavourable sign.

## Prognosis.

The question of prognosis in relation to hypertrophy mostly resolves itself into this: whether the compensation which it establishes is adequate and efficient, and how far it promises to be durable. The danger that the hypertrophy may go beyond the requirements of the occasion which has called for it does not, in my opinion, need consideration.

Compensation is efficient when there are no symptoms of embarrassment of the circulation, and when the heart responds to all ordinary calls upon it without undue shortness of breath or respiratory distress. The effects of exertion are an important criterion, due allowance being made for the greater liability to breathlessness which is natural to some individuals, or is produced by bodily conformation or which results from a sedentary mode of life.

But the sounds of the heart usually give notice when it is overtaxed by the resistance to the onward movement of the blood. The interval between the first and second sound may be prolonged, the systole requiring more time than under ordinary circumstances to complete itself. So long as the normal proportion between the systolic and diastolic pauses is not disturbed, there is no indication that the heart is unequal to its work or is suffering from the stress put upon it: but when the systolic interval between the first and second sounds is lengthened at the expense of the diastolic, so that the sounds are equidistant, the period of repose and reconstitution of the muscular fibres of the ventricle is shortened, and their nutrition must in time suffer. During systole the blood is squeezed out of the walls of the heart, and it is during the diastolic relaxation that it obtains free access to the cardiac fibres.

Another evidence that the heart is yielding to the strain of overwork is reduplication of the first sound. That is, as has been already said, due to want of synchronism between the two ventricles in the act of contraction, or rather in arriving at that point in their contraction when their valves and tendinous cords and muscular walls are all made tense. This reduplication is at first very slight, the two sounds are separated by the briefest possible interval, and are distinct one from the other only at one spot, just to the inner side of the apex; elsewhere there is only a slurring or prolongation of the first sound. Later the sounds of the right and left ventricles are quite distinct, and the duplex first sound is recognized over a considerable area, usually in the direction of the ensiform cartilage, but sometimes upwards. One variety of the cantering rhythm or *bruit de galop* is produced by this doubling of the first sound, where the successive sounds are one-one, two. Sometimes the dislocation of the ventricular first sound is so considerable that it is a task of extreme difficulty to identify the sounds of the heart at all, and associate them with the systole or diastole respectively so as to say which is first and which second. The most striking and confusing examples are met with in aortic stenosis and pericarditis. The prognosis becomes serious when the first sound is broken up in any considerable degree.

But when the cardiac hypertrophy has been brought about by high arterial tension, whether associated with renal disease, or lead poisoning, or other cause, there must be taken into consideration the possibility that the powerful heart may rupture diseased vessels in the brain, and if the arteries are conspicuously degenerated it is better for the patient that the heart also should undergo some degree of degeneration; and sometimes this takes place, so that the patient escapes cerebral hæmorrhage, and lives longer, though he succumbs in the end to cardiac failure.

## TREATMENT.

Treatment for hypertrophy, as such, appears to be out of place. The functional vigour and energy of the overgrown and overstrong heart could no doubt be reduced by various means—low diet, enforced rest, and such drugs as aconite—but unless it is clear that the hypertrophy has gone beyond the requirements of the condition which has given rise to it, the advantage of this procedure would be more than doubtful. Even in the attempt to relieve the incidents of hypertrophy, palpitation, throbbing sensations in the chest, præcordial oppression, the employment of direct cardiac depressants is rarely of service, and is at times attended with danger. In aortic stenosis, for example, I have known aconite, given with a view of quieting tumultuous action of the heart, so far reduce the contractile energy of the left ventricle that it was no longer able to cope with the obstruction, and death quickly followed from cardiac asthenia, the pulse becoming imperceptible, the extremities livid, and the surface of the body cold and damp. This would be less likely to occur where the cause of the hypertrophy was obstruction in the peripheral circulation, as the arteries and capillaries are relaxed by such agents as depress the action of the heart.

The treatment of the chief causes of hypertrophy, aortic disease and high arterial tension, have already been discussed elsewhere, so that what we have to consider here is not the treatment of hypertrophy or its causes, but treatment suggested by the hypertrophy. We shall recognize, for example, the necessity of diminishing the volume and improving the quality of the blood by appropriate diet and hygiene, and, if necessary, by tonics. We shall recognize, also, the desirability of diminishing the resistance to the onward movement of the blood in the arterio-capillary network by care in diet again, by aperients, and by eliminants of various kinds. In some cases, the resistance in the peripheral circulation may be further lessened with advantage by the physiological relaxants of the arterioles and capillaries, such as nitroglycerine and the nitrites. By these means the work thrown upon the heart is reduced, and, if necessary, the heart may be strengthened by such remedies as strychnine and digitalis.

All these measures are specially required when the hypertrophy is no longer quite equal to the task which it had originally been developed to perform, and reduplication and other modifications of the sounds are present. It is now that the incidents of hypertrophy, palpitation and the like, are most commonly complained of, and they will be best alleviated or removed by the measures just sketched, by relieving the heart of work on the one hand, and by helping it on the other.

# CHAPTER XX.

## DILATATION.

**ETIOLOGY—VALVULAR DISEASE, EXERTION, STRAIN, RENAL DISEASE, ACUTE BACTERIAL INFECTIONS—PHYSICAL SIGNS—SYMPTOMS—PROGNOSIS—TREATMENT.**

THE word "dilatation" requires no explanation as applied to the cavities of the heart. Individual cavities may be dilated, as, for example, the left auricle in mitral stenosis or regurgitation, the right ventricle in pulmonary emphysema or mitral disease; but when spoken of as a form of heart disease, dilatation usually means dilatation of the left ventricle, mostly with, but sometimes without, dilatation of the right ventricle. Together with the expansion of the cavity of the ventricle there may be more or less thickening of its walls, representing an attempt at hypertrophy, compensatory of the dilatation itself, or of the difficulty in the circulation which has led to it. The walls of the heart may have an approximately normal thickness, which will really imply a certain degree of hypertrophy, or they may be distinctly thinned. The parietes may have a normal colour, consistence, and structure, or they may be pale, flabby, and degenerated, or dense and tough from fibroid substitution. But even more important than the anatomical condition is the physiological or functional condition, the special characteristic of which is that the ventricle does not complete its systole, but only expels a portion of its contents.

Dilatation of the heart may be contrasted with hypertrophy rather than compared with it. Hypertrophy is compensatory and an evidence of vigour; dilatation is, for the most part, a confession of failure on the part of the heart muscle and an aggravation of other causes of interference with the circulation which may be in operation. In hypertrophy the augmented mass and increased strength of the muscular walls enable the ventricles to complete their contraction in the face of difficulty. The result of dilatation is that the ventricles habitually fail to expel the whole of their contents. Very frequently it is only a very small proportion of the blood which is projected into the great arteries. In well-marked cases the chambers of the heart are always full, and little blood being received and expelled, there is a stagnation in the auricles and ventricles. It has seemed to me that the imperfect emptying of the ventricles has not always been fully realized as the special feature of dilatation, but it will be seen that if a dilated ventricle launched the whole of its contents into the arterial circulation, the amount being much larger, the rate of movement of blood would be greatly accelerated, whereas the contrary is the case.

A distinction must be drawn between the dilatation due to inherent weakness of the muscular walls of the heart and that attending valvular disease.

## Etiology.

**Valvular Disease.**—The dilatation attending aortic regurgitation belongs to a different category from primary dilatation, as has already been shown, and, instead of aggravating the difficulties of the circulation, it is a part of the compensatory arrangement. It is clear that if a certain proportion of the blood projected into the aorta at each systole returns to the ventricle during diastole, it is an advantage, and indeed a necessity, that the capacity of the ventricle should be increased, so that, in spite of the reflux, a normal amount of blood may remain in the arteries and be distributed to the tissues. The dilatation, however, in aortic regurgitation is accompanied by hypertrophy which enables the ventricle to contract perfectly, so that the characteristic of dilatation—the partial and imperfect emptying of the ventricle—is not present.

It is probable, again, that the dilatation of the left ventricle met with in mitral regurgitation may have a similar compensatory effect. It would seem to be an advantage, since some of the blood regurgitates into the auricle, that the ventricle should contain sufficient to allow for this, and yet discharge a due amount into the aorta. In dilatation consecutive to mitral regurgitation, moreover, there is a certain degree of hypertrophy, and the systole is carried through. The dilatation of mitral regurgitation stands, then, on a totally different footing from primary dilatation.

The mode of production of dilatation of the heart is highly complex; it is usually understood to be the result of a gradual yielding of the walls of the ventricles, either from their own inherent weakness or from undue resistance to the onward course of the blood. It is often supposed also, when dilatation exists, that it is an established and more or less unvarying or progressive condition. Both these ideas require modification.

**Exertion.**—All violent or protracted exertion is attended with temporary dilatation of the heart, which may go so far, even in strong and healthy persons, as to give rise to temporary murmurs. Loud murmurs so produced may be heard at the apex, over the tricuspid area and over the pulmonic area, in individuals who have no evidence of cardiac weakness at the time, and who develop no valvular or other cardiac disease for many years afterwards. A personal friend always had a loud, systolic, pulmonic murmur after hunting, which sometimes, when there had been a severe run, lasted two or three days. It is, again, not very uncommon for young and strong men to return from climbing in Switzerland with more or less dilatation of the heart, which may persist for weeks. This is usually when little exercise has been taken during the year, and considerable ascents or very long walking excursions have been made without sufficient preliminary training. Boat-races no doubt give rise to temporary dilatation, and it may be met with as a result of training for races. It might, perhaps, be better to speak of distension of the cavities of the heart in these instances, rather than of dilatation.

In violent exercise the pulse in becoming extremely frequent also becomes extremely soft and short; the arterioles and capillaries are relaxed in order to facilitate the rapid movement of the blood which is necessary to supply fuel and oxygen to the muscles during exertion, and the arterial tension is low. The resistance to be overcome by the ventricles is thus reduced to a minimum, which diminishes the liability to over-distension.

But the circumstances which are capable of producing a temporary distension of the ventricles in a sound and vigorous state of the organ will be competent to give rise to dilatation when it is weak and flabby, and when other conditions are present which tend to dilatation, and it is more likely that the weakly ventricles give way from time to time under stress and fail to recover perfectly, than that the yielding is gradual and continuous.

**Overstrain and Degenerative Change.**—Acute dilatation of the heart is more common than is generally supposed.

In a very large proportion of the cases admitted into hospital suffering from symptoms due to cardiac dilatation, there has been an acute aggravation of the affection from work or exposure, and under treatment a considerable diminution in the size and capacity of the heart is commonly observed. But cases occur in which there is ground for supposing that dilatation has been induced at once in a heart not previously affected. The following are examples selected as illustrations.

A gentleman at the age of 70, in vigorous health and capable of any ordinary amount of exercise, overtook a labourer pushing a heavily laden wheelbarrow uphill, who had to stop and rest every few yards. Proud of his strength, he told the man to stand aside, and himself wheeled the barrow for some distance at a good pace. He lost his breath and found that he did not recover it as he expected, but that he continued to pant and to be conscious of violent action of the heart, accompanied by a sense of oppression in the chest. He got home with difficulty, the least exertion was attended with shortness of breath, and he could not rest at night. After a few days he sent for his medical man, when the physical signs of dilatation of the heart were found to be present. Mitral insufficiency was quickly established, and when I saw him considerable dropsy existed. He died shortly afterwards.

A gentleman, aged about 55, remarkably strong and active, who was said to have had a slight attack of pleurisy shortly before, ran quickly up a long flight of stairs in the City. On arriving at the top he was found gasping for breath, unable to speak and scarcely able to stand. He was soon sufficiently recovered to be sent home, and a few days later he was brought by his medical attendant to my consulting-room, chiefly in order that I might aid in enforcing the rest and care which were considered necessary. The patient admitted that he was weak and soon out of breath, but declared that he was quite equal to business. The pulse was irregular in force and frequency, the apex beat of the heart diffuse, devoid of the impulse or thrust, and displaced downwards to the sixth space and outwards beyond the nipple line, and the other physical signs of a considerable degree of dilatation were present. With great reluctance a certain amount of rest and treatment was submitted to, and the heart and pulse became stronger and steadier, and the apex beat came in towards its normal situation about an inch.

Two months later the patient ran down from a committee-room in the House of Commons for a bag of papers which he had forgotten, and back again. An attack of the same kind as that just described came on, and this time lasted longer. The evidences of dilatation of the left ventricle were more marked, and œdema of the ankles soon came on. The patient was kept in his room, and as far as practicable at rest in bed or on a couch. Improvement was again obtained, but much more slowly than before, and as my visits were the chief restraint upon him, after a brief attendance at short intervals, further consultations were put off indefinitely.

Within a few days the exertion of going downstairs and a serious imprudence in diet brought on a return of symptoms, and the œdema of the lower extremities was shortly complicated by thrombosis of the deep femoral vein of the left side, which extended along the iliac vein to the vena cava and down the right iliac and femoral veins. A tedious illness followed, which finally proved fatal by extension of the thrombosis to the renal veins, the heart itself appearing to improve somewhat.

Another case was that of a boy who was admitted into St. Mary's Hospital with extreme dilatation of both ventricles. He had had no previous illness, but had been underfed. Most Londoners will be familiar with the appearance of lads in the scanty attire of the cinder-path, who are making use of the streets as a training-ground for races, usually in the dusk of the evening, after working hours; perhaps, also, this time is chosen to avoid police interference. I have myself often been astonished at the pace and endurance of these athletes-under-difficulties. The patient had been training in this way, and had persevered in spite of shortness of breath, till severe symptoms set in. He died soon after admission, and the ventricles were found to be enormously dilated.

**Renal Disease.**—A certain degree of dilatation of the left ventricle usually occurs at the onset of acute renal disease, under the combined influence of the resistance in the peripheral circulation and of the enfeeblement of the heart.

It is very striking in watching the course of a case of what is commonly termed "large white kidney," in which the patient survives the dropsical stage and the kidney tends to approximate that of the "contracted granular." At the outset the heart is greatly dilated, the apex beat is not palpable, and the first sound is short and feeble. The pulse is only of moderate tension, as there is little force in the cardiac systole. After the lapse of about six months the dropsy may all subside, and the pulse will then be found to be one of higher tension with the vessel in a state of hypertonus. The heart will have, to a great extent, recovered from its dilatation, and will have undergone very marked hypertrophy, and the apex beat will be easily felt and forcible. The patient will then be liable to die from uræmic convulsions as in chronic interstitial nephritis.

In cases which are from the outset of the type of "granular kidney," associated with very high arterial tension, dilatation of the heart is seldom met with, though the hypertrophy of the left ventricle is often enormous. This is what one would expect, as here the increase of the peripheral resistance and of the strain on the heart is gradual, so that the heart has time to hypertrophy, to cope with the extra work thrown on it, whereas in acute nephritis a severe strain is suddenly put upon it which it is unable to meet, and thus dilatation of the left ventricle occurs.

**Acute Bacterial Infections.**—In acute rheumatism and chorea there is usually a certain degree of cardiac dilatation, which is often extreme in cases of acute pericarditis. Attention has been called to this in the chapter on pericarditis, so it will not be further discussed here. In pneumonia the right ventricle is especially liable to become dilated under the combined effects of the extra strain thrown on it by the obstruction to the flow of blood through the lungs and the damage to the cardiac muscle by the action of the bacterial toxins.

Influenza is a common cause of cardiac dilatation which is liable to be overlooked and to be a source of trouble after the acute illness has subsided, as the patient is apt to go about and resume his ordinary avocations too soon after the attack, and increase or perpetuate the dilatation.

Undue exertion at an early period after any acute bacterial infection, *e.g.* enteric fever, is liable to induce cardiac dilatation, as the heart muscle will have suffered a varying degree of injury from the toxins evolved by the micro-organisms, and will not be able to stand any extra strain, even if it has not given out during the illness itself.

**Psychological Influences.**—Another cause of dilatation of the heart is anxiety. The influence of prolonged mental depression upon the heart, as experienced by the sensation of aching, oppression, and weight which attends grief and anxiety, which were considered to point to the heart as the seat of emotion generally, is indicative of an injurious effect upon this organ. The combination of overwork, excitement, worry, and trouble, often met with in City life, especially on the Stock Exchange or in mercantile or financial circles during a commercial or financial crisis, is responsible for many cases of cardiac dilatation among men, and domestic anxieties—grief on account of children who have died or given trouble, etc.,—may have the same effect among women.

**Injudicious Régime.**—Among the special causes of dilatation of the heart—acting, no doubt, on pre-existing tendencies—which have come under my notice, are injudicious hydropathic treatment, the so-called Banting method of reducing obesity, and inhalation of the fumes of Himrod's powder for the relief of asthma.

In one case a gentleman suffering from dyspeptic symptoms, probably due to cardiac weakness and consequent sluggish circulation in the abdominal viscera, underwent a routine treatment by baths, wet cold packs, and compresses, under which attacks of dyspnœa came on and œdema set in. He had previously been under the care of competent observers, who had not found any serious degree of dilatation. The dropsy advanced in spite of treatment, and when I saw the patient it was considerable, and the physical signs gave evidence of extreme dilatation and thinning of the left ventricle. Death occurred suddenly during a paroxysm of dyspnœa.

Another patient came straight to my consulting-room from a hydropathic institution, where he had undergone vigorous treatment for digestive and liver derangements, attributed to long residence in India. He was very anæmic, and breathless; the heart was greatly dilated and its action irregular, and there was incipient œdema. Fortunately he recovered.

One of the most extreme cases of dilatation I have ever met with was in the case of a lady who had undergone an amateur course of Banting treatment for obesity. She had lost some of her fat, but had become extremely breathless, so that to walk across a room or put on an article of clothing with the assistance of her maid caused her to pant and gasp for breath in a very painful way. The pulse was weak, small, and very irregular; no impulse or apex beat could be felt, and the size of the heart, as mapped out according to the deep dulness, was incredibly large, had not the results of percussion been confirmed by the sounds being audible over the entire area of dulness, and, later, by a feeble apex beat in the seventh space near the mid-axillary line. Apparently habitual high arterial tension had been exaggerated by an exclusively nitrogenous diet, and, under it, the ventricle had given way.

It may, perhaps, be well to add that in the treatment of obesity by beefsteak and copious draughts of hot water there has not been, according to my experience, increase of arterial tension, but the reverse.

The following case is the most serious of several attributable to Himrod's powder:—

In December, 1883, I saw, with Dr. Andrews, of Hampstead, a gentleman, aged about thirty-six, apparently of sturdy constitution, who, after an attack of bronchitis, suffered from severe nocturnal attacks of asthmatic dyspnœa. A month at Hastings had apparently restored his health; but, after a fortnight of work in London, his nocturnal asthma and shortness of breath were as bad as ever. For the asthmatic attacks he had inhaled immoderately the fumes of Himrod's powder, obtaining relief for the time, but with disastrous after-effects. The whole house was reeking with the odour of the fumes at the time of our consultation. Dr. Andrews had witnessed the rapid development of the condition of the heart which existed. The area of cardiac dulness was greatly increased; no apex beat was recognizable; there was a doubtful systolic murmur (mitral) in the region of the apex, a loud systolic murmur (tricuspid) near the ensiform cartilage, and a faint systolic aortic murmur. Tricuspid incompetence was further distinctly manifested by great enlargement of the liver, and by marked jugular pulsation. There was nothing in the patient's habits, or mode of life, or previous history which was at all calculated to give rise to dilatation of the heart, and I had the less hesitation in attributing it to the solanaceous fumes, from having seen similar effects in other cases. In about a fortnight, after free purgation by calomel and the administration of digitalis, the patient was much better, free from asthma, and able to walk upstairs, while the liver had gone down to its usual size. The heart remained very large, gave no defined apex beat and only a diffuse general impulse, while a high-pitched mitral murmur, a louder tricuspid murmur of low pitch, and a faint aortic murmur, all systolic, were audible. The action of the heart was curious; now and then there was a sudden bump against the palm of the hand placed over the right ventricle, and it was found that the beats of the heart were in pairs, only the first of which was accompanied by a systolic apex murmur, the second having a loud first and second sound, but scarcely reaching the pulse. With both beats the loud tricuspid murmur was present. The improvement continued, so that the patient resumed his duties before the end of January, and attended regularly to business through the month of February. In March came another relapse which led to dropsy, and the patient died early in April. Fortunately an examination of the body was permitted, notes of which are as follows:—

There was much œdema of the legs and right arm, but no fluid in the abdomen. The heart was enormous, measuring six inches and a half from base to apex, and sixteen and a half in circumference. It was flabby, pale, fatty looking, not lacerable. The right auricle was greatly dilated and very thin, the wall being translucent at one part; the appendix was filled up by solid clot and stained black by blood. The tricuspid orifice took four fingers easily; there was no roughness. The right ventricle was enormously dilated, and would almost have held a duck's egg; the walls were thin, soft, and flabby, the valve stained black; the flaps were thin and the cords delicate. The pulmonary artery and valves were normal. The left auricle was not at all dilated, the appendix contrasting with the right, and compared with the other cavities curiously small. The mitral orifice would admit two fingers. The left ventricle, like the right, was enormously dilated, and looked as if it would hold a fist: the walls were thin, mottled, and flabby, but not lacerable; the papillary muscles were small, the mitral valve and cords quite normal, and remarkably free from thickening. The aorta was very small and the valves normal.

## Physical Signs.

The pulse in advanced dilatation of the heart is usually irregular in rhythm and unequal in force of beat, and is sudden, short, unsustained, and usually easily compressed. The artery at the wrist may be large or small; it will be specially large when there has been antecedent high tension which has dilated the arteries. The significance of a pulse of this character is not absolute, as all these characters may be present when there is no recognizable change in the walls, cavities, or valves of the heart, apparently from disordered nervous influence only. The pulse, again, need not be irregular in advanced dilatation of the heart so long as the patient is in repose and the breathing is tranquil and easy. The regularity, however, is easily disturbed by exertion or effort, or by bronchitis, or merely by deep breathing. In moderate and slight dilatation the pulse may be regular, but, while irregularity is the rule, there is no such constant relation between the degree of regularity or irregularity of the pulse and the amount of dilatation of the heart as to make one diagnostic of the other.

**The Heart.**—In the examination of the heart, inspection and particularly palpation will be of the greatest importance. The visual examination will be directed to the situation and character of the apex beat and to the impulse of the right ventricle. Retraction or bulging of the intercostal spaces, elsewhere than at the visible apex beat, will be noted.

The apex will be displaced outwards and downwards, and it may be visible over a large area. Very commonly it cannot be seen at all, and the point of maximum apparent impulse does not necessarily belong to the true apex. The right ventricle impulse will be diffuse, if recognizable at all, and as a rule it is inconspicuous.

Palpation in most cases of dilatation furnishes information which contributes more to precision of idea as to the actual state of the heart than any other branch of physical exploration. The right hand should be applied closely over the entire cardiac region, the palm over the right ventricle, the fingers, spread out and close together alternately, over the apex region. Distinct impulse over the right ventricle, while it indicates more or less obstruction in the pulmonary circulation, indicates also some degree of vigour in this ventricle available for compensatory work. A mere vibration has a converse significance. The first object of attention, however, will be the identification of the point of maximum impulse in the apex region, and a careful estimation of the area over which the apex beat extends, and of its force and character; whether, for example, it is a mere concussion of the chest wall or a more or less distinct thrust at any point. Sometimes the word "slapping" is employed to describe the impulse or apex beat characteristic of dilatation. Further exploration will be made by pressing the fingers into the intercostal spaces around and beyond the point of maximum impulse, and it must be borne in mind that this impulse may not be the real apex beat, but the impulse of the right ventricle. Sometimes impulse is detected much above the normal situation, in the fourth space perhaps as far outwards as the anterior axillary fold or behind it, or it may be concealed by the female mamma. It may be the left edge of the right ventricle resting on the inter-ventricular septum which is here felt, or a part of the rounded apex of the left ventricle. According as the apex is capable of giving a distinct thrust or communicates only a diffuse shock, and, according as the beat is well-defined and steady, or vaguely felt over a considerable area, will be the estimate of the degree of dilatation and of the thickness or thinness of the heart wall. Not unfrequently neither impulse nor apex beat can be detected, or the impulse is so vague that it cannot be localized; unless this is due to overlapping lung, it indicates great weakness of the muscular walls of the heart.

By deep percussion the outline of the heart can be more or less accurately mapped out. It is more rounded in the apex region than normal, and the area of dulness is greatly extended to the left. When no impulse of any kind can be felt we may have to depend entirely on percussion for information as to the size of the heart. I have found continuous deep dulness outwards as far as the mid-axillary line and downwards to the seventh space, shown to be cardiac by the intensity of the sounds at the extreme limits, and, when the heart had gained strength, by an apex beat recognizable by palpation at the farthest point.

Auscultation.—The characteristic modification of the sounds of the heart produced by dilatation is that the left ventricle first sound becomes short; usually it is also sharper than normal. Probably from this change in the character of the left ventricle first sound it is almost always audible in the aortic area, contrasting in this respect with hypertrophy. It is audible also to the left of the apex beat. When no impulse or apex beat can be felt, the sounds, and especially the first, must be made use of to ascertain how far to the left, the left border and apex of the heart have been carried by the dilatation, and in what degree the enlargement is due to dilatation or hypertrophy. Percussion, of course, maps out the deep dulness, and shows approximately the limit of the heart and its extension to the left, but the point of maximum intensity of the sounds and the area over which they are audible will corroborate or correct the idea formed as to the size of the heart from percussion, and percussion yields no information whatever as to the kind of enlargement, but leaves it to be supplied by the character of the sounds on auscultation.

Not uncommonly dilatation of the left ventricle gives rise to a systolic apex murmur, obviously due to mitral incompetence. This is induced by imperfect accomplishment of the constriction of the orifice, which is part of the normal contraction of the ventricle, and which co-operates with the curtains of the valves in preventing regurgitation into the auricle. Mitral valvular disease is attended with precisely the same combination of conditions—incompetence of the valve and dilatation of the ventricle—and of physical signs—a systolic murmur and displacement of the apex beat with increased cardiac dulness. The prognosis is different in the two cases, and it is therefore important to distinguish between them. This cannot always be done by means of physical signs alone, but they may give important information.

The presence of the left ventricle first sound and its peculiar character in primary dilatation, and its partial or complete replacement by the murmur in a valve lesion will sometimes be of service in differential diagnosis. The age of the patient, and the history of the case, will be of great help, and the mode of onset of the symptoms and their causation should be carefully inquired into. If the patient is middle-aged and the symptoms date from some imprudent over-exertion, the presumption will be in favour of primary dilatation. If there is a history of acute rheumatism, there will be little doubt as to the diagnosis, especially if the patient be a child or young adolescent, and there is evidence of compensatory hypertrophy of the right ventricle.

There is nothing in dilatation of the cavities of the heart to affect specially and directly the second sound, but, in proportion as this condition of the ventricles impairs the propulsive energy of the systole the second sound will be enfeebled, and the aortic second sound is usually weak as compared with the left ventricle first sound. The relative loudness of the sounds therefore enters into the considerations from which may be calculated the efficiency of the ventricle.

Very important information is often supplied by observation of the intervals between the first and second and the second and first sounds, the short and long pauses respectively. When, with dilatation of the left ventricle there is resistance in the arterioles and capillaries, which is very commonly the case, the interval between the first and second sound may be prolonged, and as this marks the duration of the systole it shows that the ventricle is endeavouring to cope with the difficulty and to complete its contraction. The short or systolic pause may be so prolonged as to equal the diastolic or long pause, and the sounds thus become equidistant, the first also having become short and sharp; the only difference between the sounds is one of emphasis or of pitch, and it is often difficult to say which is which. The sounds may be compared, when the heart is acting slowly, to the ticking of a clock; when rapidly, to the puffing of a distant locomotive.

On the other hand, the first and second sounds may be approximated, and as we cannot suppose that a dilated and enfeebled ventricle completes its systole in a shorter time than normal, the only possible explanation is, that it is quickly brought up short by the resistance in the arterial system and expels but a small proportion of its contents. This abbreviation of the systolic pause is therefore a serious indication of failure of the ventricles, and when carried to an extreme, so that the second sound follows the first immediately and almost seems to overtake it, is significant of immediate danger.

In two successive attacks of symptoms due to dilatation of the heart, when the degree of dilatation appears to be exactly the same, a difference in the length of the systolic interval is sometimes the chief, if not the only, point which makes a difference in the prognosis. The first and second sounds are spaced in the first attack, which is survived, and approximated in the second, which proves fatal.

## Symptoms.

The symptoms which attend the earlier stages of dilatation are extremely varied and often very vague. An imperfect and fluctuating supply of blood to the brain will give rise to impairment of bodily and mental energy, and to irresolution and vacillation of purpose; the memory is liable to fail, especially in regard to recent events, and the power of sustained attention and consecutive thought is diminished. The frame of mind will often be despondent, and the temper may be irritable. There may be attacks of giddiness or faintness. Sleep is usually disturbed, and sometimes almost absent, and, whether the nights are good or bad, there may be slumber at any period of the day, the patient dropping off to sleep even over his morning newspaper. For the same reason, viz. the irregular and imperfect blood supply and the back pressure in the veins, digestion and the action of the liver will be deranged. The appetite is bad, and food is followed by discomfort and by flatulent distension, which latter again reacts on the heart, and gives rise to oppression, or palpitation, or irregular action. The bowels are usually torpid. The urine is deficient in amount and high coloured, and there is often an habitual deposit of urates. Turbidity of the urine day after day, whatever the food and drink, or weather, or mode of life, should direct attention to the state of the circulation.

There is no one, and scarcely any combination, of the symptoms enumerated, however, which may not occur independently of weakness and dilatation of the heart, especially in states of system attended with high tension; and it would be waste of time to attempt to disentangle those directly due to the state of the heart from those which are merely accidentally associated with it.

The special symptom which calls attention to the heart as the probable starting-point of a number of ailments is breathlessness on slight exertion, but even this may be produced by other causes—by anæmia, for example; after middle age, pernicious anæmia may often give rise to extreme breathlessness, which may excite a suspicion of heart disease. High arterial tension alone, which has not yet given rise to dilatation, simple debility, sedentary habits, with a tendency to corpulence, may also cause shortness of breath. These facts are mentioned in order to warn against a too ready inference that dilatation of the heart exists simply because the breath is short. An interesting fact in connection with breathlessness due to dilatation of the heart is that it is often relieved by exercise of the voice. I have met with several instances in which a clergyman has climbed into the pulpit with the utmost difficulty, and has not only preached a sermon comfortably, but has been all the better for it. A sense of breathlessness coming on during repose, and inciting the patient to make frequent deep inspirations, is usually a symptom of nervous depression, and has no necessary relation to heart disease. For the most part, as the disease advances, symptoms arise which are indicative of back pressure in the systemic veins, a gradually advancing œdema of the legs, congestion of the lungs, etc.

In an extreme case the patient will be dropsical, œdema invading the thighs, loins, and abdominal parietes, as well as the legs, and there may be fluid in the abdomen, and perhaps in one or both pleural cavities. The feet and legs will be cold and pale, or purple and livid, especially if hanging down; the hands also will be cold, and are often crimson or purplish, and the nails of a deep or dusky tint, instead of a bright pink. A white patch on the hand, produced by pressure, is very slowly invaded by returning colour. The sufferer is probably unable to lie down in bed, and is propped up by pillows, or he must have his legs down, and therefore spends day and night seated in his chair. Remarkable exceptions, however, are met with in this respect, some sufferers, while extremely ill, being able to lie down without distress. The face is pale, and perhaps puffy, especially under the eyes, with injected capillaries over the cheeks, and wears an expression of distress, and the eyes are watery. The lips are pale or bluish; the breathing is more or less laboured, even in repose, and the sufferer constantly supplements his reflex respiration by voluntary deep breaths. When he speaks it is in fragmentary sentences, and with evident effort and aggravation of the respiratory distress. The least movement brings on shortness of breath, which is often painful, even to witness. The pulse is frequent, irregular, and probably greatly deficient in tension. The urine will be scanty, of a deep colour, and high specific gravity; it most commonly throws down a copious deposit of brickdust lithates, and it may contain albumen, the amount of which may vary from day to day. The appetite will be bad, and there may be nausea; the tongue may be furred, the bowels constipated or irregular. One of the most distressing symptoms is sleeplessness, and when, after hours of weary shifting of position, the sufferer is overcome by fatigue and drops off, he has painful dreams, and wakes suddenly in affright and suffocation for lack of voluntary help to his respiration. The longest and best sleep will be obtained while sitting in a chair, and sometimes by day rather than in the night.

The jugulars will be found full, but not, as a rule, greatly distended or pulsating forcibly. The liver will be enlarged, coming down sometimes as low as the umbilicus, and extending across the epigastrium into the left hypochondrium. It will often be jogged by the right ventricle, but does not usually exhibit true expansile pulsation. The jugular distension and pulsation, as was pointed out by Mackenzie of Burnley, may be greatly exaggerated by pressure on the enlarged liver. There may be fluid in the peritoneal or pleural cavities, more commonly not, and there will, in most cases, be physical signs of œdema and congestion of the lungs; occasionally the percussion note may be good and the entry of air free and unattended with adventitious sounds of any kind to the very base of both lungs.

## Prognosis.

We may consider first the most serious case where the symptoms present are such as have just been described. We are called upon to answer the question, Has the patient a chance of recovering from the condition described, or will he die?

The first element in the judgment to be formed will be the urgency of the symptoms, and special importance will attach to two of the series—the nausea and loss of appetite and the sleeplessness—from the effects which they have on the patient's strength. Frequent vomiting of food is of very grave import, not only because the patient does not get the benefit of the nourishment, but because it shows that the stasis in the abdominal circulation has reached a point which interferes seriously with the digestive secretions. Attacks of faintness and of extreme exhaustion, or of severe dyspnœa, are also of serious import.

It is not always when the dropsy is excessive that the condition of the patient is worst. From the late appearance or entire absence of dropsy in fatty degeneration of the heart, in aortic disease, and mitral stenosis, it would appear that a certain degree of pressure in the arterial system is required to co-operate with the back pressure in the venous system for the full development of dropsical effusion; and when the œdema remains moderate in amount, while other symptoms—such as breathlessness, faintness, and muscular weakness, the latter especially—indicate great cardiac inefficiency, it may be because the left ventricle propels the blood with very little force. Degeneration may be a factor in the case. A frequent, short, unsustained pulse and heart-beat, without much œdema, may thus indicate a more grave condition than extreme dropsy. Long-continued excessive frequency of the pulse is an unfavourable sign.

The urgency of the symptoms being about the same, a greater degree of dilatation, as indicated by a more extended area of dulness, by marked displacement of and diffuseness and weakness of the apex beat, will add gravity to the prognosis. A further unfavourable indication will be approximation of the first and second sounds.

When the symptoms and physical signs have been well weighed, the first question to be asked in view of prognosis is whether there has been any adequate exciting cause of the symptoms. If there has been recognizable over-exertion or excitement, or grave anxiety—any mental or bodily strain—or if there has been a chill, giving rise to bronchitis or other affection of the lungs, or deranging seriously the liver and digestive organs, it may be hoped by means of rest and treatment to undo the ill-effects and restore the balance. If, on the other hand, the symptoms have crept on gradually without traceable cause of the kind mentioned, and especially when due care has been exercised, and there has been no habitual error of regimen or neglect of bowels, the probabilities are that the symptoms are the outcome of conditions which cannot be reversed—of radical inherent weakness of the heart.

The previous mode of life, active or sedentary, careful or imprudent, and especially the habits with regard to alcoholic stimulants, will have a very important bearing on the probable issue of the attack, as will also the general soundness and the absence or existence of disease of any other important organs, especially of the kidneys and liver. The patient's cheerfulness, hopefulness, and courage under his sufferings, or his despondency, will make powerfully for or against him, not only as direct influences, but because the state of mind is often an index of the state of the system.

Another inquiry of great prognostic weight will be as to the patient's family history. It is through this that we obtain an idea of his vital tenacity, of the trustworthiness of his tissues, and of the special liabilities to cardio-vascular degeneration. There are few tendencies which run more strongly in families than those which are manifested in the heart and vascular system, whether to high arterial tension with the effects on the vessels and heart, which follow from this, or to dilatation and weakness, or to degeneration, and a prognosis, otherwise not unfavourable, might have to be instantly revised on learning that the father, an uncle, or a brother, had died at about the patient's age from heart disease. Finally, the response to treatment will speedily afford an indication of the utmost value.

### Treatment.

**Mild Cases.**—In view of the tendency to dilatation in acute rheumatism and influenza, and after any acute bacterial infection when the heart muscle has been more or less damaged by toxins, a period of rest, with avoidance of any undue exertion, is advisable after any acute illness. Loss of tone of the cardiac muscle, with a certain degree of dilatation of, and, it may be, irritability of, the heart, is especially liable to occur after an attack of influenza, and is frequently associated with mental depression and loss of nerve tone. This class of case is usually much benefited by the "Schott" treatment of baths, as the daily routine, enforced period of rest, the sedative effect of the baths, the change of air and scene, with absence of excitement and mental exertion, is highly beneficial. It is by no means essential that the patient should go to Nauheim, as the treatment can be carried out at his own home or at various bathing stations in England, *e.g.* Bath, Buxton, Harrogate, and other places, or, if the patient wishes to go abroad, at numerous other health resorts; in France, for instance, as pointed out by Huchard, at Chatel Guyon, Salins Moutiers, Royat, etc., and at various places in Germany. This hydrotherapeutic treatment is usually only necessary in cases in which there is an element of neurosis, cardiac irritability, or mental depression, when the psychological element must be taken into consideration.

In slight cases of dilatation and loss of tone, a complete holiday from work, with change of air to a bracing climate, will usually suffice. Mild cardiac tonics may be given, and gentle exercise taken, the duration of which should be gradually increased day by day. At first, rest in the recumbent position for at least half an hour before meals should be insisted on.

**Severe Cases.**—In the treatment of advanced symptoms

due to dilatation of the heart, we have to deal at the same time with defective propulsive power on the part of the ventricle, and damming back of blood in the venous system —the former being the primary and principal difficulty— and the indications are to relieve the ventricles of work and give them strength, and at the same time to deplete the venous engorgement.

This last object must, indeed, be taken first.

Venesection, the most effectual means of relieving the right side of the heart, is rarely applicable in acute dilatation. It is conceivable that under some pulmonary complications resulting from chill, the engorgement of the right ventricle and auricle might be such as to make blood-letting the less of two dangers; but, the initial fault being weakness of one or both ventricles, we cannot trust the heart to adjust itself to a rapid change of any kind, and the right ventricle may not be in a condition to take advantage of the relief afforded it. Usually, however, the venous engorgement is developed slowly, and the indications for venesection do not arise.

The application of six or eight leeches over the liver is safer, and it will usually effect all that can be done by direct abstraction of blood. The indication for this local bleeding is enlargement of the liver, and, when this is considerable, it rarely fails to afford striking relief. Frequently, for example, the patient, who has previously been tortured by sleeplessness, will sleep at once and sometimes for a night or two afterwards. The reason for selecting the hepatic region for the application of the leeches is simply that pain and tenderness felt there are relieved; it is not supposed that blood is drawn from the liver, or that the same amount abstracted elsewhere would not be equally efficacious. The leeches should be followed by a hot fomentation, which, besides encouraging the bleeding, will bring blood to the surface. When the liver is not enlarged, and especially if the right ventricle impulse and sounds are weak, there is no advantage to be gained by leeching.

Concurrently with the application of leeches a purgative will be given, which will deplete the portal system at the same time that the leeching depletes the systemic veins. Afterwards this will be the principal means of keeping down the venous engorgement. In a large majority of cases, indeed, we have to depend entirely upon purgatives for this purpose, as abstraction of blood by any method is inadmissible. It is not a matter of indifference what purgatives are employed. The object of a purgative is not simply to carry off as much fluid as possible and so drain the tissues. This may be the case, perhaps, in ascites from cirrhosis of the liver; but in heart disease of any kind, and especially in dilatation, much more is to be gained by rectifying the balance of the circulation: the kidneys will then often resume their function and remove the excess of liquid.

Purgatives, then, may be made to contribute to this; and before considering them further we must refer to the first object of treatment, the relief of the heart from work and the increase of its vigour. Of these we can be much more sure of the first than of the second; we can more easily and certainly diminish the resistance in the arterioles and capillaries than we can lend strength and efficiency to the action of the heart, and, without removing the obstruction in the peripheral circulation, it might only do harm to incite the heart—weakened as its structures are—to greater effort to overcome it. Mercurial purgatives have this effect of diminishing arterio-capillary resistance and of lowering arterial tension, and therefore of relieving the heart. This is a fact of clinical experience and observation, and its explanation is a matter of secondary importance, but the hypothesis by which, as it seems to me, it is best explained, is that mercury influences the liver metabolism and promotes the elimination of impurities which, when retained in the blood, give rise to resistance in the capillaries. But, whatever the explanation, the fact that the arterial tension is notably lowered by mercurial aperients is one which is confirmed by daily experience. It is remarkable how frequently the statement recurs in works on heart disease that other remedies often fail to act until a dose of calomel or other mercurial preparation has been given.

Mercurial purgatives, then, have the double effect of depleting the portal system, which relieves the enlargement of the liver and the distension of the right side of the heart, and of diminishing the resistance in the peripheral circulation, and so relieving the left ventricle of stress. Very commonly the best of testimony as to the beneficial character of the result is given by refreshing sleep. The disadvantage, if such it be, that less fluid is carried off than by hydragogue cathartics is often compensated by an increased flow of urine; and elaterium, gamboge, pulv. jalap. co., and the like, when repeated, give rise to great exhaustion.

Calomel, then, or blue pill or grey powder, should be given in doses of from 1 to 5 grains, according to the urgency of the case, with colocynth and hyoscyamus or rhubarb, followed by some mild saline. After one or more full doses at the outset, a moderate dose may be given every third or fourth night. The acid tartrate of potash will often co-operate beneficially, both by its action on the bowels and on the kidneys.

The heart being relieved of work may be urged to more vigorous contraction by digitalis, strophanthus, spartein, squills, caffein, convallaria, apocyanum, the special heart tonics, with which strychnine may usually be combined with advantage. In a case of extreme suffering, digitalis may be given with ammonia, ether, and nux vomica; in a more chronic stage, with iron, strychnine, and perhaps nitric or hydrochloric acid. Sometimes an effect can be obtained by giving diuretin or caffein in a cachet, at the same time with digitalis in a mixture, when singly neither seems to be efficacious. Squills, again, may be given with digitalis as in the well-known pill with mercury, or in some liquid combination. Next to digitalis stands strophanthus, which is a most valuable alternative when digitalis seems to produce sickness, as is sometimes the case, or when it fails to exercise a favourable influence on the heart. Sulphate of spartein I have seen to be of great service when digitalis and strophanthus appeared to have exhausted their influence. Of convallaria I have little to say. Apocyanum has, in one or two cases, seemed to carry off dropsy in a remarkable way, but one patient died suddenly when apparently just well.

It is not necessary to go into greater detail with regard to these remedies. Throughout a case of the kind the medical man has to fight, so to speak, with both hands, and continuous watchfulness will be necessary to meet the vicissitudes which occur, and many changes in method may be required, while the same principles are held in view.

The prognosis, as has been said, will be greatly influenced by the response to treatment. This will be energetic, especially in the matter of purgatives, in proportion as the symptoms are urgent, and if no favourable effect is produced, the prospect of recovery is very poor. Very commonly improvement takes place up to a certain point, and then progress seems to come to an end. This is a trying stage both to the patient and to the medical man. Change of remedies and new combinations must be tried, both in regard of the aperient and of the tonic, not frequently and capriciously, but with careful study of the results and due allowance of time for obtaining them. Sometimes it does good to suspend all medicines for a few days and start afresh. When the œdema of the legs is considerable, it may be of the greatest service to drain the fluid from the legs. The good result of removing an ascitic accumulation, should this be present, may be still more striking. Even a moderate amount of effusion in the pleural cavity, such as we should not think of dealing with under ordinary circumstances, should be aspirated. A straw may turn the balance either way, and a very slight obstacle may prevent the heart from regaining control over the circulation. It is not always desirable to postpone the removal of fluid till the particular conjuncture described arrives; it may be an urgent necessity at a very early period. Usually, however, it is prudent to give remedies a chance before resorting to puncture or paracentesis. As regards the method of drainage to be employed, Southey's tubes are, in my opinion, much the best, whether for œdema or ascites, but particularly in case of ascites, as the too rapid removal of the fluid is inadvisable.

**Dropsy.**—It has been found that in Bright's disease with œdema and ascites the dropsical fluids are rich in chlorides. Normally, the proportion of chlorides in the blood and urine is a stable quantity, and any excess of chlorides ingested is eliminated in the urine. In Bright's disease there is usually deficient elimination of salts in the urine and an excess in the blood. It is argued, therefore, that when the kidneys are diseased, and there is defective elimination of salts, the accumulation of salts, more especially chlorides in the blood, favours the production of dropsy. Widal, indeed, claims that he can in certain cases of Bright's disease provoke or abolish dropsy at will, simply by the administration or withholding of sodium chloride in the diet. Though this is not altogether proved in the case of cardiac dropsy, it is advisable, in view of these observations, to eliminate from the diet common salt and other chlorides, as far as possible.

The feeding of the patient through the long course of

treatment will be a task of extreme difficulty. We have to contend with nausea and distaste for food amounting to disgust; sometimes the sufferer positively cannot swallow anything requiring mastication. The object to be held in view is to keep down the volume of the blood while maintaining its quality. A small amount of solid or semi-solid food should be taken about every three hours. When the patient is not too ill to take his meals at the accustomed times it is a great encouragement to him to be allowed to do so, and he may then eat what he can of fish, fowl, tender meat, and milk puddings. When the appetite is small the regular meals may be supplemented by intermediate nourishment, such as a beaten-up egg, a little milk, or perhaps a small cup of beef-tea, or a little beef or chicken jelly, or meat extract. Soups and jellies have the disadvantage of containing little proteid and much liquid, and many extractives and salts, but they are stimulants to the flagging heart. Potted meat sandwiches are a great resource, and the pulp of raw beefsteak can be given in this form, disguised by cooked meat or concentrated gravy. A German method of treatment is to feed patients suffering from cardiac dropsy entirely on raw ham.

The amount of fluid must be restricted as far as possible, especially that taken with food. Stimulants are usually necessary, but should be kept within limits known to and defined by the medical man. The patient is under a great temptation to resort to them for the relief of faintness, exhaustion, and nausea. Cream of tartar drink may be taken to quench thirst between meals, and in some cases a copious draught of hot water once or twice a day will run through the system rapidly and wash out the organs and tissues without augmenting permanently the volume of the blood or adding to the dropsy. When this is tried it must be ascertained definitely that the amount of urine is correspondingly increased.

A question which arises in almost every severe case is whether the patient must be urged to remain in bed or allowed to get up. Bed is undoubtedly the best place for him at first, during what may be called the crisis of the attack, for many reasons; the rest and warmth protect the heart from the strain of exertion and changes of temperature. On the other hand, the dyspnœa is usually worse in the recumbent posture, even with the shoulders raised, and may be intolerable unless the legs are allowed to hang down; not unfrequently it is simply impossible for the patient to remain in bed. A suitable chair, therefore, is necessary, with support for the elbows, shoulders, and head, which can be taken advantage of in turn in the frequent changes of position to which the patient has recourse to ease his breathing or elude discomfort, and the quickness and ingenuity of the medical man or nurse in devising expedients may greatly alleviate his sufferings. A bed table or other form of support, upon which the patient may rest his arms or elbows and head when leaning forwards while sitting in his chair, will often be useful. A patient will frequently sleep better in this position than in any other. Perhaps the most common state of things is that the patient is up during the day, and tries to spend more or less of the night in bed. When he cannot at once bear to go to bed at night, he may undress and sit in his chair wrapped in blankets near the bed, when he will often, after a time, be able to lie down and sleep.

Small doses of morphia may be given hypodermically to enable the patient to get a little sleep and relief from his sufferings. Little benefit can be expected at this stage from the administration of cardiac tonics which will have been freely given at an earlier period. The heart is past recovery, and all that can be done is to treat symptoms as they arise and give temporary relief as far as is possible.

# CHAPTER XXI.

## STRUCTURAL CHANGE IN THE RIGHT VENTRICLE.

PHYSIOLOGICAL DILATATION—HYPERTROPHY AND DILATATION—DEGENERATION OF THE MUSCULAR WALLS.

DILATATION and hypertrophy of the right ventricle are perhaps the most common of all the structural changes to which the heart is subject. Some primary dilatation accompanies all severe exertion, and when the exertion has been inordinate it may be considerable and persist for some time, but unless the muscular fibres have undergone degeneration from age or abuse of alcohol, or a sedentary life, or from recent febrile disease, or diphtheria, there is a wonderful power of recovery. If over-exertion is habitual the dilatation will be neutralized by hypertrophy. In all cases of valvular disease of the left ventricle or of lung disease, such as bronchitis, emphysema, etc., which give rise to obstruction in the pulmonary circulation, dilatation and hypertrophy of the right ventricle follow as a necessary physiological result, as has already been explained in a previous chapter.

Dilatation and hypertrophy of the right ventricle are thus, for the most part, pathological in name only, and are really compensatory adjustments which neutralize more or less perfectly the effects of valvular or other disease of the left side of the heart, and when compensation is effectual become an indication of the degree of severity of the original disease.

## Physical Signs and Symptoms.

**Hypertrophy or Dilatation** of the right ventricle carries the apex of the heart to the left and increases the horizontal dimensions of the heart. The apex beat may be found at or beyond the vertical nipple line, not unfrequently in the anterior or even mid-axillary line, when there is also enlargement of the left ventricle. The character of the apex beat depends more on the left ventricle than the right, but with much dilatation of the right ventricle it is usually diffuse. The area of cardiac dulness will be increased, and, on percussion, it may be found that the area of dulness extends to the right or considerably beyond the right margin of the sternum and upwards to the second rib, in consequence of the dilatation of the right auricle, which usually coexists with the dilatation of the ventricle, which is evident from its pulsation in the epigastrium.

The degree of hypertrophy is estimated by the force of the right ventricle impulse as communicated to the hand applied over the lower left costal cartilages and the epigastrium, and also by the degree of accentuation of the pulmonic second sound. It is the degree of hypertrophy which is of vital importance, as on this depends the efficiency of compensation.

The symptoms usually associated with the changes in the right ventricle just described are pulmonary congestion, venous stasis, and dropsy, but these are not so much the effects of dilatation of the right ventricle as the final results of the original disease of the left ventricle or lungs, which the right ventricle has been unable to combat efficiently.

It has seemed to me that our ideas of the effects of disease of the right ventricle have been too much based upon a study of the symptoms which attend affections of this ventricle secondary to disease of the left ventricle or its valves, which therefore are really attributable to the original disease.

Undoubtedly the supervention of dilatation of the right ventricle and of reflux through the tricuspid orifice allows back pressure to be brought to bear upon the veins, but this only intensifies pre-existing effects and symptoms, and makes no change in their character.

We are perhaps justified in assuming that the venous back pressure, to which insufficiency of the tricuspid valve will give rise, will in some degree produce the same results, whatever the state of the left side of the heart, and whether or not the tricuspid regurgitation has been caused by obstruction in the pulmonary circulation; but the conditions are fundamentally different when the tricuspid reflux is primary. It is not impossible, for example, that a sound and strong left ventricle may come to the aid of the right ventricle, just as the right ventricle so constantly comes to the aid of the left, notwithstanding the great length of the systemic as compared with the pulmonic circuit and the weak blood pressure in the systemic veins. The pressure which will cause the blood to spurt for two or three feet in venesection might carry a current through the capillaries of the lungs aided by the respiratory movements and the valves of the pulmonary artery.

It has, moreover, seemed to me that weakness of the right ventricle—the left ventricle being in a normal condition—has in some cases given rise to symptoms due rather to inadequate supply of blood to the left side of the heart than to damming back of blood in the veins. I have, for example, met with several instances of primary tricuspid regurgitation, either as a constant condition or coming on under very slight provocation. When any effect of this has been traceable it has not been breathlessness on exertion, but tendency to syncope. Perhaps this is what we ought to expect, since the occurrence of tricuspid regurgitation in the breathlessness of violent exertion has been regarded as a safety-valve action, by lowering the pressure in the pulmonic circulation. A difference of symptoms ought to attend mitral and tricuspid insufficiency, one giving rise to turgescence and high pressure in the pulmonary circulation, the other to deficient supply of blood and low pressure. If mitral disease produces pulmonary symptoms, tricuspid disease may well produce systemic symptoms.

In a few cases which have come under my notice, in which the right ventricle has appeared to be predominantly or almost exclusively affected by asthenia or degeneration, the effects have been similar to those of tricuspid regurgitation.

A master in a public school, who had been accustomed to vigorous exercise, received a severe blow on the chest. He had for some time great pain in the cardiac region, and when he walked he soon felt faint. When I saw him some time after the injury he had had slight but distinct syncopal attacks. On examination, no valvular disease was present, and the heart was of normal size. There was a fair apex push in the normal situation, and the left ventricle first sound and the aortic second sound were normal in character. No right ventricle impulse, however, could be detected, and its first sound and the pulmonic second sound were very weak.

What had happened exactly cannot be stated, but from the contrast between the action and sounds of the two sides of the heart, it seemed as if the right ventricle had been in some way injured, and that its contractile energy was impaired.

The patient regained the power of taking exercise, and with this the sounds of the right ventricle became normal.

A patient, aged 72, who had never had a day's illness in his life, consulted me in 1879, complaining of failing vigour, giddiness on running to catch a 'bus, tendency to fall asleep in the day. He was constipated; the pulse, which was not more than 60, was sometimes tense, sometimes soft. The heart sounds generally were weak, the aortic second accentuated. In April, 1881, symptoms, which had previously been relieved, returned, and it was now found that over all parts of the right ventricle, and even over the pulmonic area, there was absolute silence. No impulse or apex beat could be detected, but at the apex the sounds were normal; the aortic second sound was accentuated. The pulse was 72, a little irregular, but fair in force and length. A month later he was much better. The pulse was 60, fair in strength and length; the left ventricle sounds were good, the right ventricle sounds faintly audible. From this time neither the right ventricle first, nor the pulmonic second sound were ever at any time audible. The pulse varied considerably both in frequency and in tension, but it was usually well sustained, indicating considerable vigour of the left ventricle, and the left ventricle sounds were good. He had from time to time severe fainting attacks, which sometimes threatened to prove fatal. He was always worse when the bowels were not kept freely open. In June, 1883, the pulse is described as large, full, and tense; the aortic second sound was accentuated at the apex and in the right second space; there were no right ventricle sounds whatever. Towards the end of 1884, when not under my care, the bowels were allowed to get confined, and he fell into a condition of torpor, with incontinence of urine and fæces. He recovered from this condition after free purgation, and was again able to go about, though his mental faculties were impaired and he was childish; but in November, 1885, thrombosis of the left middle cerebral artery took place, giving rise to hemiplegia and aphasia, of which he died.

The entire absence of right ventricle sounds in this case was very remarkable, and I cannot doubt that there was a very feeble action of this ventricle. As it seemed to me impossible that the pulmonary circulation could be maintained without its aid, I formed a very unfavourable prognosis; and when this was belied I watched the case with extreme care, first to make sure that my observation was not at fault, and next in order that I might arrive at some comprehension of the problem presented by the facts. The conclusion appeared to be unavoidable that the left ventricle was carrying on the circulation through the lungs; it was throughout capable of maintaining high tension in the arteries. The amount of blood passing through the pulmonary vessels under these conditions and reaching the left auricle would be easily influenced, and would vary greatly, and the fluctuating supply of blood to the left ventricle would account for the varying character of the pulse.

One of the most serious effeots of weakness of the right ventricle is met with in disease of the mitral valve. When the mitral valve is incompetent, or from thickening and shrinking of the curtains and tendinous cords becomes stenosed, the right ventricle is for a time the rampart by which the reflux of blood is arrested, or increased pressure in the left auricle is maintained to promote a more rapid flow through the narrowed orifice. When we hear an apex murmur telling of mitral regurgitation or stenosis, the murmur itself gives no trustworthy information as to the severity of the lesion. We gather this mainly from the effects upon the right ventricle. The first of these is accentuation of the pulmonic second sound, indicating increased pressure in the pulmonary circulation, and following on this hypertrophy of the right ventricle, by means of which the obstruction to the passage of blood through the lungs is overcome. It is by the augmented strength of the right ventricle that the mitral leakage or obstruction is neutralized and a working equilibrium established. The greater the regurgitation or stenosis the greater the amount of hypertrophy required to compensate for it. The change in the right ventricle thus becomes, together with the accompanying changes in the left ventricle, a measure of the regurgitation or stenosis.

When, therefore, we detect a mitral murmur, we at once examine the right ventricle in order to gather from its condition information as to the amount of reflux or obstruction which is not yielded by the murmur itself. This is specially the case when symptoms of failing compensation have set in. But if the right ventricle is in a state of degeneration or great weakness, as may be the case in lesions established late in life, these indications fail us altogether. The absence of dilatation and hypertrophy, instead of denoting comparatively slight regurgitation or stenosis, shows that the right ventricle is incapable of coping with it. There is no right ventricle impulse, and the pulmonic second sound instead of being accentuated is weak, while dropsy and other evidences of serious stasis and back pressure in the venous system are prematurely developed for lack of hypertrophy or compensatory effort on the part of the right ventricle.

Under these circumstances the prognosis is extremely grave. The right ventricle is unable to come to the aid of the left, the mechanism of compensation makes default, and the back pressure bears at once upon the venous system. The fulcrum for some of our most efficacious therapeutic measures is missing. We dare not open a vein however great the respiratory embarrassment and cyanosis; the effect of leeching over the liver is less certainly good, and a dose of calomel is not well borne. Recovery is rare, and twice it has happened in my experience that during apparent convalescence, when an unfavourable prognosis seemed to have been belied, the patient has died suddenly when beginning to walk about, and the right ventricle has been found degenerated at the autopsy.

Similar conditions result from time to time from adhesion of the pericardium. The right ventricle suffers proportionately more than the left from pericarditis, as its walls are relatively very thin, and when the muscle is damaged by myocarditis the ventricle readily dilates. Again, the right ventricle is much more hampered by adhesion of the pericardium than the left, partly because its superficial area is relatively large, but chiefly because of the thinness of its walls; and when the adhesions are general, and especially if there is also adherence of the pericardium to the chest wall and diaphragm, efficient contraction of this ventricle must be impossible. Cases are not uncommon in which there is valvular disease, mitral or aortic, but from the size of the heart, the position and character of the apex beat and impulse, the persistence of sounds in spite of the murmurs, there are grounds for concluding that the valvular lesion is not very severe. There is, however, a premature development of symptoms. Under such circumstances, we may often confidently infer adhesion of the pericardium when it cannot be demonstrated with any certainty by physical signs. This has already been discussed in the chapter on adherent pericardium.

The right ventricle is undoubtedly sometimes the cause of sudden death, and when the heart is embarrassed or stopped by pressure upwards of the diaphragm by a distended stomach or colon, it must be on the right ventricle that the pressure takes effect. This part of the heart rests upon the diaphragm, and will be directly compressed when it is pushed up. Probably it is the diastole which is mostly interfered with, and it would seem that the proper expansion and filling of the ventricle must be impossible when the pressure upon it is such that the heart is carried up bodily by the diaphragm, especially when the ventricle is dilated and over-distended. A melancholy illustration of this occurred in my experience in the case of an eminent artist. He was suffering from mitral stenosis and regurgitation, and had overthrown the compensation established by hypertrophy of the right ventricle by serious imprudence in the form of over-exertion and exposure undertaken to remedy the effects of overwork. There was an extreme degree of distension of the right side of the heart, with tricuspid regurgitation, and he suffered from sleeplessness and dyspnœa, so that his misery was insupportable, and life was despaired of. The application of leeches over the liver, which was enormously swollen, and the administration of calomel, at once gave him sleep, and by a repetition of the leeches and regular employment of mercurial aperients, with the usual heart tonics, he so far recovered as to be able to leave his room, and his convalescence seemed to be assured.

One morning, after a hearty breakfast in bed, the nurse was about to wash his face and hands as usual, but he impatiently bade her give him the basin, and stand aside. He sat up in bed with the basin between his knees, and when the time came for washing his face, bent forwards over it. The pressure upwards of a full stomach caused by this movement brought the weak right ventricle to a standstill, and the patient fell back dead.

One cannot help being reminded, in relating this incident, of the rough and ready, but effectual, way in which a man is brought to who faints after the severe exertion of a boat race. He is seated on the ground, and his body is bent forcibly forwards, so that his head almost comes to the ground between his knees, or, if he has fallen forwards over his oar, it is done while he is in the boat. The *modus operandi* of the remedy is pressure on the distended right heart, and, when emetics are resorted to in bronchitis, which has gone on to the production of cyanosis, the good effect is due, not only to the emptying of the bronchial tubes, but to unloading of the right auricle and ventricle by compression in the act of vomiting.

## CHAPTER XXII.

## DISEASE OF THE CORONARY ARTERIES.

ATHEROMA OR SCLEROSIS—ENDARTERITIS—THROMBOSIS—EMBOLISM—ANEURYSM.

DISEASE of the coronary arteries is very common, and is of the first importance, inasmuch as they constitute the sole blood supply to the heart, and obstruction to the flow of blood through them from disease of their walls may be a cause of sudden death, or give rise to degenerative change in the cardiac muscle which eventually occasions heart failure.

Atheroma or sclerosis is the commonest affection of the coronary arteries. The terms "atheroma" and "sclerosis" are employed indiscriminately to denote the same affection, though, strictly speaking, atheroma etymologically means "a gruel-like condition," and sclerosis "a hardening."

Probably this confusing nomenclature has originated from the presence in the aorta of patches of softening and ulceration, whereas arteries when affected are hard, firm, and inelastic to the touch. Hence the term "atheroma" is commonly employed to denote degenerative changes in the aorta, and "sclerosis" similar changes in the smaller arteries. Pathologically, however, and to a great extent etiologically, the conditions are identical.

The general question of atheroma is discussed in a later chapter. For the present we are chiefly concerned with the effect on the heart of degenerative changes in the coronary vessels.

**Morbid Anatomy.**—The coronary arteries are thickened, inelastic, and hard. Their lumen may be partially obstructed by small whitish, opaque projections, so that on section they have the appearance of a signet ring, with the signet turned inwards, or the lumen may be almost occluded by a uniform thickening which involves the whole

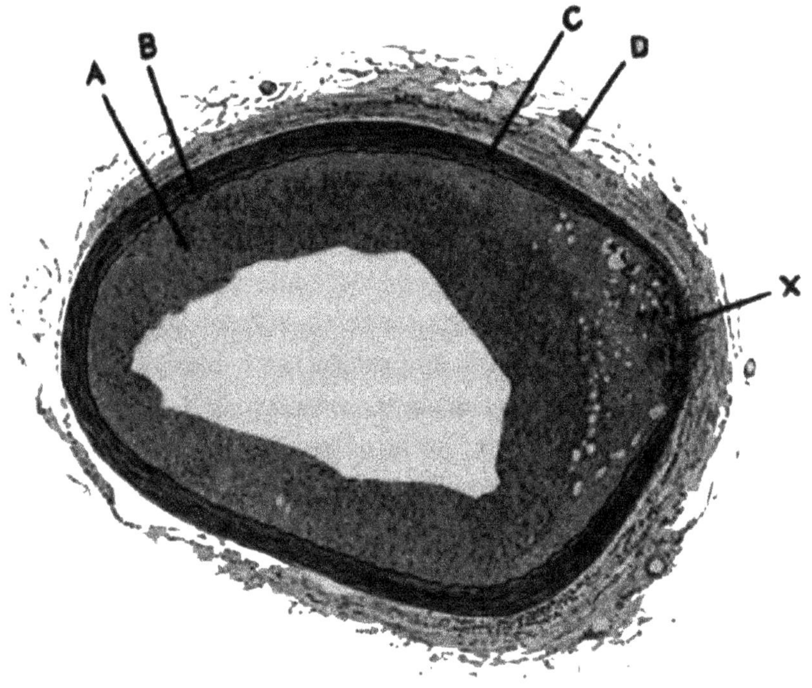


Fig. 19A.—Section of coronary artery showing advanced sclerosis. A, greatly thickened intima; B, internal elastic lamina; C, muscular coat; D, adventitia. At X the muscular coat is almost destroyed, and patches of calcification are seen in the degenerated tissue beneath.

circumference. On microscopic examination of a section through one of these projections, it is seen to consist of a swelling immediately beneath the endothelium, which is pushed inwards; externally it is usually limited by the internal elastic lamina. The muscular coat beyond this may be atrophied from pressure, or may in advanced disease be involved in the degenerative process and to a great extent destroyed. The swelling is seen to consist of amorphous non-staining débris, in which may be distinguished strands of hyaline degenerated tissue, and small atrophic nuclei of cells which vary greatly in number in different stages of the disease. (*Vide* Fig. 19A.) Frequently calcareous patches are present from deposit of lime salts in the degenerated tissue.

The condition would seem to suggest necrosis of the subendothelial tissue either from toxic influences or from imperfect nutrition, followed by swelling of the necrotic tissue and a futile attempt at repair, the latter being evidenced by the presence of the cellular infiltration, which appears to consist of atrophic connective tissue cells.

Huchard regards endarteritis obliterans of the vasa vasorum, which may be due to a variety of causes, as the most important etiological factor in this primary necrosis. Some consider that proliferation of connective tissue cells beneath the endothelium is the first stage in the process, occurring as a result of irritation due to intermittent strain, or to some toxic substance, and that necrosis of this newly formed tissue follows. Be this as it may, the important point is, that narrowing of the lumen of the coronary arteries and its branches results, and consequently obstruction to the flow of blood through them; moreover, even in the absence of pronounced obstruction, the rigidity and loss of elasticity in the vessels and the presence of calcareous plates in their walls seriously impair the circulation in the heart. Hence may result sudden death, angina pectoris, and various degenerative changes in the heart muscle described in the following chapters.

**Endarteritis obliterans** of syphilitic origin, or possibly due to other toxins, may affect the coronary arteries.

In this affection there is active proliferation of the cells of the endothelium which is not followed by degenerative changes, so that there is uniform thickening of the vessel with narrowing of its lumen, and actual obliteration may ensue in some of the smaller branches of the coronary artery. It is frequently accompanied by periarteritis or thickening of the adventitia.

**Thrombosis.**—This usually occurs in association with sclerosis of the coronary arteries, the diseased condition of the vessel wall and the narrowing of its lumen contributing to the result. Obstruction at the mouth of the coronary artery from atheroma of the aorta involving its orifice, or from a thrombus attached to a diseased aortic valve, may also be a contributory factor. Slowing of the blood stream in a failing heart is also an important cause.

*Infarction.*—There are anastomoses between the main trunks of the coronary arteries, but there are no anastomoses between the smaller branches after they have entered the myocardium. The intramuscular branches are therefore "terminal arteries" in Cohnheim's sense of the word, and infarction results when they are occluded by thrombosis or embolism.

Infarcts of the heart are not typically wedge-shaped, as in the kidney or lung, but are somewhat irregular in outline, those I have seen being oblong, tapering at the distal end. They are usually anæmic, of a pale yellowish colour, sometimes surrounded by a zone of hyperæmia. Microscopically they show coagulation necrosis of the portion of muscle cut off from its blood supply. They may break down and give rise to an aneurism or to rupture of the heart, or they may be gradually absorbed and replaced by fibrous tissue.

Thrombosis of one of the main trunks of the coronary artery may be a cause of rapid death. Cases are, however, on record which show that thrombosis of a large branch may occur without causing death. This may be explained by the fact that there are anastomoses between the main branches of the coronary arteries, and if the thrombosis is gradual in onset, sufficient time may elapse for efficient collateral circulation to be established. Much will, of course, depend on the size of the thrombus and its situation, and whether or not it blocks the mouth of an anastomosing branch.

There are no characteristic physical signs or symptoms by which thrombosis of the coronary vessels can be diagnosed.

It is probably of much commoner occurrence than is generally supposed, and it is possible that it may cause attacks of angina pectoris or præcordial pain, and be responsible for a certain proportion of cases of sudden death which are put down to other causes, such as fatty degeneration of the heart, etc. A systematic investigation of the coronary arteries throughout their course is not commonly made at post-mortem examinations, and my attention was drawn to the subject in investigating a case of Bright's disease in which the heart was enormously hypertrophied, where I found two infarcts in the wall of the left ventricle, with extensive thrombosis of two branches of the left coronary artery. The thrombosis was not evident till I laid open the walls of the vessel throughout their course in searching for an explanation of the infarcts. The patient died from uræmia, and not from the coronary thrombosis, which from the microscopic appearances of the infarcts had apparently taken place some little time before.

**Embolism.**—This is far less common, according to Welch,* than thrombosis. It may occur in pernicious endocarditis from detachment of a fragment of an affected valve, or possibly in atheromatous degeneration of the aorta, from detachment of a portion of a thrombus adherent to the diseased surface. Embolism of the coronary arteries gives rise to results similar to those of thrombosis described

* Allbutt's "System of Medicine," vol. vi. p. 281.

above, namely, sudden death or infarction, according as a main branch or an intramuscular branch is affected; but whereas death due to thrombosis may be preceded by premonitory symptoms from the more gradual nature of the onset of thrombosis, death due to embolism must, when it occurs, be absolutely sudden.

Aneurysm of the coronary arteries is rare. It may result from local weakening of the vessel by atheroma or syphilitic disease, or from acute softening of the arterial wall due to lodgment of septic emboli on its inner aspect in pernicious endocarditis.

Huchard* gives an account of eleven cases which he has collected from international literature. In all except two the aneurysms were associated with atheromatous degeneration of the coronary vessels. In the remaining two the patients were young, 21 and 22; the aneurysms were multiple; pyrexia was present in one case of obscure origin, in the other the patient had suffered from malarial fever. In nine of the cases sudden death occurred from rupture of the coronary aneurysm.

In the St. Mary's Hospital Museum is a specimen with thirteen small aneurysms of the coronary artery of embolic origin, from a case of pernicious endocarditis in a girl aged ten.

There are no symptoms or physical signs by which aneurysm of the coronary arteries can be diagnosed during life. They must, however, necessarily impair the circulation in the heart, and most commonly they rupture and cause sudden death.

* "Mal. du Cœur," vol. i. pp. 232 *et seq.*

# CHAPTER XXIII.

## AFFECTIONS OF THE MYOCARDIUM.

ACUTE MYOCARDITIS—FIBROID CHANGE—ETIOLOGY AND MORBID ANATOMY—SYPHILITIC AFFECTIONS OF THE MYOCARDIUM—PHYSICAL SIGNS AND SYMPTOMS OF FIBROSIS—DIAGNOSIS—PROGNOSIS—TREATMENT.

ACUTE interstitial myocarditis occurs most commonly in association with pericarditis or endocarditis. It is not simply due to direct extension of the inflammatory process from the pericardium or endocardium along the connective tissue network to the subjacent muscular substance, but, as Poynton* has shown, in rheumatic pericarditis and endocarditis there is usually a general "carditis," a term suggested by the late Dr. Sturges, and implying inflammation of the heart throughout its substance.

**Morbid Anatomy.**—The inflammatory changes are usually best marked in cases of subacute pericarditis that prove fatal. On microscopic examination, the nuclei in the interstitial tissue are seen to be increased in number owing to exudation of leucocytes between the muscle fibres and proliferation of the connective tissue cells. In pernicious endocarditis large masses of micrococci, surrounded by an inflammatory zone of polynuclear leucocytes, may sometimes be seen in the substance of the heart wall as shown in the illustration (Fig. 20), where the muscle fibres in the neighbourhood are destroyed and broken up. The

* *Med. Chi. Trans.*, May, 1899.

muscular fibres are affected in varying degree, those near the surface, as a rule, more than those in the deeper layers. Of some, nothing will remain but a mass of granular material; others have lost their striation, and are swollen and opaque; others are in a state of cloudy swelling, and some may appear to be little altered. The changes will be more marked and general in proportion to the duration and severity of the inflammation.

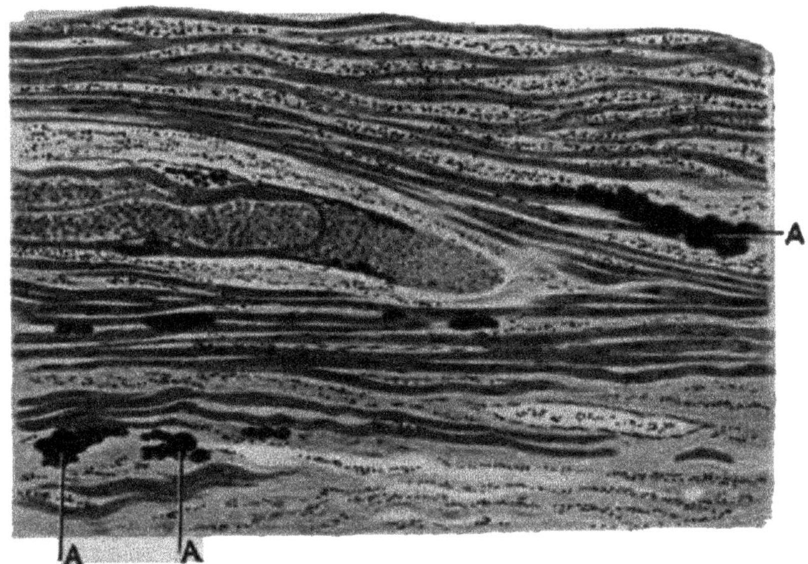


FIG. 20.—SECTION OF HEART MUSCLE FROM A CASE OF PERNICIOUS ENDOCARDITIS, SHOWING ACUTE INTERSTITIAL MYOCARDITIS. MASSES OF MICRO-ORGANISMS ARE SEEN AT A, A, A, AND THERE IS WIDESPREAD INFILTRATION OF POLYNUCLEAR LEUCOCYTES WITH DESTRUCTION OF MUSCLE FIBRES.

**Physical Signs.**—In the early stages, acute myocarditis gives rise to no definite physical signs or symptoms by which its existence can be diagnosed with any degree of certainty. When present, the physical signs will be those indicative of progressive cardiac dilatation or asthenia, or of both combined. The signs of cardiac dilatation will be, increase in the area of cardiac dulness with displacement of the apex beat downwards and outwards, and weakening of the first sound, the impulse becoming, at the same time, diffuse and tapping in character. The signs of cardiac asthenia will be feebleness or loss of the apex beat, with weak and short heart sounds, and a frequent, short, and easily compressible pulse. When acute myocarditis occurs in association with pericarditis of rheumatic origin, the cardiac dilatation is rapid and considerable, and signs of cardiac weakness and embarrassment appear early in the course of the disease.

**Prognosis.**—The prognosis depends on the extent to which the cardiac muscle is affected by the inflammatory process. Myocarditis is, however, almost invariably associated with pericarditis or endocarditis, affecting the prognosis in these affections very materially. This has already been referred to in the chapter on pericarditis, where the prognosis of the combined affections is fully discussed. After the acute attack has subsided, the muscle fibres which have been destroyed are replaced by fibrous tissue, which leads to serious weakening of the heart wall. Consequently, the heart will be liable to break down under any unusual exertion, and the various symptoms associated with fibroid changes in the heart walls may set in at a later period.

**Treatment.**—There is no special treatment beyond that for the pericarditis and rheumatism usually associated with it.

**Cloudy Swelling.**—Under the head of myocardial inflammation are included the changes in the cardiac muscle, known as "cloudy swelling," or albuminoid degeneration, which occur in certain diseases attended by high and prolonged fever, such as septicæmia, pneumonia, enteric fever, scarlet fever, rheumatism, etc. Cloudy swelling is not confined to the heart, but is found at the same time in the liver, kidney, and spleen, and appears to be due, mainly, if not entirely, to toxins evolved by the micro-organisms which are responsible for the disease. The changes differ from those found in acute interstitial myocarditis just described, inasmuch as they are mainly confined to the muscular fibres.

**Morbid Anatomy.**—The interstitial tissue is not as a rule affected, though some cellular exudation may be present, the changes being chiefly manifest in the muscle fibres. These are swollen, their striation is indistinguishable, and they are rendered opaque by the fine granules which pervade their substance and obscure their nuclei. The granules are composed of an albuminoid material, soluble in acetic acid, after treatment with which the muscular fibres seem to almost regain their normal appearance. The condition of cloudy swelling is frequently followed by fatty degeneration of the muscle fibres, if the fever is prolonged or the toxæmia is severe.

**Physical Signs and Symptoms.**—The physical signs and symptoms are those of progressive cardiac asthenia. The first sound of the heart becomes gradually weaker and shorter, and the apex beat more and more feeble till it is scarcely perceptible. There is seldom any marked dilatation of the ventricles in the earlier stages, as is the case in the interstitial myocarditis of rheumatism. The pulse is increased in frequency, easily compressible, and often markedly dichrotic.

**Prognosis.**—The prognosis is that of the disease to which the cardiac condition is secondary.

**Treatment.**—Stimulants such as brandy or ether may be necessary, together with strychnine, which is usually more effective when given hypodermically. Sometimes digitalis in small doses is of benefit during convalescence, but it should not be given while fever is present, as the damaged muscle fibres are not in a condition to profit by increase of tone, and the increase of peripheral resistance would entail more work on the heart.

## Fibroid Change in the Heart Walls.

Two main varieties of fibroid change in the heart wall may be distinguished—

(1) A substitution of fibrous tissue for muscle fibres which have been damaged or destroyed by disease.

(2) A patchy or diffuse fibrosis of the heart associated with marked degenerative changes in the coronary vessels. The question as to whether this fibroid change is a direct result of disease of the coronary vessels, or whether it is the result of a chronic interstitial inflammation, or whether some of these cases should be classified in Group I., will be discussed later.

**Etiology.**—1. In the process of repair, cicatricial fibrous tissue may take the place of muscle fibres destroyed by acute myocarditis due to some acute bacterial infection, by gummata, or by acute softening the result of embolism or thrombosis of branches of the coronary arteries.

Huchard * gives a remarkable illustration of areas of dense fibrosis in the heart wall, produced experimentally by Mollard,† by repeated inoculations of diphtheria toxin, the fibrous tissue having been formed in the process of repair to replace the muscle fibres which have been destroyed by the toxin. This important experimental evidence shows that acute toxæmias may be responsible, if the patient recovers, for areas of dense patchy fibrosis, which later on may give rise to apparently unaccountable symptoms of myocardial weakness. In a very extreme case of fibrosis of the heart, which I mounted for the St. Mary's Hospital Museum, and which is figured in the text (Fig. 21), about two-thirds of the heart wall consists of dense fibrous tissue. The endocardium was also of a dense white opaque colour,

* "Maladies du Cœur," vol. i. p. 214.

† "Sclérose du Myocarde," *Ann. de l'Institut Pasteur*, 1897.

and the mitral valve were thickened and rigid, though there

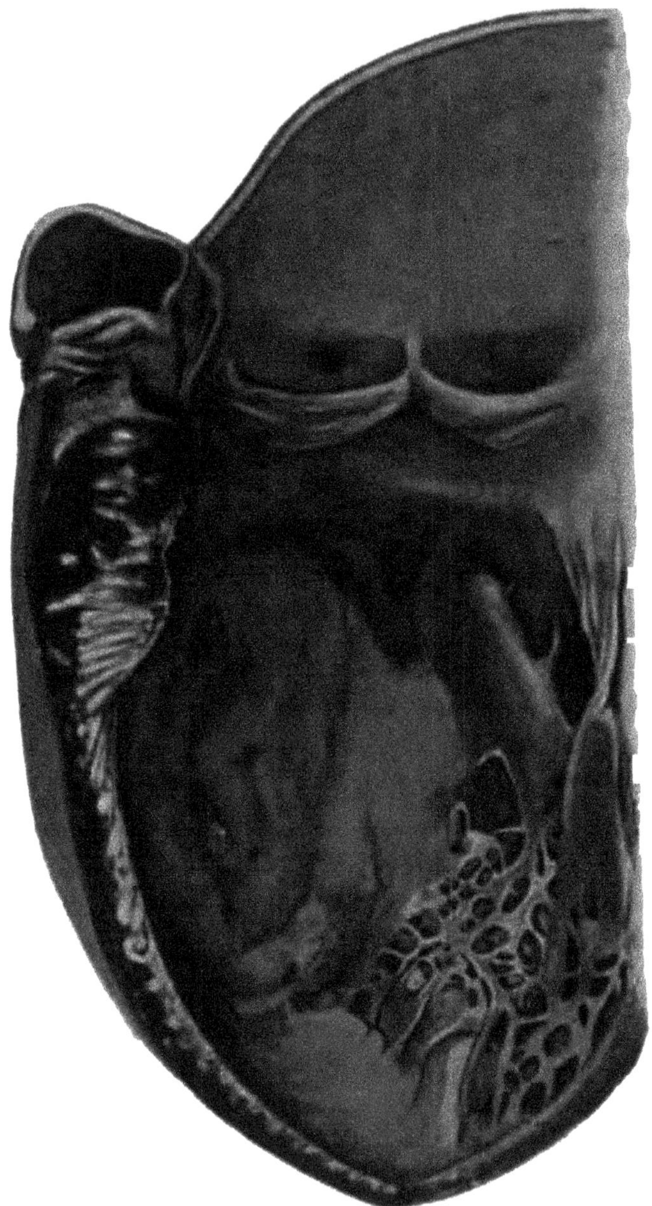

FIG. 21.—HEART SHOWING AN EXTREME DEGREE OF FIBROSIS OF THE WALLS AND ENDOCARDIUM.

was no actual loss of substance. The coronary arteries were patent, and not rigid or thickened. The heart was dilated, but not hypertrophied. Microscopically, the white opaque tissue, of which the bulk of the heart wall consists, was seen to consist of very dense old fibrous tissue, in which here and there were seen muscular fibres isolated from their fellows, some in a fair state of preservation. The vessels were not obliterated or markedly narrowed. The condition suggests that this cicatricial fibrous tissue has replaced muscular fibres destroyed at one time by a severe toxæmia, possibly the result of acute endocarditis, with accompanying myocarditis. The heart was obtained from a woman aged 61, who was brought in dead to St. Mary's Hospital, having succumbed to a sudden syncopal attack. Unfortunately, therefore, no history could be obtained.

2. Weigert drew attention to what he considers an important cause of fibroid changes in the heart wall, namely, sclerosis of the coronary arteries. He states that when the cardiac circulation is slowly interfered with by sclerosis of the coronary arteries, atrophy of the muscle fibres takes place without destruction of connective tissue, and that the shrunken and atrophied fibres are gradually replaced by fibrous tissue.

Huchard * also considers that obliterative lesions or endarteritis of the coronary arteries are the most common cause of patchy fibrosis, or, as he terms it, of "sclérose dystrophique." He holds that the fibrosis is the result of a primary degenerative change in the muscle fibres due to their deprivation of nutriment, and that this necrosis of the muscle fibres sets up an irritative proliferation in their neighbourhood, with resulting formation of fibrous tissue. He gives illustrations † of patchy fibrosis in the heart wall with obliterated vessels in their neighbourhood, and states that "there is never well-marked sclerosis without accompanying endarteritis." ‡

* "Maladies du Cœur," vol. i. † Ibid., pp. 215, 240, 241.
‡ Ibid., p. 242.

He considers that a diagnosis can be made between chronic myocarditis and what he terms "sclérose dystrophique." In both affections symptoms of myocardial weakness will be a prominent feature, namely, dyspnœa on exertion, feebleness of the apex beat and the first sound, enlargement of the area of cardiac dulness, and perhaps congestion of the bases of the lungs from dilatation and back working. Certain symptoms, however, will be peculiar to "sclérose dystrophique," for inasmuch as it is due to sclerosis of the cardiac vessels, there will be evidence of vascular degeneration elsewhere, or of high arterial tension, which is usually associated with it, namely, thickening of the radials, dilatation of the aorta, tortuous degenerated brachials, and possibly cerebral hæmorrhage may occur.

In addition, there may be angina pectoris from the narrowing of the coronary arteries.

Lindsay Steven,* in a paper on the subject, gives a series of twenty-one cases of cardiac fibrosis, which bear out Weigert's observations, and in a later communication,† discussing the difficult question as to why obstruction to the coronary circulation should in some cases give rise to fatty degeneration and in others to fibrosis, comes to the following conclusion :—

"In cases where the main coronary artery is slowly obstructed, and at last completely occluded at its origin, generalized fatty degeneration is likely to occur, and the cause is similar to that in profound anæmia, namely, deterioration in the supply of blood to the whole organ.

"When smaller branches are slowly obstructed but the main branches remain patent, slight fatty degeneration may result with localized fibrosis."

He bases his conclusions on a study of twenty-one cases, in nine of which fatty degeneration was present as well as fibrosis. In nearly all his cases the heart was hypertrophied,

* *Journal of Path. and Bact.*, 1894. † *Lancet*, 1887, vol. ii.

nd in nine there was chronic interstitial nephritis and in seven atheroma of the aorta.

It is easy to conceive, and we have ample evidence that sclerosis of the coronary arteries may give rise to fatty degeneration and atrophy of the muscle fibres by interference with their nutrition, but it is difficult to understand how it can give rise to fibrosis, though the two conditions are undoubtedly very frequently associated. Huchard considers that the narrowing of the coronary arteries causes death of the muscle fibres supplied by its terminal branches, and that this necrobiosis sets up an irritative inflammation in the adjoining areas.

Some authors consider that fibroid change in the heart is the result of chronic inflammation. Bristowe applied the term "cirrhosis" of the heart to this condition, and Friedreich and Lancereaux speak of chronic interstitial myocarditis as responsible for cardiac fibrosis.

Gibson * includes under the head of chronic myocarditis all conditions in which there is general or local increase of fibrous tissue in the myocardium. Among the causes he includes—

(1) Factors modifying the condition of the blood, *e.g.* lithæmia, glycæmia, and faulty conditions of the blood arising from defective metabolism.

(2) Infective diseases such as enteric fever, also syphilis.

(3) All changes in the coronary arteries, whether affecting their walls or lumen.

Huchard considers that a true chronic interstitial myocarditis is rare, if, indeed, it occurs, as he holds that destruction of muscle fibres precedes fibrosis, and that this is most commonly dependent on sclerosis of the coronary vessels.

In examining hypertrophied hearts from cases of

* "Diseases of the Heart and Aorta," p. 681.

Bright's disease, in which there was slight diffuse interstitial change or fibrosis, I have found that the most marked change was in the muscle fibres, namely, swelling, absence of staining, and breaking up of the nuclei (karyorhexis), as in Fig. 22, at the poles of which in the muscle fibres were granules of brown pigment, similar to those seen in brown atrophy of the heart. In these cases death had occurred from cerebral hæmorrhage, and not from heart failure.

In other cases of hypertrophied hearts associated with

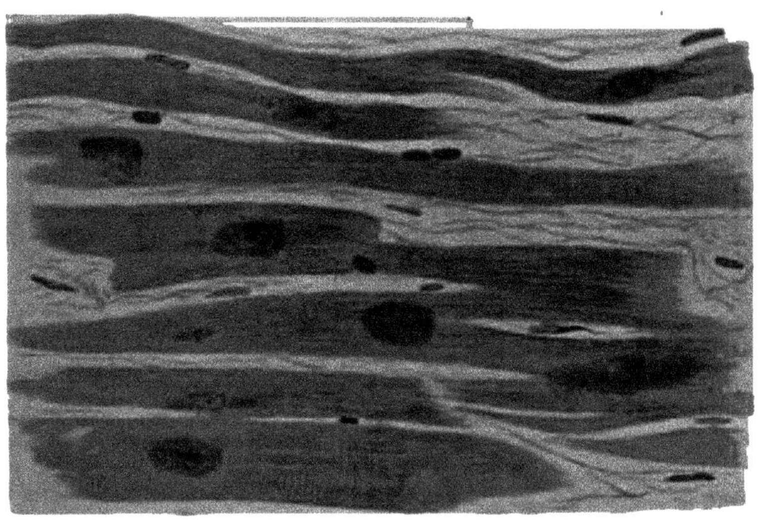

FIG. 22.—SECTION OF MUSCLE FROM HYPERTROPHIED HEART, SHOWING SWELLING, LOSS OF STAINING REACTION, AND BREAKING UP OF NUCLEI, WITH DEPOSIT OF GRANULES OF BROWN PIGMENT AT THEIR POLES.

high arterial tension and general arterio-sclerosis, not attributable to Bright's disease, in which death occurred from heart failure, I have found similar changes in the muscle fibres, with areas of patchy fibrosis, as seen in Fig. 23. These would come under Huchard's category of "sclérose dystrophique," as they were associated with atheroma of the coronary arteries and general arterio-sclerosis.

Possibly, in some cases of cardiac fibrosis associated with atheroma of the coronary arteries, destruction of muscle fibres and substitution of fibrous tissue for them occurs at an earlier date than the degenerative changes in the vessels, as a result of some acute toxæmia. Later on the vessels are affected, and sclerosis of the coronary arteries takes place, which would tend to cause fatty degeneration in muscle fibres previously undamaged, and thus explain the presence of fibrosis and fatty degeneration side by

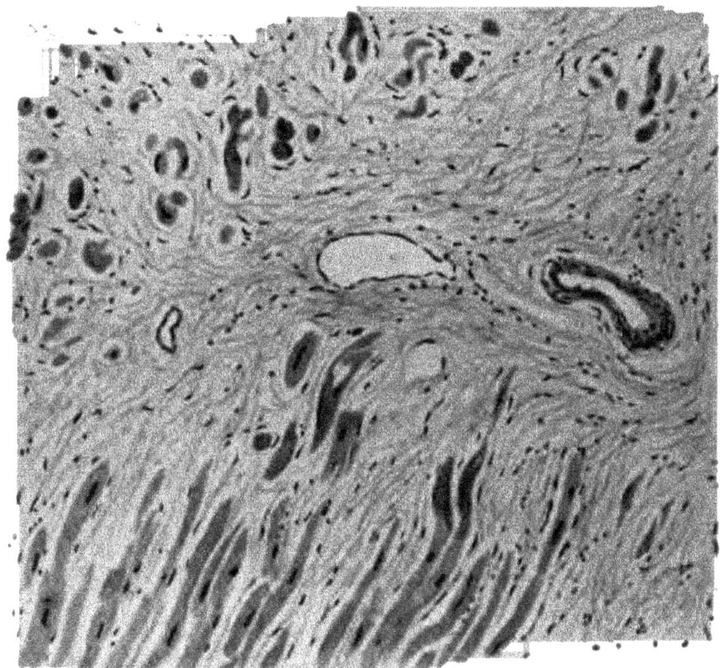

FIG. 23.—SECTION OF HEART WALL, SHOWING AREA OF FIBROSIS ASSOCIATED WITH ATHEROMA OF THE CORONARY ARTERIES.

side in the same heart, as drawn attention to by Lindsay Steven.

It is probable that syphilis is an etiological factor in a certain proportion of cases, fibrosis resulting either from cicatrization of gummata, or possibly occurring in association with endarteritis and periarteritis of the coronary vessels.

The illustration (Fig. 24) is a striking instance of fibrosis associated with extreme narrowing of the smaller branches of the coronary arteries, the lumen of which was almost obliterated. The specimen came from a woman aged 37, who died suddenly. The heart was hypertrophied, and the aorta was atheromatous, but there was no kidney disease. The age of the patient and the condition of the vessels, which is that of endarteritis obliterans, strongly suggest syphilis as the cause.

Syphilitic affections of the heart wall are not very

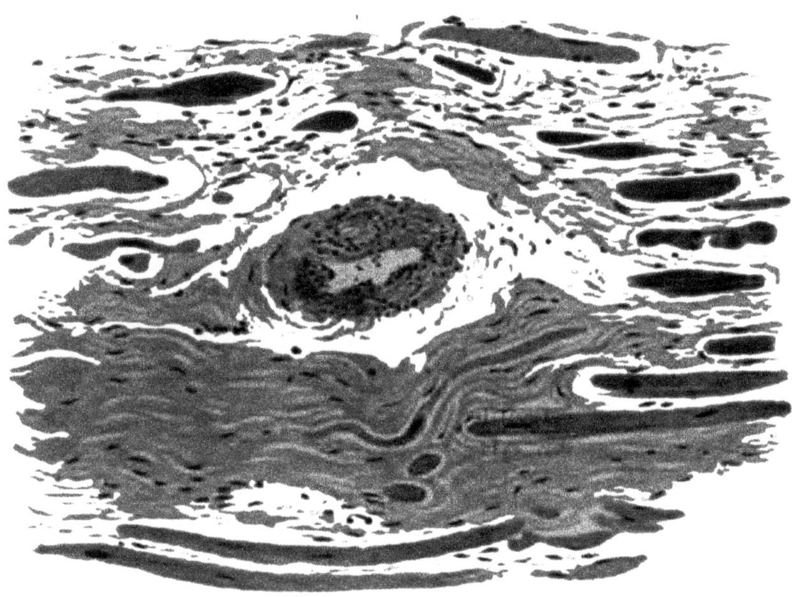

FIG. 24.—SECTION OF HEART WALL, SHOWING FIBROSIS ASSOCIATED WITH ENDARTERITIS OBLITERANS PROBABLY OF SYPHILITIC ORIGIN.

common, but are doubtless frequently overlooked. Sidney Phillips,* in a paper on this subject, recorded twenty-five cases described by various authors, together with some which had come under his own observation. In the majority of these cases gummata were the lesions found, and the diagnosis was only made on the post-mortem table.

**Physical Signs and Symptoms.**—In cases associated with coronary sclerosis and general vascular degeneration, the

* *Lancet*, 1897, vol. i. p. 223.

patient, usually middle-aged or elderly, may complain of breathlessness, palpitation, præcordial oppression, or of anginoid pains. He will usually be a man who has lived well, or who has led an arduous and strenuous life. The arterial tension will be high and the radial vessel thickened somewhat. The heart will be hypertrophied to a varying degree. There will usually be breathlessness on exertion, and possibly slight œdema of the legs, which subsides after a night's rest in bed. The pulse may be irregular, and the arterial tension moderate or low, because of the failing power of the heart. A sudden syncopal attack may prove fatal before any symptoms of a nature to cause anxiety have arisen. This is especially liable to occur in cases where there is marked narrowing of the coronary arteries or rigidity due to degenerative changes, and the sudden death is to be attributed to this cause and resulting ischemia of the heart rather than to the fibroid changes in the cardiac muscle. Cerebral hæmorrhage is liable to occur, as degenerative changes are frequently present in the cerebral vessels. Cheyne-Stokes respiration may develop in association with this, and is often pronounced and persistent.

In other cases there may be distressing dyspnœa at night of the type of uræmic asthma.

When cardiac fibrosis is the result of cicatrization after damage to the muscle by some severe toxæmia, there may be at a later date dilatation of the heart, for which there is no apparent cause; dropsy may set in, with engorgement of the lungs and other symptoms of back working and right ventricle failure, and the condition of cardiac fibrosis is not suspected during life.

**Diagnosis.**—As may be gathered from what has been previously said, the diagnosis of this condition is one of considerable difficulty, and is to a great extent a matter of inference during life, and can only be determined with certainty by a post-mortem examination. When, however, in association with evidence of vascular degeneration, the heart is hypertrophied, and there are breathlessness, anginal pains, a tendency to syncopal or apoplectiform attacks, with a failing pulse, one may suspect fibrosis; but there are no characteristic features by which this can be diagnosed from other degenerative changes in the heart muscle.

**Prognosis.**—This is necessarily unfavourable, inasmuch as cardiac fibrosis is usually associated with degenerative changes in the vascular system as a whole, and in the coronary and cerebral vessels in particular. Because of the associated sclerosis of the coronary arteries, death may result from sudden syncope without previous warning, or anginal attacks may set in, one of which eventually proves fatal. Cerebral hæmorrhage is liable to occur, giving rise to hemiplegia, and is frequently associated with Cheyne-Stokes respiration of a pronounced and distressing type. This may develop in the absence of cerebral hæmorrhage, and is always of serious prognostic significance.

Frequency or irregularity of pulse usually are unfavourable indications, if persistent, and not due to reflex causes; but in one case in which irregularity was present to a marked degree, with breathlessness on exertion and slight œdema of the legs, the patient, after a month's rest in bed, regained his health, and by care in his mode of life survived for six years, though the pulse remained irregular all the time. Eventually he succumbed to a sudden syncopal attack.

In another case, apparently similar at the outset, the patient, three months after he sought medical advice, had an attack of cerebral hæmorrhage, associated with Cheyne-Stokes respiration. He began to recover some power in the affected side, but a month later had another attack of cerebral hæmorrhage, which proved fatal.

Possibly, in fibrosis associated with syphilitic endarteritis, the prognosis is more favourable if an early diagnosis could be made and suitable treatment carried out, but this is scarcely possible in the majority of cases, and even on careful microscopic examination post-mortem it is difficult to be sure of a syphilitic origin.

According to the statistics of the cases collected by Sidney Phillips, gummata usually give rise to no definite physical signs or symptoms, and death is liable to occur from a sudden syncopal attack, or possibly rupture of the heart. Aneurysm of the heart may be a result of a gumma, or, in the most favourable cases, cicatrization, with a resulting patch of fibrosis.

Apart from syphilis, the cases in which the prognosis is most favourable are those in which the fibrosis is the result of cicatrization after damage to the heart muscle by acute myocarditis. It is probable that in many cases no symptoms arise until later on in life, when possibly degenerative changes may set in in the previously undamaged muscle, associated with sclerosis of the coronary vessels. In other cases, where the lesion is severe, cardiac dilatation may result, for which there is no apparent cause, and which resists all treatment, and it is only on careful microscopical examination of the heart muscle post mortem that the explanation is manifest.

Treatment.—This must be directed to relieving the heart of work as far as possible. Moderation in food and drink, and regularity of meals must be enjoined, to avoid undue variations of blood pressure; and measures must be taken for the lowering of arterial tension if this be excessive. For this purpose mercurial purgatives combined with colocynth and hyoscyamus should be given once a week, or oftener if required, and vaso-dilators, such as erythrol tetranitrate or liquor trinitrin, should be administered, and continued for a long period if necessary. Rest in bed must be insisted on when warning symptoms such as breathlessness on slight exertion, or œdema of the extremities are

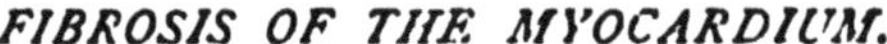

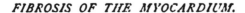

present. Iodide of potassium is useful not only in syphilitic fibrosis, but in all cases where there is general thickening of the arteries and evidence of atheroma. Cardiac tonics, such as strychnine, nux vomica, and arsenic, may often be given with marked benefit, but digitalis and its congeners are seldom indicated.

## CHAPTER XXIV.

## AFFECTIONS OF THE MYOCARDIUM (*Continued*).

DISTINCTION BETWEEN FATTY INFILTRATION OF OBESITY AND FATTY DEGENERATION—CAUSATION OF FATTY DEGENERATION — SYMPTOMS — SPONTANEOUS RUPTURE OF THE HEART—PHYSICAL SIGNS—DIAGNOSIS—PROGNOSIS—TREATMENT—ANEURYSM AND NEW GROWTHS OF THE HEART.

### Fatty Degeneration.

No form of heart disease is regarded with so much apprehension as fatty degeneration. More than any other, it carries with it the danger of sudden death and the liability to angina pectoris, and, although happily it is not very common, it would be a most important acquisition to be able to make the diagnosis with certainty at an early period.

It must be understood from the first that fatty infiltration or the fat-laden heart of obesity does not come under the designation of fatty degeneration, and it may be dismissed from further consideration with a few words. In advanced life there is a tendency to the formation of adipose tissue beneath the visceral pericardium, especially along the course of the coronary arteries. In obese persons and those addicted to alcohol, more especially beer drinkers, the amount may become considerable, so that the entire heart may be encased in fat, and adipose deposit may penetrate between the muscular fibres. When such is the case, the heart will be hampered in its action, and a further source of embarrassment will be present in fatty deposit on the surface of the diaphragm and in the omentum.

**Fatty Infiltration.**—In fatty infiltration there is a deposit of fat between the muscle fibres, which may be traced, on careful examination, as a down-growth from the overlying layer of fat around the heart. There is no deposit of fatty material in the muscular fibres themselves, as is the case in fatty degeneration. It is possible that compression of muscle fibres by intervening fat may lead to atrophy of some of them, and it is of course possible that there may be fatty degeneration as well as fatty infiltration, but the two are quite distinct processes, and are due to different causes.

Distressing shortness of breath may be produced by such fatty deposit and infiltration, and not uncommonly there is a certain degree of œdema about the ankles and along the tibiæ at night, especially in hot or relaxing weather. Such patients are especially liable to succumb to acute infections such as pneumonia, typhoid fever, etc., and usually take anæsthetics badly. The condition, however, is not attended with the same danger as actual degeneration of the muscular fibres or with the characteristic symptoms.

**Fatty Degeneration: Morbid Anatomy.**—Virchow taught that in the liver the presence of fat in the cells might be merely the result of physiological infiltration, but that in the heart the appearance of fatty globules in the muscle fibres was invariably due to a retrogressive change in which there was actual conversion of the degenerated protoplasm into fat. Hence the term "fatty degeneration."

In 1901 Rosenfeld * carried out a series of experiments on animals, tending to show that in the heart, as in the liver, the fat found in the interior of the muscle fibres is

* *Cent. fur Inn. Med.*, 1901, p. 145.

really an infiltration, and is not formed from the degenerated protoplasm, but brought from fat stores elsewhere in the body and deposited in the damaged muscle.

The presence of fat in the cardiac muscle fibres, however, even though it be due to infiltration, and not a degeneration in Virchow's sense of the term, is pathological, the result of a retrogressive morbid change, and, to avoid confusion, the term "fatty degeneration" will here be retained to denote this condition.

In advanced fatty degeneration the heart substance will be pale and softer than normal, so that the finger can be readily thrust into it; the musculi papillares will usually have a streaky appearance, the so-called "tabby-cat" striation, due to pale strands of fattily degenerated muscular substance, being interspersed among healthy fibres.

Microscopically, on staining with osmic acid, it will be seen that the deposits of fat are in the muscle fibres themselves, and not between them. The tiny globules of fat first make their appearance at the poles of the muscle nuclei, but eventually the degenerative process extends throughout the muscle fibre, so that it loses its striated appearance, and is seen to be filled with globules of fat.

When unstained, the granular appearance of the degenerated fibres might be mistaken for the condition of "cloudy swelling" or albuminoid degeneration; but the distinction is readily made by treating the section with acetic acid, which does not affect fat globules, but dissolves the albuminoid granules, or by staining with osmic acid, which gives quite characteristic appearances.

## Etiology.

1. Sclerosis of the coronary arteries or obstruction of these vessels by endarteritis is one of the most important causes of fatty degeneration. The heart—perpetually at

work—cannot afford to be mulcted of its full supply of blood. When, from any cause, this is defective, the wear and tear of the muscular fibres, which must go on, is not repaired, and their structure breaks down. Whether the fatty granules and globules which are found within the sarcolemma are deposited there, or are derived from the atrophied sarcous elements, is not a matter of great consequence. The important point is that the primary change is atrophy of the muscle substance, the invasion of the fibres by fatty matter being secondary to this and consequent upon it.

Disease of the coronary arteries, being thus a cause of fatty degeneration of the heart, the existence of conditions which may lead to the implication of the coronary arteries or their orifices in morbid processes, will warrant a suspicion that any cardiac weakness which may be recognized is the result of degeneration. For example, an aortic murmur coming on after middle age may not indicate serious valvular lesion, but, as it is probably the result of atheromatous changes in the valves or arterial walls in close proximity to the orifices of the coronary arteries, there is reason to apprehend that the disease may cause obstruction here or may have extended to the vessels themselves, and progressive weakness of the heart, were this to supervene, would be attributable to degenerative change in its walls.

Acute aortitis, again, may in the same way give rise to blocking of the mouths of the coronary arteries. A like apprehension attaches to syphilitic disease of the aorta and its valves, which is not uncommon in early middle life, and especially to endarteritis obliterans affecting the coronary arteries.

2. Apart from disease of the coronary arteries, there is a large and varied group of causes which may give rise to fatty degeneration of the heart, comprising—

(*a*) Certain poisons: phosphorus, arsenic, and phlorizin.

(*b*) Acute yellow atrophy of the liver.

(c) Acute or prolonged toxæmia of bacterial origin, e.g. typhoid fever, diphtheria, erysipelas, pneumonia, and long-continued suppuration.

True fatty degeneration is by no means always present in these affections, and the morbid change commonly found is limited to so-called "cloudy swelling," or albuminoid degeneration.

(d) Carcinoma, phthisis, diabetes, and pernicious anæmia.

Fatty change in the heart may thus be due to toxins present in the blood, either ingested or of bacterial origin, or to deterioration in the quality of the blood from morbid processes elsewhere in the body. Consequently, the clinical features in this group, apart from the signs of increasing cardiac asthenia, do not specially point to the heart as the seat of disease, but are those of the primary affection.

It is otherwise with the more serious form of fatty degeneration associated with disease of the coronary arteries, in which anginoid attacks and sudden death from syncope are liable to occur.

It is a disputed point whether the sclerosis and narrowing of the coronary vessels or the fatty change in the muscle fibres is immediately responsible for the sudden cardiac failure in these cases.

Huchard * attributes the symptoms in angina pectoris entirely to the coronary sclerosis. Gibson † and Douglas Powell ‡ admit the importance of fatty degeneration as a possible cause of angina and sudden syncope. Pratt, § in a recent paper on the causes of cardiac insufficiency, concludes with the somewhat sweeping statement "that there is no evidence to show that fatty metamorphosis of the heart produces cardiac insufficiency," adding, "that in the light of our present knowledge, anatomical considerations,

* "Maladies du Cœur," vol. ii. p. 1.

† "Diseases of the Heart and Aorta," p. 765.

‡ Allbutt's "System of Medicine," vol. v. p. 891.

§ Bull. "John Hopkins Hospital," vol. xv. p. 102.

especially coronary sclerosis and interstitial myocarditis, must be regarded as the most common causes of heart failure."

He bases his conclusions partly on a series of pathological investigations carried out by himself, and partly on experiments on animals performed by Welch, Balint, Hasenfeld, and Fenyvessy. As the fatty change in these experiments was induced by phosphorous poisoning, which is an acute process due to an irritant poison, whereas the fatty degeneration under discussion is very slow in its onset and due to deficient blood supply, this evidence can scarcely be admitted. In spite also of the conclusions he draws from his own observations, it is impossible to accept the statement that fatty degeneration cannot be a cause of cardiac failure.

The fatty change, even if it be an infiltration, as argued by Rosenfeld, and not a "degeneration" in Virchow's sense of the term, is unquestionably a serious pathological condition, and the fat deposited in place of contractile protoplasm must necessarily impair the efficiency of the muscular fibres. That it is a serious lesion is further demonstrated by the fact that spontaneous rupture of the heart may occur.

It is not denied that sclerosis and narrowing of the coronary arteries is the most important and serious lesion, inasmuch as the fatty change is secondary to and dependent on this; but it is impossible to determine whether syncopal attacks and sudden death in these cases are due to ischemia of the heart from coronary stenosis, or to inability of the fat-laden, atrophied muscle to respond to the call when extra work is thrown upon it. The latter is, at any rate, quite sufficient, and it can be recognized clinically. The former can only be inferred. Many of the symptoms and physical signs of fatty degeneration associated with coronary stenosis, as will be seen later, can scarcely be ascribed directly to the vascular lesion, but are significant of failing muscular power of the heart.

## SYMPTOMS.

There is little that is characteristic in the symptoms unless we consider angina pectoris to be such, and definitely associate it with fatty degeneration of the heart. The relation between the two is undoubtedly very frequent but is not constant, and angina is therefore reserved for special and separate consideration.

In a large proportion of cases the subject of this affection has had no ailment which has led him to consult a medical man when he is overtaken by sudden death during exertion or excitement, or after a full meal. Or, the excitement and exertion may be passed through safely and death follow some hours later, next day even. Among the causes which precipitate a sudden fatal termination, dilatation of the stomach is frequent. Digestion is usually imperfect from advancing years, or as a result of sluggish circulation due to the state of the heart, and the tone of the muscular coats of the stomach is impaired, allowing of passive distension by the contained gases, the products of fermentation. The upward expansion of the stomach is moreover often facilitated by a weak and relaxed condition of the diaphragm, so that the upper line of gastric resonance can not unfrequently be traced horizontally across from the root of the ensiform cartilage to the usual situation of the apex beat in the fifth space. Such a condition is attended with immediate danger when there is degeneration of the heart walls, and may cause sudden death by pressure on the heart, long before this would have resulted from the state of the heart alone.

Rupture of the heart is one mode of termination, and this may take place on very slight provocation. Sometimes the patient has been engaged in his usual avocation up to the moment of its occurrence. In one case which came under my observation, an old gentleman of quiet retired habits, with nothing beyond the weakness incident to age, was heard to knock at the wall against which his bed was placed, and was found dead, the bedclothes scarcely being disturbed. A neat slit was found in the left ventricle near the apex close to and parallel with the septum. In another case in which very advanced fatty degeneration of the heart was found to be present at the autopsy, associated with extreme stenosis of the coronary arteries, the diameter of which was less than a millimetre, spontaneous rupture took place during an attack of biliary colic. There had been no history of attacks of angina or any warning symptoms.

The bearing of such occurrences on prognosis is direct and simple. No doubt in many cases of sudden death there have been warnings which the patient has ignored or has not spoken of. These will sometimes be acknowledged in the course of examination when they have not been mentioned spontaneously.

When the course of the disease has been sufficiently chronic to permit of the recognition of symptoms, which in my experience is chiefly when the degeneration is secondary to change in the coronary arteries, they will be such as are produced by a slackening circulation, and they are not so different from those attending dilatation as to permit of any distinction being drawn between the two conditions in an early stage, without physical examination. There may, perhaps, be greater fluctuations in dilatation, though even in degeneration there may be great temporary improvement under care and treatment. In advanced stages characteristic differences make their appearance. The symptoms of advanced dilatation have already been described; those attending degeneration are evidences of heart failure of another kind. A noteworthy point is that well-marked dropsy is rare, and probably never occurs in uncomplicated degeneration. The significance of this is that the special effect of the disease is defective pressure in the arterial system; and it is to this are due the syncopal, apoplectic, and epileptiform attacks, which, together with the angina pectoris, are the most characteristic later effects of fatty degeneration.

The syncopal attacks vary greatly in intensity. So far as they have come under my observation, they have been marked rather by duration than intensity, and have rarely been so complete as to be attended with absence of consciousness; they have usually been accompanied by prolonged coldness of the extremities and of the surface. I have not met with instances of sudden and complete loss of consciousness and immediate recovery as in dilatation. These fainting attacks are very significant, and are often premonitory of fatal syncope.

The apoplectiform seizures are very remarkable, and in the absence of history and without examination they are not distinguishable from the apoplectic condition resulting from cerebral hæmorrhage. The patient is unconscious; the respiration, if he is allowed to lie flat on his back, may be stertorous—though stertor, after the teaching of Dr. Bowles, ought to be eliminated from the symptomatology of apoplexy—and there may be hemiplegia, but this will be fugitive. Cheyne-Stokes breathing, which was first observed in connection with fatty degeneration of the heart, has not been present in the few cases which I have actually seen in the apoplectiform state, while I have met with it in a very large number of cases of uræmic coma and in connection with serious consequences of high arterial tension. On examination of the pulse and heart, however, it will be clear that there cannot have been sufficient pressure in the arteries to rupture even the most degenerate vessel, and, on the other hand, thrombosis or embolism is not competent to produce unconsciousness of the character and duration of these attacks. According to my experience, the patient is never quite the same after an apoplectiform attack; he is feebler in mind and body, and sometimes increasingly liable to syncopal attacks.

The epileptiform attacks are not often violent, but resemble *petit mal* rather than a typical epileptic fit; while, however, the convulsion may not be so severe, there is profound unconsciousness—not like epileptic coma, but of a syncopal character—and the pulse may be extremely infrequent, sometimes less than twenty in the minute. In my judgment, the heart failure manifested by the slow pulse and the consequent arrest of the cerebral circulation are the cause of the fits, and it is not the epileptiform attack that affects the action of the heart.

By the time any of these forms of attack occur the diagnosis of fatty heart is usually sufficiently clear; but when they are associated with a very slow pulse, in which the strength and volume of the pulse and the degree of impulse of which the heart is capable preclude the idea of fatty degeneration, they are probably to be referred to the condition of Bradycardia known as Stokes-Adams disease, which is discussed in a later chapter.

An important question is whether there is anything characteristic in the appearance of a patient suffering from fatty degeneration of the heart? A greasy state of the skin with a sallow pallor of the face has been described, and if such a condition has supervened upon a previously healthy complexion the change would have significance, but nothing of the kind is present in a large majority of the cases. Many of the subjects of the disease retain the look of health for a long time, and even up to the moment when the heart ceases to beat. The degeneration may be due to a local cause—obstruction of the coronary arteries; and, even if a tendency to general deterioration of the tissues is present, the change mostly advances so much more rapidly in the heart than elsewhere, that there is no time for it to become conspicuous in the skin. The picture appears to have been drawn from cases of a universal chronic degeneration of vessels and heart. The arcus senilis again, which has been said to indicate the existence of cardio-vascular degeneration, has no such significance.

## Physical Signs.

**The Pulse.**—The most constant and significant feature of the pulse is that it is short and unsustained. The size of the artery at the wrist and the condition of its walls may vary greatly. When the arterial coats are healthy they are apt to feel extremely thin. The pulse rate may be regular and about normal, or extremely irregular both in force and time, and it may be frequent or slow. A very slow pulse with extreme low tension is most characteristic, but then it is the most rare.

**The Heart.**—The physical signs may be described as negative. Unless degeneration has attacked a heart already enlarged the size will be normal. If the fatty change is at all advanced, impulse can neither be seen nor felt, or, if perceptible, it is only as a faint vibration. A heart in this condition is incapable either of giving a distinct push or of maintaining continuous pressure in the arteries. The sounds are weak, sometimes so weak as to be almost inaudible; but except that the first is short, there is nothing abnormal about them; the intervals, again, are usually normal. The very absence of physical signs, such as murmur, or conspicuous modification of the sounds or intervals, or disturbance of the relation between the two sides of the heart, or increase of dimensions, when symptoms of serious slackening of the circulation are present, and especially when there have been anginal, or syncopal, or apoplectic attacks, adds gravity to the case.

But a weak, short, unsustained pulse is common as a constitutional peculiarity, or may at any period of life be simply a result of general debility, and impulse and apex beat may be entirely absent, and the sounds may be short and weak. In young people there is no danger of such weakness being taken to be indicative of degeneration of the heart, but it may arouse anxiety after middle age, especially if there is also irregularity in its action.

It is important to be able to distinguish between functional weakness of this kind and weakness arising from organic disease. Usually this is accomplished by making the patient walk briskly. A few steps will often be sufficient. If the heart is sound it rises to the occasion. The pulse, and beat, and sounds are all more distinct, and strong, and regular, whereas the fatty heart "goes to pieces," and the pulse becomes irregular and shorter than ever, or may even disappear.

Until the disease is far advanced the diagnosis of fatty degeneration of the heart is not easy, and is scarcely to be made without more than one opportunity of examination.

## Prognosis.

When the diagnosis has once been made, the prognosis, for the most part, can contemplate only one result; a fatal termination is merely a question of time and circumstance. Excluding cases in which death has been sudden without warning, the shortest period in my experience over which characteristic symptoms have extended, together with recognized physical signs, has been about six weeks; several patients have survived the diagnosis two years before justifying it by dying suddenly. But circumstance as well as time enters into the question; a slight effort, or a fall, a little hurry or excitement, too hearty a meal, an attack of flatulent indigestion or constipation, a chill, may hurry on the fatal termination; and on the other hand, judicious care may postpone it till the heart is completely worn out and comes to a standstill, or senile gangrene may result from the combined effects of cardiac and arterial degeneration.

The question must be asked, Is fatty degeneration of the heart ever cured or arrested? If the fatty change which may result from typhoid fever and other toxæmias is to be included under the term, the answer must undoubtedly be Yes. The heart may ultimately regain structural soundness and functional vigour when during the fever the first sound has been completely lost and the impulse has been scarcely perceptible; and when degeneration has been the result of other forms of blood poisoning or deterioration, it ought to be possible, and now and then to occur, that recovery of the heart should follow a return to a healthy state of the blood.

Twelve years before his death I came to the conclusion that a gentleman, aged at the time about 55, was suffering from fatty degeneration of the heart. Spare in habit, strictly moderate in eating and drinking, regular in taking exercise, and a great pedestrian, he rapidly lost strength without recognizable cause, became breathless on very slight exertion, so that he could scarcely walk slowly a hundred yards without actually stopping, either to get his breath, or on account of anginoid pain. On one occasion at least, while sitting in his chair he became suddenly pale and unconscious, his head fell on his chest, and the jaw dropped. With this change in his health, the pulse and heart were extremely weak. He would never relinquish exercise, but continued to walk, however slowly and at whatever cost of pain and distress, every day, exercising great self-command and measuring his strength very exactly. Little by little he gained ground, and attained fair health, but was capable of very little in the way of work, though never at any time were his intellectual faculties at all affected. Eventually he died suddenly in bed.

This case may have been an instance of arrest and partial recovery, but unfortunately no autopsy was obtainable.

## Treatment.

It must be acknowledged at the outset that it is not in our power to modify in the least degree the condition of the cardiac muscular fibre when far advanced in fatty degeneration, and that we can do very little, if anything, to arrest the progress of the deterioration when it has reached a stage at which it is recognizable either through symptoms or by physical signs. Even at a very early period we should doubt the possibility of reversing a process which in some cases is an inherited tendency to natural decay at a given time of life, in others an effect of imperfect blood supply due to narrowing of the coronary arteries.

If, indeed, the degeneration has been the result of acute disease, such as typhoid fever, time and care will bring about a restoration of the muscular fibres; but this is not fatty degeneration of the same nature as that due to coronary sclerosis, but is rather a secondary consequence of the condition of so-called cloudy swelling, which is a result of prolonged toxæmia.

When, again, the condition is not true degeneration of the muscular fibres, but a fatty heart, due to a sedentary life, with privation of fresh air and neglect of exercise, together with undue indulgence in alcoholic drinks and in the pleasures of the table, there is not then, at any rate till an advanced stage, true fatty degeneration, but a deposit of fat between the muscular fibres or fatty infiltration. In such cases careful dieting and graduated exercise, such as the Œrtel treatment, may reverse the degenerative tendency and even cause a gradual absorption of the fatty tissue already deposited in and around the heart as well as elsewhere.

While, however, acknowledging the limitation of therapeutics in dealing with the organic change, we are not altogether powerless to avert its consequences, and by so doing to prolong life. We see from time to time, on post-mortem examination, the heart so far gone in fatty change that it is scarcely recognizable as muscle, either to the naked eye or under the microscope. Such change must have been long in progress, and the subject of it must have lived for months if not for years, while the slightest obstruction in either pulmonary or systemic circulation would have brought the heart to a standstill, and a shock, a fall, or an indigestible meal, would have been fatal. We meet with cases of this kind during life, in which the decay of the mental and bodily powers is so slow as to be almost imperceptible, or in which thrombosis of one cerebral vessel after another brings the patient to a state of dementia or bed-ridden paralysis from general or local cerebral softening. Or the immediate cause of death may be senile gangrene. It is not that results such as those just named are desirable—death would be preferable were we allowed to choose—but cases of the kind serve, with others, to show that prolongation of life is possible when the central organ of the circulation can barely keep the blood in motion, and to illustrate the conditions under which this is observed. These conditions are a gradual diminution of mental and bodily activity, together with attention to diet and regulation of the bowels. The setting in of softening of the brain, or an attack of paralysis, not unfrequently seems to put an end to cardiac symptoms and to prolong life; the sufferer is no longer his own master; he cannot undertake business or go about, his food is under orders, and the action of the bowels is known to others besides himself.

If, in an early stage of fatty degeneration of the heart, the same command over the patient's mode of life and the same knowledge of the state of his secretions were attainable, not only might life be made longer by many years, but much suffering which is seen to arise out of this form of disease might be averted. It is unnecessary, and it would be impossible to enter into particulars with regard to the amount of work and exercise to be permitted, or the quantity and kind of food to be allowed; the latter may, and indeed in most cases must, be liberal and varied, but precautions must be taken against an inordinate appetite, and it is always safest to let some judicious relative or attendant who knows his likings and what suits him, help the patient at meals, and decide for him what dishes and what quantity will be good for him, acting under the advice of the medical man.

Proper regulation of the bowels is of the utmost importance. As years increase people are apt to become less observant, and to take it for granted that, so long as the habitual regularity in going to stool obtains, the action of the bowels is satisfactory and efficient, whereas it may be that the evacuation is much too small in amount. Accumulation thus gradually takes place, and it is not uncommon for a second daily call to relieve the bowels, resulting from this, to be regarded as evidence of improvement in their action. The statements of patients, then, with regard to this function, are not always trustworthy, and the testimony of a competent observer, or inspection by the medical man, is necessary. The quantity of fæcal matters which may unconsciously accumulate in the colon is astonishing, and the prevention of such an occurrence is essential to the well-doing of a patient whose heart is organically weak. For the regulation of the bowels mild aloetic aperients are best, with pil hydrarg. and colocynth occasionally in small doses, if there is arterial tension. Any tendency to flatulent distension of the stomach must be counteracted, as far as possible, by careful dieting and the administration of alkalies and carminatives. Bitter tonics may be given, and massage or gentle exercise is often of great service. Extremes of heat and cold should be avoided, and a dry, bracing, healthy spot in the country should be selected as a residence.

Aneurysm of the heart is of rare occurrence, and seldom gives rise to any physical signs or symptoms by which it can be diagnosed during life. It usually affects the left ventricle. It results from local destruction or weakening of a portion of the heart wall, which may be due to breaking down of a gumma, abscess from a septic embolus, softening from thrombosis, or embolism of a branch of the coronary artery.

It is usually lined by laminated clot, and varies in size. In one instance I have seen, the aneurysm was situated in the lower half of the wall of the left ventricle, and was three inches in diameter. It was completely filled up with layers of laminated clot. It gave rise to no distinctive physical signs or symptoms during life, and did not appear to be the immediate cause of death.

**New growths** of the heart are rarely, if ever, primary. Secondary growths are also very uncommon; but nodules of sarcomatous or carcinomatous growths in the heart wall are occasionally met with secondary to growths in other organs.

# CHAPTER XXV.

## ANGINA PECTORIS.

CHARACTERISTICS OF TRUE ANGINA—ASSOCIATED SYMPTOMS—EXCITING CAUSES OF PAROXYSMS—ETIOLOGY AND MORBID ANATOMY—DISCUSSION OF THEORIES ADVANCED TO EXPLAIN THE PAIN—DIAGNOSIS—PROGNOSIS—TREATMENT.

WHILE heart disease generally is remarkable for the almost entire freedom from pain—so that when patients come complaining of pain in the cardiac region, it is a presumption against the existence of any serious organic lesion rather than an indication of any such change—there is one form of pain in and around the heart, angina pectoris, which is very definite and constant in its significance of disease and danger. The term "angina pectoris," or pain in the chest, has come to have a specialized meaning, and is commonly employed to denote a complex group of symptoms associated with certain grave pathological changes in the heart and coronary arteries.

As an account of the distinctive features of "angina pectoris" involves a discussion of the associated symptoms, it will be more convenient to describe these first, and to defer the consideration of the etiology and morbid anatomy to a later period.

### CHARACTERISTICS OF TRUE ANGINA PECTORIS: ASSOCIATED SYMPTOMS.

In a typical attack of angina there is intense pain in some part of the cardiac region, most frequently behind the sternum, with radiation down the left arm, but occasionally across the upper part of the chest, in the left breast, or in the neighbourhood of the ensiform cartilage. Accompanying the pain is a sense of utter helplessness and extreme fear and dread. The patient keeps still, not daring to move, and feels as if he were in the act of dying. He will say afterwards that if the pain had lasted another moment he must have died. In no other condition is the physical agony of dying realized in the same degree. The two elements of pain and sense of impending death coexist in a true paroxysm of angina, and are almost equally characteristic.

The pain differs in character and situation and in intensity in different cases. Some sufferers will say it is indescribable—nothing in their previous experience suggests even a comparison; others speak of the pain as severe cramp in the heart, or as if the heart were gripped by an iron claw; while pain of a shooting, neuralgic character, sometimes intermittent, sometimes persistent, seems to radiate from the chest to the left shoulder, down the inner side of the arm to the forearm, and the ring and little fingers. Occasionally there is a sensation as of the wrist being grasped so tightly as to cause pain. With the pain in the heart there may be pain down both arms or shooting up into the left side of the neck, very rarely in the right arm only. Occasionally the pain may be felt first in the wrist or arm and seem to travel up to the chest, or may come in the inner side of the arm as a kind of warning of an attack. Another description of the pain is that it feels as if the sternum were being crushed back to the spine, or, again, as if the whole chest were being held in a vice. In other cases the pain is compared to a bar of iron across the upper part of the chest; in others, again, to a ton weight upon the lower part of the chest. The ramifications of the cardiac plexus and its communications with other nerves make the radiation of pain in all the various directions enumerated comprehensible, and the nerve of Wrisberg has been specially instanced as explaining the pain in the left arm, but no explanation can be given why in one case the pain is felt in one part of the cardiac region, and has some particular character, and takes a given direction down one arm or both or through to the back, while in another case the seat, character, and extension of the pain are quite different. It is not a pressure effect on the plexus outside the heart, neither heart nor aorta being necessarily enlarged, and fusiform dilatation of the arch of the aorta is common without anginoid pain; there can be no stretching or mechanical irritation of the nerve-ramifications beneath the endocardium at all comparable to that which takes place in acute dilatation of the heart. It seems to me that the pain is a danger signal given by the sensory nerves of the heart. The radiation of irritation giving rise to its extension takes place in the spinal cord, as will be shown in the next chapter.

An interesting point is that at the end of a paroxysm there is usually flatulent eructation from the stomach. The attacks are therefore very commonly attributed to flatulence, and distension of the stomach by food or gases may undoubtedly be, and often actually is, an exciting cause, but more frequently the sensation as of wind on the stomach is only a part of the general commotion, and is due to communicated or sympathetic irritation of the gastric distribution of the vagus, the cardiac branches of which are primarily implicated. The escape of gas from the stomach is often a signal that the paroxysm is over rather than the means of bringing it to an end. Occasionally there is a vehement desire to pass urine, although the bladder may at the time be empty.

The duration of the attacks is very varied; sometimes it can be reckoned in seconds. Most frequently, perhaps, a paroxysm will last a few minutes, but I have known a patient sit in the same position almost through an entire night, not venturing to make the slightest movement and scarcely seeming to breathe, while the perspiration rolled off his forehead and came through his clothes. According to my experience, it is when the attack comes on in the night, without provocation by exertion or exposure, that it is protracted. When it is started by exertion it generally ceases soon after the exertion is left off.

While it would not be justifiable to say that a patient was the subject of angina pectoris unless he had had one or more paroxysms of intense radiating pain, associated with a sense of immediately impending death, it must be admitted that attacks of true angina occur which fall short of the typical development. For example, when a patient has been taught prudence by one or more bad attacks, he may, by standing still on the first warning, or by taking remedies, cut short the paroxysm, which will then have been represented only by the initial pain in the breast or arm without the mortal dread. It is possible, therefore, that before any characteristic attack has occurred, pains of a similar kind and intensity, disregarded by the patient or relieved by rubbing the chest or arm, may have the same significance as a fully developed paroxysm.

Again, a patient who has had attacks of true angina may cease to suffer pain, but may have attacks of what he calls faintness, in one of which he ultimately dies. These, which have lost their title to the name angina, have an equally serious significance. They are sometimes called angina pectoris sine dolore.

The aspect of the patient is one of extreme anxiety or alarm. He is usually pale and often livid round the mouth, but it is said that sometimes the colour does not change. A cold perspiration usually bursts out on the forehead, and may be so copious as to drip off the face. The pulse, in the rare instances in which I have had the opportunity of examining it during a paroxysm, has been irregular, small, and weak. In some cases it has been reported to be very small from contraction or spasm of the arteries. In others, again, it has scarcely been affected at all.

**Exciting Causes of a Paroxysm.**—Great importance attaches to the exciting cause of the paroxysms. In the first instance they are almost always brought on by exertion. The patient, while walking perhaps more sharply than usual, or uphill, or against a wind, is more or less suddenly arrested by pain in the chest, with a feeling as if the heart were about to stop and he to fall down dead. On standing still the pain gradually passes off, and he is able to resume his walk, but only feebly and gently. For a while the attacks only occur when provoked by exertion, but more and more easily as time goes on, and they tend to become more severe. They are more readily induced when a walk is taken, or any imprudent exertion, such as stooping, drawing on boots, pulling open a drawer, pushing up a window, is made soon after a meal, especially after breakfast. External cold, again, predisposes to an attack, and exercise, which can be taken with impunity in mild weather, brings on a paroxysm if the air is cold and damp. Attacks, again, may be brought on by indigestion or constipation, apparently either through reflex disturbance of the heart, or as a result of pressure from the distended stomach or colon carrying the diaphragm upwards and obstructing mechanically the action of the heart and the expansion of the lungs.

They are also liable to occur during the night, and may be induced in various ways. On first lying down, the contact of cold sheets may have this effect by causing contraction of the peripheral arterioles, and thus throwing increased work on the heart; the exertion of undressing may predispose to an attack, or the upward pressure of the abdominal viscera, on assuming the horizontal position, may embarrass the heart. An attack may come on after sleep when the vigour of the circulation has run down, and when possibly also evolution of gases in the stomach, and distension of this viscus or of the colon, have given rise to pressure on the diaphragm.

It is clear that the great exciting cause is a demand for increased effort on the part of the heart to which it is not equal, or occasionally the cause may be interference with the movements of the heart by a dilated stomach and colon.

## Etiology and Morbid Anatomy.

The conditions of the heart associated with angina pectoris are varied, but perhaps the most remarkable and significant point in the relations between heart disease and angina is that angina does not attend the chain of events through which stenosis or incompetence of the mitral valve proves fatal, and is not among the symptoms which arise out of the valve lesion and its effects upon the heart. This fact was duly emphasized by Walshe, in his classical work on the heart, and no exception to it has occurred in my experience. I have, indeed, known instances in which, after attacks of angina had occurred at intervals for many months, mitral regurgitation has supervened with dilatation of the left ventricle, and concurrently with the establishment of so-called mitral symptoms—pressure in the pulmonary circulation, dilatation of the right side of the heart, and dropsy—the angina has ceased. In these particular circumstances Balfour's view, that the giving way of the mitral valve may be an advantage to the sufferer from aortic disease, is perhaps justified, or it is possible that in such cases breathlessness may compel the cessation from exertion before the condition which gives rise to pain is reached.

Aortic stenosis may be attended with true angina, as may also aortic incompetence or combination of the two conditions of the aortic valve. In association with aortic valvular disease angina may be met with in early adult life, and may continue for many years without proving fatal. The sense of impending death is, however, not so fully pronounced in aortic cases, though the pain may be very severe.

**Injury to the root of the aorta** has been known to give rise to angina. I have had a case under observation for several years, in which a severe crush of the chest gave rise to a double aortic murmur and to distressing attacks of angina. For a time the attacks came on very frequently, even while the patient was kept in bed, and they continued to occur on very slight provocation, requiring frequent recourse to nitro-glycerine, which the patient took in considerable quantity. There was scarcely any compensatory hypertrophy and dilatation in this patient, and he was never able to work.

In **aortitis** affecting the root of the aorta there is usually angina, the attacks at first slight, increasing in intensity and duration, and coming on more frequently as the disease advances. The heart rapidly becomes weaker without notable enlargement, the impulse more feeble, the sounds weak and short. Both the angina and the weakness of the heart point to interference with the coronary circulation, and the orifices of the coronary arteries are found small and contracted by the swelling of the walls of the aorta.

**Gout.**—Attacks of pain in the region of the heart may occur in gouty subjects. Frequently they are merely reflex due to gastric disturbances. True angina, when it is met with, is to be attributed not directly to the gout, but to the degenerative vascular lesions to which gout predisposes, and which may affect the aorta or coronary arteries.

**Bacterial Infections.**—Angina has followed recovery from plague in two cases I have seen, and was experienced on slight exertion for several years, and a characteristic attack of angina has been described to me as having occurred in intermittent fever.

**Fatty Degeneration of the Heart.**—In a very large proportion of cases in which angina proves fatal the heart is found, when examined after death, to be in a more or less advanced stage of fatty degeneration. The fatty change may be so far advanced that the fingers sink into the walls of the heart on slight pressure, and scarcely any sound muscular fibres can be found on microscopic examination. Sometimes it may appear to be comparatively slight, and only evident to the naked eye as yellow patches or striæ in the ventricular walls and in the musculi papillaries, but microscopic examination shows widespread fatty degeneration and fat globules in fibres that appear to be normal to the naked eye. The heart may be normal in size or perhaps greatly dilated, or there may be a considerable degree of hypertrophy. The coronary arteries will invariably be found to be diseased. Sometimes they can be dissected out as hard, rigid, calcareous tubes from the auricular grooves, and frequently their walls are so thickened that the lumen is almost obliterated.

**Fibrosis.**—In some instances the morbid condition found is fibrosis, general or local, associated with coronary sclerosis, or possibly the result of myocarditis.

There may be little or no change recognizable in the walls of the heart, and the coronaries at first sight may appear to be healthy, especially when the first attack has proved fatal or death has supervened after a few paroxysms. It is probable, however, that in such cases, on careful examination, obliteration of a branch of the coronary artery by endarteritis or its obstruction by an embolus or thrombus will be discovered.

**Angina Vasomotoria.**—Angina is also met with in a certain proportion of cases of high arterial tension associated with general arterio sclerosis, in which the maintenance of a high degree of pressure in the circulation precludes the existence of any marked degree of fatty degeneration in the cardiac muscle. In this class of cases the paroxysms of angina appear to depend on increased arterio-capillary resistance, which raises the blood pressure and throws extra work on the heart. To this group the term "angina vasomotoria" may be conveniently applied to distinguish them from cases in which fatty degeneration of the heart is pronounced, and inherent cardiac weakness is the prominent feature. The heart is hypertrophied and may be capable of powerful contraction, and the circulation in the coronaries may be sufficient for ordinary needs, but when the arterial tension is further raised by exertion or increase of peripheral resistance attacks of angina are induced. I have thought it well to make special allusion to this form of angina, which has been termed "vasomotoria," as the prognosis is less serious, and more satisfactory results can be obtained from suitable treatment than in cases in which angina is associated with fatty degeneration of the cardiac muscle. The attacks of angina cannot, of course, be attributed simply to the high arterial tension, which is met with in an extreme degree, without angina, in chronic Bright's disease and various other conditions. The real underlying cause will be found to be partial occlusion of the mouth of the coronary arteries by degenerative changes in the aorta, or sclerosis of the coronary vessels, which are results of the high arterial tension. There will not, as a rule, be extreme stenosis of the coronary vessels such as may be present in fatty hearts, but rather thickening and rigidity, and it may be calcification of their walls, the loss of contractility, which must have seriously impaired the circulation in the heart during life.

*Conclusions.*—It will be seen from a review of the above-mentioned etiological factors that interference with the flow of blood through the coronary arteries from disease of their walls, from thrombosis or embolism, or from narrowing of their orifice by atheromatous changes in the aorta, is by far the commonest cause of true angina pectoris, and is the only constant pathological lesion found post-mortem. In fatty or fibroid degeneration of the heart, with which angina is frequently associated, sclerosis of the coronary vessels is present, and in the aortic lesions to which reference has been made above there is either atheromatous degeneration of the aorta, which may involve the orifice of one or both coronary arteries, or the coronaries themselves are diseased. In cases of angina following acute bacterial infections, it may be that acute arteritis is set up in the coronary arteries, or in the vasa vasorum supplying them, which will subsequently lead to degenerative changes in the coronary vessels from impaired nutrition. Of this, however, we have no direct proof. Huchard,* after a very comprehensive enumeration and a masterly discussion of all the possible causes of angina, sums up in the following words, "Il n'y a pas plusieurs angines de poitrine, il n'y a qu'une seule, l'angine coronarienne." He† admits, however, that in tobacco poisoning there may be attacks of true angina without coronary sclerosis. These he attributes to temporary spasm of the coronary arteries.

## THEORIES ADVANCED TO EXPLAIN THE PAIN.

Numerous theories have been advanced to explain the pain of "angina pectoris."

**Stretching of the Heart Muscle Fibres.**—It might be supposed that mechanical stretching of the muscle fibres in the endeavour to overcome resistance in the circulation would give rise to pain, but acute dilatation of the heart may occur under various conditions without giving rise to angina.

**Neuralgia.**—It has been suggested that the pain might be due to cardiac neuralgia, but the nature of the attacks and of the exciting causes which induce them are scarcely

* "Maladies du Cœur," vol. ii, p. 183.

† Ibid., p. 105.

compatible with this theory. Angina, moreover, is far more common in men than women, whereas the converse is the case with neuralgia.

**Impairment of Contractility of the Heart Muscle.**—Mackenzie,* in a paper on the cause of angina, gives an interesting series of pulse tracings, two of which, taken during an attack of angina, show the presence of the "pulsus alternans," that is, a large beat regularly alternating with a small beat. This pulse is not necessarily associated with angina, but is frequently met with in other conditions. He regards the "pulsus alternans" as evidence of impairment of the contractile power of the heart muscle, and states that in cases of angina, the same exciting cause—extra strain on the heart—may provoke both angina pectoris and the alternating action of the heart, and that both may disappear with removal of the cause. He therefore concludes that angina pectoris will be found to be associated with impairment of the function of contractility of the heart.

**Spasm of the Heart.**—The condition of the heart during the attacks has been supposed to be one of spasm, but there are many objections to this view, and ideas as to what is meant by spasm of the heart in the anginal paroxysm by those who have employed the term have been diverse and vague. If by spasm of the heart is understood tonic contraction or an unrelaxing systole, this is certainly not the condition present. The heart has never been found in this state after death, and in most cases is incapable of such contraction from the state of its walls. No pulse would be possible were the heart in a spasm of this kind, and the pulse, though small and often irregular, can usually be felt. It has, indeed, in some cases been apparently unaffected by the paroxysm.

But by spasm may be meant an irregular and partial contraction like cramp in voluntary muscles, or a fibrillar

* *B.M.J.*, vol. ii. 1905, p. 845.

contraction, such as is sometimes induced by faradic currents in muscle under experiment. The late Dr. Matthews Duncan, in the last conversation I had the honour to hold with him, suggested that the state of the heart in angina pectoris might be like hour-glass contraction of the uterus. He had at that time experienced the pain.

Views of this kind cannot be proved to be wrong, but objections might be raised, and the central fact and essential significance of angina is that stress is put upon the heart, to which, for the moment, it is unequal.

One of the main causes of such stress is resistance in the peripheral circulation, or, in other words, high arterial tension, and we owe to Lauder Brunton the knowledge that in many attacks of angina there is an aggravation of habitual high tension by a general contraction of the arterioles. But the habitual state of the arterial circulation may be one of relaxed arterioles and capillaries and low tension, so that the heart has no abnormal resistance to overcome. Here sudden general arterial spasm would put the heart to greater stress than if the habitual tension were high, since the contrast between the work demanded would be greater.

Huchard considers that the attacks of anginoid pain are due to ischemia of the heart, either from spasm of the coronary arteries, or from the relatively deficient blood supply through the narrowed vessels when exertion or increase of arterial tension demands increased blood supply to the heart. He compares the condition of the heart to that of the limbs in "claudication intermittante."

This explanation is by far the most satisfactory that has yet been advanced, and the cases Huchard instances of true angina occurring in patients suffering from the rare condition of claudication intermittante are of great interest. Whether actual spasm of the coronary arteries occurs must be problematical, and, indeed, from the thickened, rigid condition of their walls in many cases, it would scarcely seem to be possible. But the suggestion that the relatively deficient blood supply to the heart muscle through the diseased coronary vessels induces a condition akin to cramp of the heart when it is called upon to do extra work will explain the occurrence of angina in all the diverse pathological conditions of the heart with which it may be associated.

We must, it seems to me, assume that it is one of the arrangements by which the adjustment of internal reactions to external conditions is secured. The existence of the patient is threatened at the moment of the attack by arrest of the heart's action, and were it not for the warning given by the pain, and the cessation of exertion thus enforced, the subject of this particular affection of the heart would die suddenly without any warning.

## Diagnosis.

Angina pectoris may be closely simulated by paroxysms of pain which are not symptomatic of disease of the heart of any kind, and are not attended with danger, and, as we usually have to depend on the account given by the patient, it is often a matter of great difficulty to distinguish between true angina and merely anginoid attacks. The difficulty will sometimes be aggravated by the fact that the patient has carefully read up the symptoms.

The age of the subject may be of assistance in determining the question. Angina is very rare before the age of forty-five, except in the case of aortic valvular disease or aneurysm or aortitis.

Sex, again, may often enable us to exclude angina without hesitation. It is extremely rare in women at any period of life in the absence of the conditions just enumerated, whereas so-called angina is a favourite complaint of neurotic ladies at all ages above thirty. What is described as "spasms" by tea-drinking female out-patients becomes angina among the educated and neurotic.

The appearance of the patient as ascertained from friends who have witnessed attacks may be valuable evidence. It does not necessarily follow that if he turns pale and has a look of alarm and suffering the paroxysms are those of true angina; but if his colour and expression show no change it will be evidence to the contrary.

The circumstances under which the early attacks come on are very significant. With rare exceptions the pain of angina is first experienced during exertion, and when it gradually increases in intensity with each successive attack and is provoked more and more readily, there can be little doubt as to its nature. If, on the other hand, the first paroxysms set in during repose, and particularly at a given interval after food, or at a particular hour of the night, the inference is equally strong that they are pseudo-anginal in character and of gastric origin. Unless the history, onset, and nature of the paroxysms are quite characteristic, and confirmatory physical signs are present, we should only make a definite diagnosis of angina when all possible explanation of the pain can be excluded.

If we leave out of the consideration neurotic and hysterical attacks, which are usually easily recognizable, the cause of the spurious angina is nearly always some functional derangement of the stomach, and evidences of disturbance of the digestion, such as occasional attacks of vomiting, habitual flatulency with eructation, will often aid in establishing the distinctive diagnosis. In many cases dilatation of the stomach may be demonstrable by percussion and succussion.

A common combination is dilatation or distension of the stomach and high arterial tension. Together they give the nearest imitation of true angina, and if the heart be at all weak a fatal result is by no means impossible in elderly subjects. Such a result may be invited if the functional derangement of the stomach and liver are ignored, and digitalis or other cardiac tonic is given or the Schott treatment adopted, or if the paroxysms are simply treated by nitrite of amyl or nitro-glycerine.

The following case may be given to illustrate these attacks of so-called "Pseudo-angina." A medical man, aged 52, consulted me for sudden and agonizing attacks of pain in the præcordial area. They were so severe that he had to sit down and lean forward, and was incapable of movement or speech while they lasted. He himself attributed them to angina pectoris, but found that trinitrin or nitrite of amyl gave no relief. He was a gouty subject, and had had several attacks of acute articular gout, and some of his medical friends attributed the anginoid pain to gout. I found, on examination, that the vessels were in good condition, the arterial tension was not high, there was no valvular disease of the heart, which was normal in size; and that the heart sounds were good. On examining the abdomen, I found that there was enormous dilatation of the stomach, and, on questioning him, ascertained that he was a heavy feeder, and was in the habit of eating large quantities of meat and drinking effervescing water with whisky at lunch and dinner. I also ascertained that the attacks of pain did not come on after exertion or exposure to cold, but usually after a full meal. Taking all these matters into consideration, I came to the conclusion that the attacks were not those of true angina pectoris. I enjoined moderation in diet, the giving up of effervescing water, and limitation in the amount of fluids taken, and prescribed a mercurial purge once a week. The attacks soon ceased, and have never recurred, and though he has since had several bouts of acute gout, he is now in good health, and it is ten years since the attacks of præcordial pain for which he consulted me.

## Prognosis.

The prognosis of angina is beset with uncertainty. We can never tell when the next attack will come on, or whether it may not be the last. We are not, however, altogether without guidance, the elements of which will be an estimate of the relative predominance of the two chief factors in the production of the attack—whether inherent weakness of the heart wall on the one hand, or, on the other.

obstruction in the circulation or other cause of embarrassment of the heart's action.

While the attacks only come on when provoked by considerable exertion or excitement, or by flatulent indigestion (not, of course, taking the patient's word for the last-named cause), the hope may be entertained that by care in avoiding all known occasions they may be postponed indefinitely. If, further, there is habitual high tension in the pulse, as in "angina vasomotoria," this is at the same time evidence of obstruction in the arterioles and capillaries which may be capable of mitigation by treatment, and of some degree of vigour in the heart, which will usually be hypertrophied. So also will be accentuation of the aortic second sound, and still more any recognizable impulse or apex beat.

The patient, of course, must not take exercise immediately after food, must never hurry or walk against a wind, and even on level ground must adapt his pace to his condition, and if compelled to go uphill must do so very gently and circumspectly.

Angina, again, in connection with aortic valvular disease, may run a very protracted course. It is when the pulse is soft and the heart is normal in dimensions, with imperceptible impulse and weak sounds, as in fatty degeneration—when, in fact, the results of careful examination are negative—that the greatest uncertainty and danger exist. The occurrence of unprovoked attacks and of nocturnal angina will emphasize this conclusion.

## TREATMENT.

The primary significance of angina pectoris is, as has been said, that the heart is unequal to the task of propelling the blood. The heart is itself always in fault, but undue resistance in the vessels may play an important part in the production of the pain. The first consideration' therefore, when the treatment of angina is undertaken, will be whether there is arterio-capillary obstruction which can be removed. The pulse will be examined carefully and repeatedly at different periods of the day, before and after food, before and after the night's rest, before and after such exercise as the patient can take with impunity. If at any time the artery is distinctly full between the beats, virtual tension exists, *i.e.* there would be tension were there adequate *vis a tergo*, and it may be concluded that obstruction is present in the arterioles and capillaries which probably contributes to the embarrassment of the enfeebled heart, the removal of which may afford relief. Not uncommonly there will be found a well-marked senile pulse, with the arteries large, tortuous, and thickened, full between the beats, but compressible, the pulse wave being sudden and unsustained. Here the loss of elasticity and expansibility of the entire arterial tree will be a cause of difficulty to the heart. The aortic trunk and its main branches being atheromatous and refusing to dilate when the blood is propelled into them, the systole encounters the peripheral resistance at once just as if the vessels were a system of rigid, inelastic tubes. Nothing can be done to remedy the degeneration of the arteries, but it may be possible to lessen the resistance in the capillary net-work which has been a chief factor in the production of the atheromatous state, and which is now adding cardiac overstrain and angina to previous ill-effects.

In some cases of angina the pulse has all the characters of high tension without advanced disease of the vessels. This will usually be in gouty subjects, and we have angina which may justly be called "gouty."

Whenever high arterial tension can be distinctly recognized in angina pectoris, there is an opening for treatment which may be palliative to a very important extent, and sometimes curative. The treatment will be such as has already been described in discussing high arterial tension. Colchicum may be given with the mercurial aperient in gouty angina, and also a mixture containing iodide and bicarbonate or citrate of potash, with gentian or some other vegetable bitter tonic, twice or three times a day. The iodide when well borne is often of remarkable service. In such cases the treatment may be pursued with confidence and with a certain degree of vigour. The diet must be strictly regulated, and the nearer it can be brought to a milk and farinaceous diet without incurring distension of the stomach and flatulent dyspepsia the better. Heavy meals must, of course, be avoided. Elimination may be furthered by a tumbler of Vichy or Evian water, or plain soft water night and morning.

When there is no conspicuous tension in the arteries, and their walls are in a state of degeneration, and when with this the walls of the heart are weak and probably fatty, while the same end is held in view and similar means are put in operation, great caution and watchfulness must be exercised. The bowels must be made to act daily, but mercurial aperients must be sparingly employed, an aloetic pill or liquorice powder, or some preparation of cascara, being given, if necessary, in the intervals.

When angina complicates disease of the aortic valves, it is difficult to say whether arterio-capillary resistance contributes in any way to its production, but if the pulse is good it will be well to give mild mercurial aperients and iodides on the assumption that such may be the case, though caution must be observed in their administration.

If the pulse in the intervals between the attacks of anginoid pain is small, short, easily compressible and destitute of tension, no good result is to be expected from eliminant treatment, and even small doses of mercury may depress the patient.

Prominence has been given to removal of arterio-capillary resistance by eliminant treatment, because when called for, it may yield more permanent relief than any other line of treatment; but arsenic and phosphorus may render very important service, and except in cases of markedly high arterial tension one or other of these should be given concurrently with eliminants. A particularly useful combination is arsenic with iodide of potassium and nux vomica. Phosphorus seems to have a specially favourable effect in angina associated with aortic regurgitation. Belladonna or cannabis indica may be useful adjuvants in some cases; quinine and nux vomica also are often of service. Nitro-glycerine or the heavier nitrites may also be required habitually, though it is best when possible to reserve their use for the anginoid attacks themselves. In the case of a medical friend the erythrol tetranitrate appeared to be of great service, enabling him to avert a fatal attack for many years.

## Treatment of the Attacks.

There remains to be considered the treatment of the attacks themselves. Formerly brandy, various combinations of ether, nitrous ether, ammonia, lavender, and camphor, were the chief drugs resorted to. Inhalation of amyl nitrite and the administration of nitro-glycerine or of sodium nitrite or erythrol tetranitrate have now almost entirely superseded these remedies.

Whatever the remedy, the patient should always carry it about with him, and have recourse to it as soon as the pain really sets in. The amyl nitrite is supplied in the convenient form of glass capsules containing five mins., enclosed in a silk bag, so that one of these can be broken in a handkerchief and the vapour inhaled. Some prefer to carry a small bottle of amyl nitrite about, to which they can have recourse when the attack threatens. Nitro-glycerine, however, taken by the mouth, appears to be more generally useful, since, though the effect is scarcely as rapid as that of inhaled amyl nitrite, it lasts much longer. Erythrol tetranitrate is even more satisfactory, as its effects are more prolonged than those of trinitrin. Tabloids of nitro-glycerine containing one min. of a one per cent. solution can be carried about, and one or two can be swallowed when necessary with very little loss of time.

In most cases nitro-glycerine has a better effect than amyl nitrite, though in rare instances nitro-glycerine appears to have no influence on the spasm to which nitrite of amyl at once gives relief. In two cases of the kind that I have seen, it has seemed to me extremely probable that the anginoid paroxysm had its origin in the right ventricle.

Occasionally when the nitrites fail we have to fall back on the old-fashioned remedies, especially when the heart failure is pronounced and the pulse tension is extremely low. Here it may do more good to help the heart by stimulants than to relieve it of work. While the paroxysms of angina are for the most part brief, the agony being such that it seems as if another moment must prove fatal, there are at times attacks of a protracted character. When the pain persists in spite of nitrites and stimulants, morphine and atropine should be administered hypodermically, and it is well to carry the needle into the substance of a muscle where the circulation is more active than in the subcutaneous cellular tissue. The initial dose should be small, but it may be necessary to employ morphine boldly. A turpentine stupe may also be applied over the region of the heart, or a mustard leaf or poultice.

It must be remembered also that the nitrites give rise to great frequency of the heart action which may be a source of distress. We should consequently employ them very cautiously when the angina is accompanied by a frequent pulse. The nitrites have been supposed to be heart tonics, but while their most prominent action is relaxation of the arterio-capillary net-work they also relax the cardiac muscular fibres.

As in so many other instances, the employment of nitroglycerine and the nitrites is not without its drawbacks. Patients often come to rely on the immunity from pain which the remedies confer and then presume upon it. Liberties are taken and imprudences are committed, so that not unfrequently sudden death is precipitated which might with care have been staved off for years. In placing the remedy in the patient's hands, therefore, emphatic words of caution must be spoken and the danger must be pointed out.

The instructions to be given with regard to exercise are extremely important. After a very severe paroxysm, however provoked, rest in bed may be necessary for some days, and even for a period of two or three weeks, if the attack has been prolonged. The heart may be left extremely weak, its action slow or faltering and irregular, and the sounds scarcely audible, and sitting up or turning in bed may be attended with giddiness or faintness or pain in the region of the heart. When such conditions are present, time must be given to the heart to recover itself, and measures must be taken to relieve flatulence and constipation, which will probably be associated with the other symptoms.

Under ordinary circumstances, however, the rule usually applicable in heart disease holds good here. Whatever exercise the patient can take without provoking an attack at the time, or prostration afterwards, he will be the better for. While, however, the exercise should be as regular as possible, in no case is it more necessary to bear in mind the fact that the capacity for exertion varies from day to day, and that the sufferer from angina can do easily one day what would be impossible for him on another. This is one of the objections to the Œrtel methods of treatment. Some of the influences which affect him we can recognize, such as wind, or severe cold, or great heat, or weather which is felt by people in health to be oppressive, or a moisture-laden atmosphere; others arise out of internal conditions, flatulence, dyspepsia, constipation, functional derangements of the liver. The patient's feelings and inclinations have thus to be taken into account, but without allowing inertia or nervousness to have undue weight. There is great room here for judgment and tact and personal knowledge of the patient's disposition. Besides the caution necessary in cold and hot weather, the liability to anginoid attacks on walking soon after food must be borne in mind, and a period of rest after meals must be enjoined, especially after that particular meal which experience in the case under treatment has shown to be worst in this respect.

## CHAPTER XXVI.

## FUNCTIONAL AFFECTIONS (SO-CALLED) OF THE HEART.

PAIN IN PRÆCORDIAL REGION—SITE OF PAIN—EXPLANATION OF REFERRED PAIN AND AREAS OF CUTANEOUS HYPERALGESIA — DISORDERS OF RHYTHM OF THE HEART — MECHANISM BY WHICH THE RHYTHM OF THE HEART IS REGULATED — INTERMITTENT AND IRREGULAR ACTION OF THE HEART — PALPITATION: TACHYCARDIA.

THE term "functional affections" is retained, not for any merit of its own but for want of a better. Under it must be discussed a variety of symptoms having the heart for their centre, but which cannot be assigned to any structural change. Taken all together they give rise to much actual suffering, and to far more nervous apprehension and fear of death than definite valvular and structural disease combined. So much is this the case that when patients come complaining of the heart, we are almost safe in concluding that the heart is disturbed by some cause outside itself and is not the seat of disease.

### CARDIAC PAIN.

Pain is one of the symptoms which frequently gives rise to apprehension of heart disease. Leaving out of the question that of angina, which has already been discussed, its most common seat is the region of the apex, but it may be felt over any part of the cardiac area, the left third space being next to the apex, the most frequent part in which pain is experienced. It is most commonly of a dull aching character, but may be sharp and stabbing or burning, and nervous women will exhaust all the epithets which can be applied to pain in their description of their sufferings. Tenderness on pressure very commonly accompanies the pain; it is superficial and is equally severe, whether the pressure is made over a rib or in an intercostal space; it is often particularly severe in the edge of the mamma when this extends into the tender area. The tenderness is quite extra-thoracic, and is felt when the heart is not even indirectly reached by the pressure.

Another special seat of tenderness is over the second rib, about an inch from the edge of the sternum, where a branch of the cervical plexus crosses the rib. Pressure here not only causes pain, but may give rise to intolerable cardiac distress.

**Explanation of Referred Pain and Areas of Hyperalgesia.**—The relationship of areas of cutaneous hyperalgesia and referred pain to visceral affections has been ably demonstrated by Mackenzie * and by Head,† and will explain most of the above phenomena. Briefly, Head's conclusions are as follows:—

As the viscera are insensitive, and from their inaccessibility to touch are incapable of developing the sense of localization, the maximum pain is not felt in the affected organ. A painful stimulus to an internal organ is conducted to the corresponding segment of the cord, where it comes into contact with the sensory nerves from the area of the body supplied by the same segment. The sensory and localizing power of the skin is enormously in excess of that

* *Med. Chron.*, Manchester, 1892, p. 293; and *Lancet*, 1895, vol. i. p. 16.
† *Brain*, 1893, pp. 1 *et seq.*; and 1894, pp. 339 *et seq.*

of the viscera, and by a psychical error of judgment the pain is referred to the corresponding segmental area of the body, instead of to the affected organ.

In neuroses of the heart, hyperæsthesia, or, as Head puts it, hyperalgesia, of the corresponding cutaneous segmental areas is a common feature, whereas in angina pectoris this is as nothing compared with the widespread agonizing referred pain.

According to Mackenzie and Head, in most affections of the heart and aorta the cutaneous areas in which hyperalgesia is present, and to which the pain is referred, are those corresponding to the first, second, third, and fourth dorsal segments, which comprise, roughly, all the front of the chest, from the second rib to the level of the nipple, the posterior and lateral surface from the level of the seventh cervical to the fourth dorsal spine, and certain areas on the inner aspect of the arms.

In angina pectoris, however, the distribution of the referred pain differs considerably from that in other affections of the heart, and it would appear that the painful stimulus to the heart is so severe that it sets up a widespread and violent commotion in the cord, so that pain may be referred upwards over certain cervical areas and downwards as low as the ninth dorsal segmental area.

**Etiology.**—Pain in the region of the heart may be due to conditions of the heart itself, to dilatation or overstrain, to an enfeebled and irritable state after a depressing illness, or to toxic influences, *e.g.* tobacco, to direct pressure upon the heart by a dilated stomach or extreme distension of the abdomen, to reflex disturbance from some visceral derangement, or to nervous or emotional states.

Taking the last-named first, it is exemplified by the sharp pain in the heart, which may be induced by a sudden shock or fright, or by powerful emotion, and by the heartache of profound or protracted grief. But, without adequate emotional influence nothing is more common than cardiac pain as an expression of nervous depression.

Reflex pains are mostly of dyspeptic origin, but may be associated with uterine derangements. The pain caused by direct pressure of the diaphragm, carried upwards by a dilated stomach or distension of the colon or intestine generally, is accompanied by oppression of the breathing, and is usually felt at the base of the heart and is aggravated on lying down.

Pain due to overstrain of the heart is commonly a diffuse ache over the cardiac area, generally accentuated in the region of the apex.

The treatment of cardiac pain will in its details vary with the cause. If due to toxic influences, these should be removed. If due to overstrain or dilatation, the treatment should be on the lines given on p. 303. But in all cases it is most important to be able to convince the patient that there is no disease. While he has the idea in his mind that he is suffering from some serious heart affection, the concentration of his attention on the heart will be sufficient to renew the pain, and his apprehensions will interfere with the recovery of his nervous equilibrium.

If due to reflex disturbances, such as derangements of the digestive organs, liver or uterus, these should be rectified by suitable diet and treatment, and, as a rule, tonics will be of service.

With the internal and general remedies the local application of belladonna as a liniment or plaster will be useful. The plaster is often more efficacious if it is applied so as to afford support or to exercise pressure on the painful part, and it is well, therefore, to apply it in strips. Counter-irritation over the tender area by a mustard-leaf or blisters is often of great service in neurotic individuals.

## DISORDERS OF RHYTHM OF THE HEART.

These may be classified under the following heads:—

1. Intermittency of the heart's action.

2. Irregularity in the force and frequency of the heart beats.

3. Abnormally rapid action of the heart, which may be temporary (palpitation) or continuous (tachycardia).

4. Abnormally slow action of the heart (bradycardia).

These will be discussed in detail under their respective headings; but it may be as well first to briefly refer to the views held as to the mechanism by which the rhythm of the heart is regulated.

## MECHANISM REGULATING THE RHYTHM OF THE HEART.

Gaskell * describes the functions of the muscular fibres of the heart as rhythmicity, excitability, contractility, conductivity, and tonicity, by virtue of which the heart is able to beat and keep up the circulation independently of nerve control, the vagus and sympathetic having only a moderating influence upon these varied functions.

The muscle fibres at the mouth of the great veins and adjoining portion of the right auricle, and the muscular tissue joining the auricles and ventricles, according to Gaskell, possess the greatest power of automatically creating a stimulus for contraction.

The fibres joining the auricle and ventricle play an important part in the conduction of the stimulus for contraction from auricle to ventricle. On applying a clamp to the auriculo-ventricular groove in a frog's heart, Gaskell states that, according to the tightness of the clamp, the ventricle may be made to respond to every second, third, or fourth contraction of the auricle.

* "Text-book of Physiology," edited by Schäfer, vol. ii.

Mackenzie,* in a valuable paper, calls attention to these facts, and to the work of Englemann and Wenckebach on disordered rhythm of the heart, and contributes a series of interesting observations on the nature of the conducting power whereby the stimulus is conveyed from auricle to ventricle. His method of investigation is to take simultaneous tracings of the jugular and carotid or radial pulses, and thus time the period which elapses between the auricular and ventricular systole.

He attaches great importance to the function of the muscle fibres connecting the auricle with the ventricle, and shows that certain forms of arrhythmia, more especially intermittent action of the heart and bradycardia, are probably due to depression of or a block in the conductivity of these fibres.

**Nervous Influences.**—Though the rhythmic action of the heart is automatic and dependent on the inherent properties of its muscular fibres, the central nervous system exercises an important controlling influence on the varied functions of the cardiac muscle through the pneumogastric and sympathetic nerves. Messages must constantly be passing to and fro along these nerves between the heart and centres in the medulla, by means of which the heart is kept informed of the condition and requirements of the body in general, and the vascular system in particular, so that the force and frequency of its beat, and the degree of tonicity of its muscle fibres, are regulated accordingly.

All are familiar with the extreme and distressing variations in the frequency of the heart beat which may be induced by sudden and violent emotions of fear or anger, or by intense excitement, which in certain diseased conditions may give rise to a fatal syncopal attack by arrest of the heart's action. Disturbances of rhythm may be occasioned by reflex impulses transmitted from the stomach

* "New Methods of Studying Affections of the Heart," *B.M.J.*, March, 1905.

or other viscera in consequence of functional derangements.

Gibson,* in his excellent account of "Nervous Affections of the Heart," gives some interesting tracings from the experimental work of Wenckebach and Cushny, which show the different effects of electrical stimuli on the rhythm of the heart, according to the region stimulated, and the time in the cardiac cycle at which they are applied.

As one of the results of these experiments, it is demonstrated that if a stimulus is applied to the heart just before the normal of contraction is due, a premature imperfect systole takes place, which is insufficient to transmit a pulse wave to the wrist, so that a beat is dropped in the radial pulse. This will explain certain forms of intermittent pulse and irregular action of the heart. The nature of the stimulus which interferes with the normal automatic contraction of the heart is not always easy to determine. Probably, when the intermittency is a temporary phenomenon, it is the result of a reflex from some gastric or other visceral disturbance. When persistent, it may perhaps be due, not to reflex nervous influences, but to a block in the conductivity of certain of the cardiac muscle fibres referred to above.

## INTERMITTENCY OF THE PULSE.

By an intermittent pulse is meant a pulse in which a beat is missing from time to time, while in the intervals it is perfectly regular. The intermission may occur at regular and definite periods every four, six, or more beats up to twenty, or the number of intervening pulsations may vary.

It is not characteristic of any form of heart affection and is rarely indicative of organic disease. An intermittent pulse may be constant and habitual, and the intermission

* "Nervous Affections of the Heart," Young Pentland, 1904.

is then more likely to occur at definite intervals; it may be occasional only, and may be attributable to some disturbing reflex cause, of which flatulent dyspepsia is the most common. In some cases the pulse is intermittent after each meal; or in others tea, coffee, or tobacco may be the special cause of the intermission. It is common also in chronic gout, and may be among the signs of fatty degeneration of the heart. In case of doubt the patient should be made to walk briskly for a minute or two, when, if the heart is really weak and degenerated, the pulse will falter, whereas, if the heart is healthy, the intermission will usually disappear. Intermittency of pulse may also be associated with nervous debility and hypochondriasis, the pulse becoming normal again when the patient regains good health. On examining the heart it is usually found that the cause of the intermission is not the actual omission of a heart beat, but the occurrence of a hurried and imperfect contraction which rapidly follows the last of the series of normal beats, and does not transmit a pulse wave to the wrist. The imperfect beat may sometimes be felt on palpation; usually only the first sound is heard on auscultation at the apex unaccompanied by a second sound. The heart beat which follows the intermission is usually more powerful than normal. While it is the rule that there is this feeble interposed heart beat, instances occur where it cannot be heard or felt, and in which the heart appears to remain quite passive. This condition will be discussed further in the chapter on bradycardia.

The patient may or may not be conscious of the intermittent action of the heart. He is more likely to be aware of it when it is symptomatic of some functional derangement than when it is habitual; he may be conscious of a vague sense of discomfort or of an unpleasant sinking sensation in the cardiac region during the intermission, or he may feel the bump of the stronger beat which usually follows the feeble and imperfect or dropped beat. In view of Gaskell's, Wenckebach's, and Mackenzie's work, referred to above, the explanation of intermittent action of the heart when persistent would seem to be that it arises from a lowering of conductivity in the muscle fibres joining the auricle and ventricle, so that the stimulus for contraction is not regularly transmitted from auricle to ventricle. Sometimes this may be attributed to cardiac sclerosis, sometimes there is no apparent cause. It may be met with in men who enjoy vigorous health and live to a good old age. When the intermittent action of the heart is only occasional, it is usually traceable to some toxic cause, such as tea, coffee, or tobacco, or to reflex gastric or other visceral disturbances, and suitable treatment for removal of the cause should then be adopted.

## Irregularity of the Heart's Action.

Irregularity of the heart's action, like intermittency, may be habitual or occasional. Habitual irregularity is commonly present in mitral incompetence and in cases of cardiac dilatation of any severity, when it is probably due to the variable supply of blood to the left ventricle, as explained in Chapter XI. It is occasionally met with in individuals in whom there is no evidence of any heart disease, and who enjoy good health and live to old age. In one instance I have known the heart's action, without any apparent cause, to be markedly irregular during a period of at least twenty years to my knowledge in a gentleman who lived to the age of seventy and enjoyed vigorous health.

Irregularity associated with excessive frequency of pulse is usually of serious prognostic significance, and may be an incident in the final stages of paroxysmal tachycardia.

Irregular action of the heart setting in after middle life

with evidence of degenerative change in the vessels is also serious, as it may be due to fibroid change in the heart associated with sclerosis of the coronary vessels.

Temporary irregularity of the cardiac action is much more common, and may be occasioned by tobacco or strong tea, by mechanical embarrassment of the heart by a distended stomach or colon, or by various reflex causes, such as gastric and liver derangements, or emotional disturbances of various kinds.

Irregularity of the cardiac action is more serious than intermission, and steps should at once be taken to remove, if possible, the exciting cause. When there is mechanical embarrassment of the heart by a distended and dilated stomach the distress at times may be severe, and there is danger of a sudden syncopal attack in elderly people in whom the heart has undergone degenerative changes.

## PALPITATION.

By palpitation is meant frequent and violent action of the heart, of which the subject is conscious; but patients will sometimes say they are suffering from palpitation when there is neither frequency nor violence recognizable in the beat of the heart or pulse by the observer, and, on the other hand, may be unconscious of extremely rapid action of the heart found on examination.

With palpitation there is usually uneasiness, sometimes pain, in the region of the heart, oppression of the respiration with frequent deep sighs and a sense of inability to fill the chest sufficiently. Often there is excitement and alarm and the patient feels giddy or faint; the face may be flushed or very pale.

When the heart is acting very rapidly, many of the beats may fail to reach the radial artery, so that the pulse becomes irregular. The reason probably is that the ventricle has not time to fill, and that consequently there is not sufficient blood propelled into the aorta to communicate a wave to the peripheral vessels. Very often the artery is small and full between the beats, there being a general excitement of the vascular system with spasm of the arterial walls. This is particularly the case in hysterical palpitation, when there will frequently also be a copious secretion of pale dilute urine.

On examination, during an access of palpitation, the heart may be felt to be hoating violently, but when the rapidity of its action is extreme a faint vibration only may be communicated to the hand. On auscultation, the first sound may be loud and short, followed immediately by a weak second sound, or, in the case of extreme frequency, the first and second sounds may be almost identical in character and equidistant, resembling very closely those of the fœtal heart, and comparable to the puffing of a distant locomotive.

**Etiology.**—Among the causes of what may be called ordinary palpitation as distinguished from tachycardia, the most important is a predisposition thereto on the part of the nerve centres governing the heart, which may be inborn or induced by modes of life or by the various circumstances which tend to lower the nervous tone or to promote nervous excitability. Palpitation is much more common in women than men, partly in virtue of the greater inherent susceptibility of the female nervous system, partly from the more emotional life of women, their greater confinement to the house, and their less vigorous exercise; but child-bearing and over-lactation are also in themselves serious predisposing causes. In men a sedentary mode of life, exciting occupations, dissipation, and excesses of all kinds, over-indulgence in tobacco, bring about a liability to palpitation. Mitral stenosis is a form of valvular disease in which attacks of palpitation are very liable to occur, the exciting cause usually being gastric disturbances.

Among the exciting causes are sudden violent impressions on the nervous system of any kind—fright, an unexpected noise, a startling incident taking place before the eyes, a powerful emotion; these will set any one's heart beating, but in a strong and healthy person the effect is of very brief duration; where the predisposition to palpitation exists they may initiate an uncontrollable attack. A similar statement applies to exertion—a brisk walk uphill causes the heart to act rapidly and powerfully under normal circumstances; in a predisposed individual the action may be exaggerated and protracted, so as to constitute an attack of palpitation.

But the characteristic palpitation of the heart starts suddenly without obvious exciting cause, while the patient is sitting quietly at work or reading, or during sleep, when he or she may wake up from a frightful dream which appears to have brought on the attack.

There is, however, as a rule, some internal exciting cause, which is most commonly gastric derangement attended or not with flatulent distension of the stomach or bowels. Other forms of peripheral irritation may act as exciting causes, such as uterine affections.

**Treatment.**—To arrest an attack of palpitation it is sometimes only necessary to take a dozen deliberate deep breaths, and it is always well to try this expedient before resorting to drugs. The remedies of most general service are combination of alkaline and carminative stimulants: bicarbonate of soda with ammonia and camphor or peppermint water is often sufficient, but compound tincture of chloroform, ether, valerian, lavender, ginger may be added or substituted; in some cases bromides are required. Undue acidity of the gastric contents is corrected, flatulence is expelled, and possibly the stimulation of the pneumogastric fibres of the mucous membrane of the stomach may have some inhibiting influence on the heart.

Digitalis appears to have little or no effect, but belladonna may be useful, especially in combination with bromide of ammonium or sodium.

For the prevention of palpitation the tone of the nervous system must be raised by the usual hygienic and medicinal means, namely, change to the seaside, or, better, to mountain health resorts, exercise, fresh air, early hours, simple wholesome food, avoidance of undue excitement of all kinds. The emplast. belladonnæ over the region of the heart appears to have some influence in preventing or moderating the attack, probably mainly due to the mechanical support.

Careful inquiry should be made as to any relation between the taking of food and the occurrence of an attack and as to the existence of functional derangements of the stomach, liver, or other organs. The abdomen should be examined to see if there is flatulent distention of the stomach, colon, or small intestine, and suitable remedies should be given for this, together with such tonics as are indicated by the general condition of the patient.

## TACHYCARDIA.

Attacks of palpitation, or rapid action of the heart, may last a few minutes or a few hours, and are usually traceable to emotional or reflex gastric disturbances, and are not of great severity.

There are, however, cases in which rapid action of the heart, with a pulse of 100 to 120, is a more or less permanent condition, and others in which attacks of extremely rapid action of the heart, with from 200 to 300 beats per minute, set in from time to time, lasting, perhaps, for several days, and eventually proving fatal. To this latter affection the term "paroxysmal tachycardia" has been applied.

## Etiology.

Occasionally one meets with individuals in good health who have normally a pulse of from 90 to 100.

Alcoholism in neurotic subjects may give rise to a permanently rapid pulse, and I have seen two instances in neurotic ladies addicted to alcohol in which a pulse of 100 to 120 was present for a considerable number of years. A retired naval officer also consulted me from time to time for some months, and when seen always had a pulse of 140, and there was every reason to believe that this rate was maintained in the intervals between his visits when he went about as usual. He was gouty, and had taken wine and spirits very freely. Eventually dropsy set in, and he died from heart failure.

In **Graves' disease** a permanent rapid pulse is one of the chief characteristics associated with enlargement of the thyroid, exophthalmos, etc.

In this affection the tachycardia is attributed by most authors to excessive secretion by the thyroid gland. In favour of this view are the clinical contrast between this disease and myxœdema, the increase in the severity of the symptoms when thyroid extract is administered, and the improvement that has followed in some cases on removal of the bulk of the enlarged thyroid.

Others consider that it is a pure neurosis, as the exciting cause can frequently be traced to some profound shock or emotional disturbance.

**Paroxysmal Tachycardia.**—This affection is characterized by attacks of extreme rapidity of the heart's action, in which the pulse rate may be from 150 to 250 per minute. The attacks may last some days, or even weeks. They may terminate fatally from syncope, or cardiac failure and exhaustion, or may suddenly cease, and be succeeded by a period in which the patient enjoys good health. They may set in without any apparent cause, and post-mortem no gross lesion of any kind is found in the valves or heart-muscle, though there may be an extreme degree of dilatation of the heart in cases in which the tachycardia has persisted for a long period.

Bristowe, quoted by Huchard, gives an account of a remarkable case in a boy aged 19 with a syphilitic history, in which the pulse ranged from 240 to 250, then became irregular, with periods in which the rate was 200 for 10 seconds, alternating with others in which it fell to 100. This lasted for 10 days, when the pulse suddenly fell to 60. Three weeks later he had a fresh attack, and the pulse rate rose to 288, but fell to 84 when he took to his bed. A month later he had a third attack, and the pulse rate rose to 308 when he was up, but fell to 64 when he lay down. This recurred on several occasions, and fifteen days later he died suddenly while playing the piano.

## Pathogeny.

The main cause of this affection must be some derangement of the nervous mechanism controlling the heart, and opinions are divided as to whether it may be due to excitation of the sympathetic or temporary paralysis of the vagus, or to some affection of the inhibitory centre in the medulla. There is little to be said in favour of the theory that it is due to stimulation of accelerator fibres in the sympathetic. It is more probable that it may be due to derangement of the inhibitory mechanism in the medulla or to interference with inhibitory impulses descending from this centre through the pneumogastric.

There is no evidence in support of bulbar disease as a cause of tachycardia, but there are cases on record in which tachycardia has apparently been due to compression of the vagus in the neck by enlarged glands, growths, or cicatricial tissue. Instances of this are quoted by Huchard.* In most cases of tachycardia gross lesions of the trunk of the vagus can be excluded, but it is possible that its fibres may be damaged after they have penetrated the myocardium, (*a*) by compression in cardiac sclerosis; (*b*) by spread of inflammation in acute myocarditis; (*c*) by the direct action of toxins in severe toxæmias, with resulting peripheral neuritis.

There is, however, no definite pathological evidence to support this surmise, and paroxysmal tachycardia is not a common sequela of acute toxæmias. It may be that increased irritability of the cardiac muscle is the more important factor, but little is really known as to the pathogeny of this obscure affection.

## TREATMENT.

In tachycardia, digitalis and the cardiac tonics generally, or the carminatives which are useful in ordinary palpitation, appear to have little or no influence on the frequency of the heart's action. Rest, mental as well as bodily, and simple diet must be insisted on, and any functional derangements of the abdominal or pelvic viscera should be corrected. The drugs which have seemed to exercise control over the heart have been bromides, in full doses, and belladonna or atropine, pushed to the limits of tolerance.

Huchard has found digitalis useful, and has had good results in three cases with large doses of quinine. He has also given ergotin with benefit.

Thymus gland has been given with the idea that it is antagonistic to the thyroid, but one would only expect benefit from this, if at all, in Graves' disease. Galvanism of the vagi has been tried, and sometimes a measure of success has been claimed for this treatment.

* "Mal. du Cœur," vol. iii. p. 866.

Barr * states that he has had satisfactory results from the administration of nitrite of amyl and nitroglycerine in two cases of paroxysmal tachycardia. It will be seen that drugs of a widely different character have been employed in the treatment of this affection, and a certain measure of success has been claimed for each in individual cases; but it cannot be said that we have any certain means of reducing the rapid action of the heart, and a certain proportion of cases defy all known methods of treatment.

* Barr, "Clin. Lect. on Paroxysmal Tachycardia," *B.M.J.*, vol. ii. 1904, p. 109.

# CHAPTER XXVII.

## DISORDERS OF RHYTHM OF THE HEART (*Continued*).

VARIETIES OF SLOW PULSE AND THEIR CAUSATION—THE CONDITION OF BRADYCARDIA KNOWN AS STOKES-ADAMS DISEASE—ETIOLOGY—SYMPTOMS—DIAGNOSIS—PROGNOSIS—TREATMENT.

### VARIETIES OF SLOW PULSE AND THEIR CAUSATION.

A CONDITION of permanent slow pulse ranging from 40 to 60 may be hereditary and compatible with good health. It is not, however, altogether free from suspicion of liability to heart failure under the stress of exertion or acute illness. Pathologically, it may be associated with cerebral tumour or meningitis (late stages), or with certain conditions of neurasthenia and with melancholia.

Extreme slowness of pulse is also met with sometimes in toxic conditions, such as lead-poisoning, when it may be attributed to protracted high arterial tension, or may follow influenza, diphtheria, or typhoid fever, the toxins of which affect the integrity of the cardiac muscular fibres. It may occasionally supervene in uræmia, and in jaundice of prolonged duration. Here, again, the slowing of the heart is attributable to toxic substances in the blood. It has been attributed in a few doubtful cases to over-dosing with digitalis and strophanthus and the like. This affection of slow heart action is to be differentiated from the apparently slow pulse met with sometimes in cardiac lesions, in which the pulse seems to be slow because all the heart-beats are not felt as a pulse at the wrist. The pulse may in such cases be irregular, as well as infrequent, but cases are not uncommon in which only every other beat reaches the radial, the rate at the heart being, say, from 80 to 100, while the pulse rate as counted at the wrist is perfectly regular, but only 40 to 50.

## STOKES-ADAMS DISEASE.

In addition to the above conditions in which true bradycardia is met with as an effect of various recognizable influences, there is a certain clinical entity characterized by a group of definite symptoms to which the name of Stokes-Adams disease has been given, from the fact that attention was first called to it by Adams in 1827, while it was subsequently described in fuller detail by Stokes in 1836.

The disease is characterized by permanent slow pulse, ranging habitually as low as 20, or from that to 30 or 40, while there are from time to time exacerbations of the infrequency associated with syncopal, epileptiform, or pseudo-apoplectiform attacks. Sometimes in the later stages there may be angina pectoris or Cheyne-Stokes breathing.

## ETIOLOGY.

The condition is almost invariably associated with senile degenerative changes in the vascular system. The patient is usually over 50 years of age, and the artery at the wrist is large, hard, cord-like, and incompressible. The walls of the vessel are thickened, and arterio-sclerosis is the prominent feature. Huchard, quoted by Osler, states that the etiology of the condition is "la sénilité arterielle," * and

* *Lancet*, August 22, 1903.

Osler endorses this opinion, although he gives three instances of the affection in young subjects in the interesting list of clinical histories of cases under his care.

While thickening of and degenerative changes in the vessels are constant and important factors in the Stokes-Adams syndrome, they cannot be said to explain the bradycardia or other phenomena.

Huchard,* commenting on the frequency of arteriosclerosis and the comparative rarity of the Stokes-Adams phenomena in association with it, suggests that the latter may be due to relative anæmia of the medulla from atheroma of the vessels supplying it. In support of this explanation, he refers to experiments by Brown-Séquard, Duret, and Conty, showing that anæmia of the bulb causes slowing of the pulse, and he instances the slow pulse met with in certain affections of the nervous system. He considers that the feeble action of the heart may be a contributory factor.

Impairment of conductivity of the muscular fibres between the auricle and ventricle has been suggested by Mackenzie of Burnley as an explanation of the slow pulse in these cases. Gaskell has shown that in the frog's heart, if a clamp is applied along the auriculo-ventricular groove, the ventricle can be made to respond to every second, third, or fourth contraction of the auricle or to remain quiescent, according to the tightness of the clamp. Mackenzie † calls attention to this, and has demonstrated, by simultaneous tracings of the auricular wave in the jugulars and the ventricular pulse in the carotids and radials, that similar phenomena may occur in the human heart. He has shown that in a case of slow pulse after influenza the ventricle failed to respond to alternate systoles of the auricle, and in a more extreme case of true bradycardia that the ventricle

* "Mal. du Cœur," vol. i. p. 410.

† *B.M.J.*, March, 1905.

only responded to every third auricular systole. He therefore attributes the slow pulse in Stokes-Adams disease to blocking of conductivity in the muscular fibres between the auricle and ventricle. According to my experience, there is always at least one pulsation in the jugulars between the beats of the pulse.

Gibson * has also published a tracing in which he demonstrates four auricular beats to one ventricular in a case of bradycardia, and he also attributes the phenomena in Stokes-Adams disease to blocking of conductivity.

Maynard † has recently published an interesting case of bradycardia, in which he noted two perceptible impulses of the right ventricle associated with subsidiary cardiac sounds interpolated between the beats of the left ventricle. He concluded that these sounds and impulses were produced in the right side of the heart during the diastolic pause of the left ventricle. This gave rise to some criticism by Gossage and Hay as to whether the assumption of an independent action of the two sides of the heart was tenable. I have, however, in one case, seen two or three distinct right ventricle beats interposed between each systole of the left ventricle. The heat of the left ventricle came at irregular intervals and was very powerful, giving a good radial pulse, but it did not always exactly coincide with a contraction of the right ventricle. I have also seen cases in which an independent beat of the right ventricle was present, associated with a pulsation in the veins of the neck, pointing to a right auricular contraction which had passed on to the right ventricle.

Though it is not possible to demonstrate the contraction of the left auricle, I think we may assume that it is present in these cases, but is not transmitted to the left ventricle from a block in conductivity. This would explain the

* "Nervous Affections of the Heart," 1904. (Fig. 23.)

† *B.M.J.*, vol. ii. 1905, pp. 847 *et seq.*

absence of the left ventricle beat, and would not entail the assumption of independent action of the two sides of the heart.

The left ventricle in this class of cases is usually hypertrophied as a result of high arterial tension, and is more subject to degenerative changes, and it is conceivable that it would require a more forcible stimulus than the thinner walled and more healthy right ventricle, or perhaps a summation of stimuli, to throw it into contraction.

## Symptoms.

Of the symptoms, the syncopal or epileptiform attacks are the most frequent and the most striking. They are characterized by sudden loss of consciousness without any warning, in which the patient usually falls to the ground, as in an epileptic fit; but there are very rarely general convulsions, usually only slight twitching of the face or extremities, or perhaps none at all, the attack resembling rather that of petit mal. In one case under my care for two years (J. F. H. B.) the patient was a retired colonel aged 74, with a pulse of 38 or 40, who had from time to time epileptiform attacks with loss of consciousness of short duration, in which he fell to the ground. He had no other symptoms, no dyspnœa or anginal attacks, and up to the day before his death he insisted on taking a daily promenade in the street.

The epileptiform attacks are accompanied by a further fall in the pulse rate, and it has been supposed that this was a consequence of the seizures. But the sudden loss of consciousness and convulsions, when they occur, are, in my judgment, due to momentary suspension of the cerebral circulation which results from a further fall in the pulse rate, already abnormally slow.

In one case which I had the opportunity of observing, loss of consciousness with slight twitching of the face took place very frequently, and occurred on more than one occasion while I was examining the heart. Each time the heart-beat, previously very slow, was suspended for a long interval. The attack then came on, and could be watched from the first. If in the act of speaking, he suddenly stopped, the expression changed, and twitchings of the face and slight general movements followed. I have, however, seen cases in which there was well-marked passive dilatation of the stomach, and have observed a diminished tendency to syncopal and epileptiform attacks when this condition was treated by dieting and other measures, suggesting that the exciting cause of the syncopal attacks was of reflex gastric origin.

## DIAGNOSIS.

The slow pulse of Stokes-Adams disease must be differentiated from the varieties of slow pulse enumerated at the beginning of this chapter, whether physiological, due to toxic substances in the blood, following on some acute bacterial infection, or associated with certain diseases of the nervous system.

The age of the patient, the condition of the vessels, the occurrence of apoplectiform and epileptiform attacks, will usually render the diagnosis an easy matter. The epileptiform attacks can be distinguished from those of true epilepsy by their association with the slow pulse and by the previous history of the case. The fact that no paralysis or apparent ill effect results from the apoplectiform seizures will readily mark them off from those due to cerebral hæmorrhage.

## PROGNOSIS.

This is necessarily grave, as sudden death may occur from syncope, from angina pectoris, or from an apoplectiform attack followed by coma, while the epileptiform seizures involve the risk of an accident at any time. As a rule, however, it does not prove very rapidly fatal, and patients may survive for many months, or even years.

## Treatment.

The condition is one in which treatment can hardly be expected to effect any great improvement. Iodide of potassium, nitroglycerine, and erythrol tetranitrate, which tend to keep down the arterial tension and make the work of the heart easier, are often of great service, and undoubtedly tend to ward off the epileptiform and apoplectiform seizures.

The frequent association of dilatation of the stomach with Bradycardia must be borne in mind, and measures for the relief of this condition will form an important part of the treatment. Recovery may take place even when Bradycardia, indistinguishable from Stokes-Adams disease, has lasted many months, and appears to be confirmed, and cases are met with in which this condition comes and goes. Treatment of any gastric complication should therefore be persevered with, and careful instructions as to diet should be given.

A light and simple diet should be enjoined in all cases, with strict moderation in animal food, if it is taken at all. Huchard advises a strict "régime lacté," as this tends to keep the arterial tension low and throws least work on the kidneys, and he points out that renal inadequacy is common in this affection.

A certain amount of gentle exercise may be taken when it is well borne and gives rise to no unfavourable symptoms, but in some cases the slightest effort is liable to bring on a cerebral attack. The amount of exercise which can be taken must be decided by experience in each individual case.

# CHAPTER XXVIII.

## ACUTE AORTITIS OR ACUTE DEGENERATIVE LESIONS OF THE AORTA.

EXPERIMENTAL EVIDENCE—ETIOLOGY—MORBID ANATOMY—PATHOGENY—PROGNOSIS—TREATMENT.

ACUTE aortitis, in its typical aspect, as described by Bizot, is a somewhat rare affection, but in lesser degrees of severity is of comparatively frequent occurrence, and has not received the attention it deserves; most affections of the aorta, even in acute infections, being usually loosely classified as "atheroma." Bizot, in 1837, and Ranvier in 1868, gave an account of the pathological, and Bucquoy and Leger, some years later, of the clinical aspects of the disease.

Gilbert and Lion, in 1889, produced acute aortitis experimentally in rabbits by inoculation of micro-organisms after first injuring the aorta with a stylet. Boinet and Romary, in 1898, succeeded in producing acute aortitis experimentally by inoculation of cultures, and also of the toxins only, of various micro-organisms, which in some instances attacked the wall of the aorta not previously injured by a stylet. They also showed that degenerative changes set in rapidly in the affected subendothelial tissue. They further showed that the administration to animals for some months of toxic substances, such as lead and uric acid, produced lesions in the intima.

Huchard,* referring to their experiments, gives a remark-

* "Maladies du Cœur," vol. ii. p. 270.

able illustration by Boinet of a section of the aorta from a case of facial erysipelas, in which typical gelatiniform plaques were present on the endothelium, and chains of streptococci were seen scattered through the middle coat.

## Morbid Anatomy.

The aorta is usually dilated, and may be fusiform or globular in shape. On laying it open it is seen to be of a patchy red or pinkish colour, and the surface is irregular and uneven for a distance of about 1½ to 2 inches from the aortic valves. The uneven surface is due to the presence of smooth, pinkish, rose-coloured, or greyish patches of varying size, termed by Bizot "gelatiniform," from their opalescent appearance. The colour of these patches may vary from a pale pink or grey to a deep red, the colouration being mainly due to post-mortem staining from dissolved hæmoglobin. In cases of less severity the change may be limited to one or more small yellow raised opaque patches, often loosely termed atheroma.

The frontispiece, drawn from a recent specimen of primary acute aortitis, well shows the appearance presented by the affected aorta.

On microscopic examination of these gelatiniform plaques or patches, the endothelium is seen to be swollen, and beneath it are necrotic patches infiltrated with flat, elongated cells, apparently due to proliferation of the connective tissue elements. The middle and outer coats are less affected, but they may be swollen and infiltrated with small round cells, which, in the adventitia, are chiefly conspicuous round the vasa vasorum.

## Etiology.

**Acute Infectious Diseases.**—Acute aortitis may occur in the course of scarlet fever, small pox, more rarely in measles, and in various affections of known bacterial origin, namely, typhoid fever, erysipelas, pneumonia, septicæmia, influenza, rheumatism, and tuberculosis.

In young children who have died of pneumonia or septicæmia, or some acute bacterial infection, I have frequently seen at the autopsy small yellow raised patches in the aorta, which may be regarded as instances of acute degenerative lesions due to the action of micro-organisms or their toxins.

Acute degenerative lesions of the aorta may also occur in severe syphilis in the secondary stage, and also in gout and lead poisoning; but in these affections the chronic degenerative change known as atheroma is more common, especially in tertiary syphilis.

## PATHOGENY.

The experimental results of Gilbert and Lion, and Boinet and Romary, referred to above, throw an important light on the pathogeny of acute aortitis, and show that it can be produced by the action of micro-organisms and their toxins.

In the instances in which the vessel wall was injured by a stylet, one must presume that the micro-organisms effected their entry at the site of the lesion by a direct frontal attack. Where acute aortitis resulted from inoculation without previous injury to the vessel, or from ingestion of toxic substances, the site of the lesion beneath the intima, and the cellular infiltration round the vasa vasorum in the adventitia, would seem to indicate that the toxins reached the affected tissue through the vasa vasorum. The immediate result appears to be necrosis of the part attacked, as there are areas of swollen degenerated amorphous tissue beneath the intima. Subsequently, there is an attempt at repair shown by the presence of flattened proliferating connective tissue cells. As the vasa vasorum normally do not penetrate the middle coat, these proliferating cells are not vascularized, so there is no formation of fibrous tissue or efficient repair, and there is a tendency to the deposition of lime salts in the affected area. In many instances of so-called atheroma of the aorta, as will be shown later in the chapter on that affection, we find vessels penetrating the media and extending down to the sub-endothelial tissue, which may be an attempt to vascularize newly formed connective tissue cells proliferated in the process of repair.

In view of the pathological changes found, which are of the nature of an acute necrosis, the term acute aortitis seems scarcely suitable, and I would suggest "acute degenerative lesions" of the aorta as a more suitable nomenclature.

## Symptoms, Physical Signs, and Diagnosis.

Throbbing of the carotids, a sense of constriction and burning pain behind the sternum, a feeling of intense oppression, accompanied by paroxysms of dyspnœa, have been described as characteristic features of this affection. The temperature is not, as a rule, raised, except as a result of a primary infection of which the aortitis may be a complication. Dilatation of the aorta frequently ensues, but as an aorta previously dilated from atheromatous degeneration may be attacked, this is not always a helpful physical sign.

Angina pectoris may be a prominent symptom, as the root of the aorta is very commonly affected, and the orifice of one of both coronary arteries may be obstructed by swelling of the adjacent tissues.

Huchard attaches considerable importance to dilatation of the aorta, and considers that a sudden onset of severe symptoms in association with this serve to render a diagnosis possible. It is, however, difficult to arrive at a diagnosis with any degree of certainty during life, and, in the absence of angina, it can rarely be made.

An interesting account of two cases of acute aortitis was published in the *Lancet* by Poynton.* One of these cases, under the care of Dr. Cheadle, at St. Mary's Hospital, I had the opportunity of observing. The following is an account of the case, abridged from Dr. Poynton's description in the *Lancet* :—

A woman aged 38 was admitted to St. Mary's Hospital, February, 1899, suffering from pain in the heart and vomiting. Two months before admission she had suffered from attacks of præcordial pain extending down the left arm. These attacks, infrequent at first, had during the last week become more severe, and were accompanied by vomiting and faintness. There was no history of syphilis. On admission she was well nourished and free from pain, but shortly afterwards she had an attack of pain in the left arm, with a feeling of faintness, which Dr. Cheadle considered to be true angina pectoris. She volunteered the statement that any sudden exertion was liable to bring on the attacks of pain. The temperature was normal, pulse 72, but at times the pulse become excited and irregular. The heart was not hypertrophied; there were no murmurs at the base, but the first sound at the apex was sharp, and was preceded occasionally by a short presystolic murmur.

At midnight three days after admission she had a severe attack of angina pectoris, accompanied by vomiting, and she died two hours later.

At the autopsy the heart was slightly dilated. The mitral valve was somewhat thickened from old endocarditis, and contained a calcareous nodule. Its orifice was slightly stenosed. Otherwise the heart appeared to be normal.

The aorta for the first two inches was extensively diseased. The intima was pinkish-red in colour, with raised patches, some of translucent appearance, others yellow, with a red flush round their bases. A few patches resembled the condition of ordinary atheroma. The appearance was that of an acute aortitis, supervening on a more chronic condition.

This is well shown in the coloured frontispiece, which was drawn from this specimen.

The orifice of the right coronary artery was slightly narrowed, but admitted a large probe. That of the left was not affected.

**Microscopical Examination**—

**Aorta.**—The intima was swollen. The vessels were distended, and

* *Lancet*, 1899, vol. i. p. 352.

around them was a free exudation of cells, which in places reached the surface of the intima. The elastic coat was also freely infiltrated with leucocytes. Where the aorta merged into the heart-wall the exudation could be traced beneath the endocardium of the left ventricle.

**Heart Muscle.**—This showed loss of striation, extensive hyaline, and fatty degeneration in many places, and the nuclei showed a feeble staining reaction. In some places between the muscle fibres there was a cellular infiltration and an appearance of active reaction. Some of the vessels showed an increase in the thickness of the outer coat, but no endarteritis or narrowing of their lumen.

Dr. Poynton points out that there was no disease of or marked obstruction of the orifices of the coronary arteries to explain the anginal attacks. He attaches great importance to the profound changes in the cardiac muscle accompanying the aortitis, and attributes death to cardiac failure from this cause.

## PROGNOSIS.

When the orifice of one of the coronary arteries is involved, and attacks of angina pectoris result, the prognosis is necessarily very grave.

In lesions of great severity affecting the arch of the aorta, there is risk of sudden death from perforation, and recently a man aged 46 was brought into St. Mary's Hospital, moribund, in whom a post-mortem examination disclosed the pericardium full of blood, and a minute perforation in the aorta only 1 mm. in diameter, the result of an acute degenerative lesion.

In lesions of minor severity the damaged area remains permanently a weak spot, and may later on in life give rise to an aneurysm, or become the seat of a calcareous deposit.

## TREATMENT.

If the affection is diagnosed, absolute rest and a light non-nitrogenous diet should be enjoined. For the attacks of angina, if present, nitrite of amyl or one or other of the nitrites may be administered. Iodide of potassium and arsenic may be given with advantage as the attack subsides.

# CHAPTER XXIX.

## ATHEROMA OR CHRONIC DEGENERATIVE LESIONS OF THE AORTA.

ETIOLOGY OF GENERAL ARTERIO-SCLEROSIS AND ATHEROMA —MORBID ANATOMY—PATHOGENY—DIFFERENT VIEWS —PHYSICAL SIGNS AND SYMPTOMS—AORTIC INCOMPETENCE DUE TO DEGENERATIVE CHANGE—ITS DISTINGUISHING FEATURES—PROGNOSIS—TREATMENT.

ATHEROMA of the aorta is a degenerative change affecting primarily the deeper layers of the vessel wall. The name is derived from the Greek word ἀθάρη or ἀθήρη, which means "gruel" or "porridge," and emphasizes the fact there is softening and breaking down of the diseased area.

It may be associated with degenerative changes affecting the general arterial system, commonly termed "arterio-sclerosis," or it may exist independently of other vascular lesions.

### ETIOLOGY.

Atheroma of the aorta is usually a disease of middle or advanced life. Many of its causes are the same as those of general arterio-sclerosis, which comprise :—

1. High arterial tension, the etiology of which has already been discussed in Chap. II. Under this heading we have chronic renal disease, gout, over-eating and drinking, particularly excessive meat-eating, associated with defective metabolism and imperfect elimination.

Heredity plays an important part, more especially in

association with the last-mentioned group of cases, in which the tendency to early vascular degeneration may be transmitted through many generations.

2. In addition to high arterial tension, which involves a constant undue strain on the walls of the whole arterial system, and is, as has already been said, a cause of general arterio-sclerosis, there is one form of intermittent strain connected with certain occupations, which affects more particularly the arch of the aorta. This has already been referred to in association with chronic endocarditis (p. 83). The occupations in question are those of the miner, collier, gravedigger, blacksmith, and hammerman, which involve violent effort in a constrained and cramped position, or exertion during which there is prolonged closure of the glottis and fixation of the chest in holding the breath, which give rise to extreme and frequent variations in the blood pressure, and excessive strain on the walls of the arch of the aorta. Hence dilatation of the aorta with associated aortic incompetence are particularly liable to result. General arterio-sclerosis is usually present as well in a marked degree.

3. Lead poisoning.

4. Diabetes and rheumatoid arthritis are mentioned by some authors as causes of arterio-sclerosis. In diabetes in young subjects I have frequently seen small patches of atheroma in the aorta, and in those past middle life extensive disease of the cerebral vessels, but in most instances the diabetes proves fatal before any extensive general arterio-sclerosis results. In rheumatoid arthritis and chronic joint affections thickening and hyperplasia of the vessels are frequently met with.

5. Alcohol and tobacco are usually included in lists of causes of arterio-sclerosis, but there is scarcely sufficient evidence to prove that they are directly responsible, though the wide variations of blood pressure to which they give

rise must have a deleterious effect apart from possible toxic influences.

Among the causes of atheroma of the aorta more particularly, as apart from general arterio-sclerosis, are—

1. **Syphilis.**—This is one of the most important causes of degenerative changes in the aorta, and may affect the aorta alone, as in many cases of aneurysm.

2. **Bacterial Infections.**—These have already been enumerated and their modes of action discussed in the chapter on acute aortitis. It is doubtful how far they should be included among the causes of chronic degenerative change, with the exception of tuberculosis, and, perhaps of rheumatism, but it is difficult to draw a hard-and-fast line between acute and chronic infections. It is possible that many instances of so-called atheroma of the aorta found in later life may be the result of an acute degenerative lesion of an early date, in which calcification or imperfect repair has taken place.

## Morbid Anatomy.

In the earlier stages the inner aspect of the arch of the aorta is studded with opaque, yellowish elevations, smooth on the surface, and varying in number, size, and shape. Later on, ulceration of the endothelial surface may take place, and irregular ragged ulcers result, or calcification of the diseased areas may occur, which may be so extensive that a portion of the aorta is converted into a rigid, inelastic, calcareous tube.

The arch of the aorta is most commonly affected, but the abdominal aorta may be attacked as well, or independently, or the whole of the thoracic and abdominal aorta may be diseased.

**Microscopic Examination.**—Microscopically, in a section from one of these irregular yellow swellings, the endothelium is seen to be pushed forward by a mass of non-staining necrotic material, in which may be distinguished elongated, spindle-shaped connective tissue cells with atrophic small nuclei, strands of swollen fibrous tissue, and in the deeper layers, elastic fibres and smooth muscle fibres, the latter undergoing hyaline degeneration. (*Vide* Fig. 25.) In more advanced cases, fat droplets, crystals of cholestrin, and areas of calcification may be present.

The degenerative process appears to start in the intima

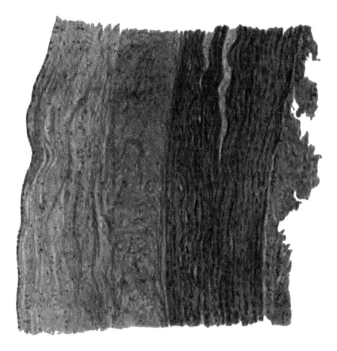

FIG. 25.—SECTION OF WALL OF AORTA, SHOWING EXTENSIVE ATHEROMA AFFECTING THE MEDIA AS WELL AS THE INTIMA.

immediately beneath the endothelium, the adjacent layers of the media being next affected, or sometimes simultaneously.

While this holds good for arteries of lesser size, in the aorta the seat of the primary degeneration may be at some point in the deeper layers of the media, particularly in aneurysm, as will be pointed out later in the chapter on this affection.

The vasa vasorum in the adventitia are usually thickened,

and may be entirely obliterated in places as the result of endarteritis, as in Fig. 26, taken from a case of advanced atheroma of the aorta in a man with a syphilitic history. Sometimes they are congested, and in their neighbourhood are extensive areas of round-celled infiltration. The cells are of the type of lymphocytes, and the appearance suggests

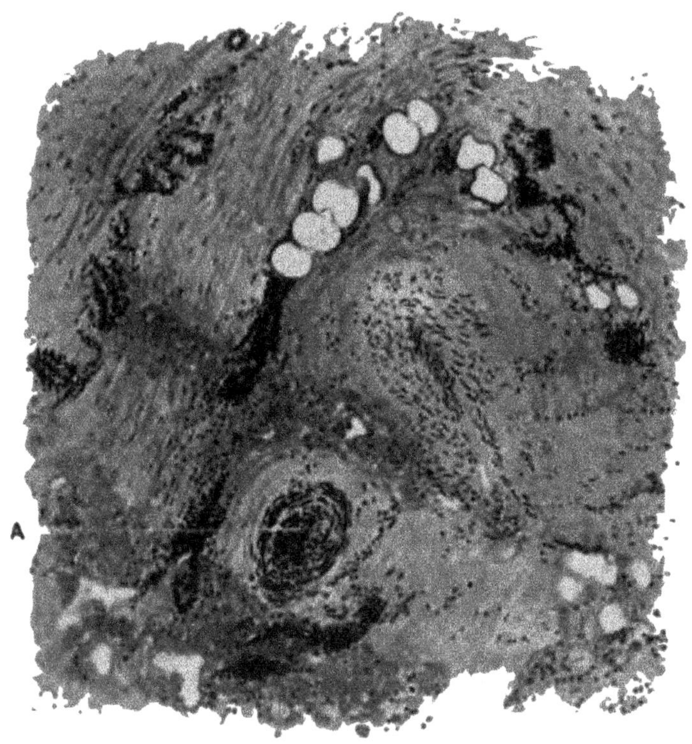


FIG. 26.—SECTION OF ADVENTITIA OF THE WALL OF THE AORTA, SHOWING ENDARTERITIS OBLITERANS OF THE VASA VASORUM. A, VESSEL COMPLETELY OBLITERATED. (x 80.)

that they are called up from the lymphatics as a first line of defence in the tissues against toxins exuding from the vessels. In addition to these lymphocytes, there may be periarteritis and proliferation of connective tissue cells, which is the second line of defence by the tissues. Whereas, normally, no vessels can be detected in the middle coat of the aorta, frequently, in cases of atheroma, numerous small vessels, offshoots from the vasa vasorum, can be seen scattered through the media, penetrating in some cases to the intima. Sometimes areas of round-celled infiltration are present in the neighbourhood of these vessels, and the middle coat is extensively disorganized and broken up. (*Vide* Fig. 27.)

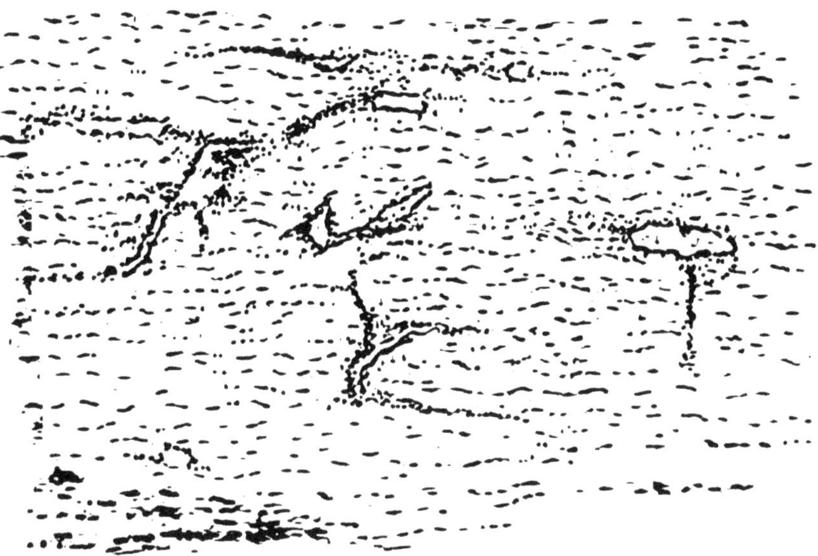

FIG. 27.—SECTION OF MIDDLE COAT OF AORTA, SHOWING NUMEROUS NEWLY FORMED VESSELS.

## PATHOGENY.

Different views are held as to the pathogeny of this condition. Some hold that the primary change is a cell proliferation in the sub-endothelial connective tissue, as a result of irritation due to strain or some toxic material in the blood stream, and that subsequently degeneration of this newly formed tissue takes place.

Thoma taught that the thickening of the intima is a secondary or compensatory process to make good the loss of tissue sustained by the media.

Neither of these views are satisfactory. On microscopical examination the most constant feature in atheroma, even in its earliest stages, is the presence of amorphous, necrotic, non-staining materal. The attempt at cell proliferation is feeble, and one never sees true fibroblasts with large healthy nuclei, which take the stain well, among the newly-formed cells; the nuclei are small and atrophic, and the half-starved cells seem to have given up the attempt to form new fibrous tissue.

The areas of atheromatous tissue do not always fit into depressions in the media, as suggested by Thoma. In the section of the atheromatous coronary artery in Fig. 19, p. 321, it will be seen that the whole of the intima is extensively diseased, and the media is only affected at the point where calcification has taken place, that is, where the disease in the intima is most advanced. In aneurysm it is true that definite atrophy and thinning of the media and a depression on its inner aspect can be made out. Here it is probable, as will be shown later in the chapter on aneurysm, that focal necrosis in the inner half of the media may be the primary change, but the condition is different to that which obtains in atheroma of the smaller vessels. It is contrary to experience that nature should attempt to repair a weak spot by evolving a mass of useless necrotic material, which is what is suggested by those who hold that the atheromatous tissue is compensatory and secondary to degenerative change in the media.

A third and more satisfactory theory is that the primary change is a degeneration or necrosis of the sub-endothelial tissue in the intima and deeper layers of the media. This may be due, among other causes, to the cutting off of nutriment by obliterative lesions of the vasa vasorum, as shown in Fig. 26 in the case of syphilis.

Huchard * attributes all forms of arterio-sclerosis and atheroma to endarteritis obliterans of the vasa vasorum, and sums up his conclusions as follows:—

* "Maladies du Cœur," vol. i. p. 163.

"1. Arterio-sclerosis or atheroma is a dystrophic sclerosis of the walls of the vessels consecutive to endarteritis obliterans of their nutrient arteries. According to H. Martin, atheroma of a vessel furnished with vasa vasorum is invariably preceded by endarteritis of its nutrient vasa vasorum.

"2. In the evolution of general arterio-sclerosis we can distinguish two periods anatomically: (*a*) development of endarteritis of the vasa vasorum; (*b*) disorders of nutrition, which are a consequence of this, and lead to general arterio-sclerosis on the one hand, and visceral sclerosis on the other. Clinically, the first period is usually latent, but the second, that of disordered nutrition, gives rise to symptoms more or less distinctive."

Huchard * meets the objection that the vasa vasorum cannot be traced to the intima, and scarcely even penetrate the media, with the statement that it is for this very reason, namely, that the intima is most distant from the source of nutriment, that the degenerative change commences in the sub-endothelial tissue; the endothelium itself, being nourished by the general blood stream, does not usually suffer.

That the more delicate endothelium of the vasa vasorum may be affected by toxins in the blood, and endarteritis result, leading to obliteration of these vessels and consequent atheroma of the aorta, is shown in Fig. 26, and has already been demonstrated by Mott † in the case of syphilis.

It is possible that other toxins also, *e.g.* lead and uric acid in gouty subjects, may act in the same way, but I do not think that obliteration of the vasa vasorum is invariably responsible for all degenerative lesions of the aorta.

It is probable that, in some cases, the areas of focal

* "Maladies du Cœur," vol. i. p. 158.

† Allbutt's "System of Medicine," vol. vi. p. 311.

necrosis in the subendothelial tissue or deeper layers of the media may be directly due to the destructive action of toxins reaching these tissues through the vasa vasorum. These toxins may be—

(*a*) Of bacterial origin.

(*b*) Metallic, *e.g.* lead.

(*c*) Autogenetic, the result of imperfect metabolism, as in cases of high arterial tension or gout.

The explanation of the presence of cellular elements, which have the appearance of atrophic fibroblasts, would seem to be that they are the result of an attempt at repair by proliferation of connective tissue cells, which fails because efficient vascularization cannot take place, since the vasa vasorum are too far distant to throw off capillary loops, which would have to traverse the media before they reached the newly formed tissue. Thus the newly formed fibroblasts are incapable of forming new fibrous tissue, and themselves degenerate in turn.

In some cases, however, numerous vessels can be seen penetrating the media and reaching almost down to the intima. This is well shown in Fig. 27. Here, I take it, we have an attempt at vacularization of newly formed tissue in the media.

This could scarcely occur if the primary lesion, causing focal necrosis, was obliteration of the vasa vasorum, but might ensue if the necrosis was an acute process due to the destructive action of toxins conveyed through the vasa vasorum, and was followed by an efficient attempt at repair when the causative toxæmia had subsided.

*Strain*, whether intermittent or continuous, is an important etiological factor in degenerative lesions of the aorta, more especially in relation to aneurysm, as will be seen later.

**Conclusions.**—Atheroma is a focal necrosis of the subendothelial tissues of the intima or the adjacent layers of the media, due either to the destructive actions of toxins conveyed by the vasa vasorum or to loss of nutriment from obliteration of the vasa vasorum by endarteritis.

The cellular elements are the result of an attempt at repair by proliferation of connective tissue cells, which fails because efficient vascularization is impossible.

The explanation of atheroma due to intermittent strain associated with arduous occupations, *if* we admit that *strain alone* can produce atheroma, may be that it is in part due to impaired nutrition of the deeper layers of the media, because the condition of over-tension and stretching of the aorta interferes with the passage of nutritive fluids through its walls, and in part to mere mechanical overstrain.

## Physical Signs and Symptoms.

Atheroma of the aorta in its early stages does not give rise to any characteristic physical signs or symptoms. The degenerative process, however, is commonly not confined to the aorta, but is associated with general arterio-sclerosis, evidence of which will be found in the thickened, rigid, uneven radials, the tortuous, irregular, and prominent brachials, which are thrown into curves at each beat of the heart. In the case of syphilis and acute toxæmias, the aorta alone may be affected. The aorta frequently becomes dilated from the yielding of its weakened walls. Sometimes there may be dulness to the right of the sternum, and slight pulsation, but this is seldom apparent except in the case of aneurysm or local dilatation. The most trustworthy sign of dilatation is the alteration in the character of the aortic second sound as heard at the aortic cartilage. This becomes low-pitched, musical, or clanging in character, and appears to be prolonged.

The aortic orifice may be stretched so as to give rise to aortic incompetence from imperfect apposition of the valves, or the aortic cusps may be damaged as a result of strain, and be involved in the degenerative process, becoming thickened, more or less rigid, and incompetent.

This form of aortic incompetence differs greatly in its characteristics from that due to acute endocarditis, discussed in a previous chapter.

Here the aortic valves have become incompetent, usually as a result of high arterial tension with which the degenerative change is commonly associated, and to which it is secondary. The amount of regurgitation is slight; the diastolic murmur is accompanied by a low-pitched, loud, ringing, second sound; the pulse is not markedly collapsing; the artery can be felt between the beats, and is usually thickened.

The arterial tension, though somewhat reduced, remains high in spite of the leakage, because the abnormally great peripheral resistance, the original cause of the high tension in the circulation, is unaltered, and the heart is usually hypertrophied, and acting powerfully. Moreover, in this class of cases, the amount of regurgitation is seldom very great. I have found the blood pressure, estimated by Riva Rocci's instrument, to range from 140 mm. to 190 mm., as contrasted with a blood pressure of 90 to 120 mm. in cases of aortic regurgitation due to acute endocarditis, in which, for reasons given in Chapter II., the mean blood pressure is usually low.

It is the indiscriminate classification of cases of aortic incompetence in which the valves have given out as a result of strain and high arterial tension, with the totally different group in which the valves have been rendered incompetent by acute endocarditis, and to a great extent destroyed, that has given rise to so much discrepancy of opinion as to the mean blood pressure or arterial tension in aortic regurgitation.

**Aneurysm.**—One of the most serious results of atheroma

of the aorta is local weakening of its wall, which may lead to the formation of an aneurysm.

**Occlusion of Coronary Arteries.**—Atheromatous change in the neighbourhood of the orifices of the coronary arteries may partially occlude one or both of them, and give rise to angina pectoris, or to fibroid change in the heart wall.

## Prognosis.

Inasmuch as atheroma is a degenerative change, is usually progressive, and may give rise to aneurysm, dilatation of the aorta, aortic incompetence, and impair the nutrition of the heart by occlusion of the coronary vessels, the prognosis is necessarily grave. As regards the duration of life, much will depend on the nature of the secondary change in the aorta to which the atheroma gives rise, and on the influences to which the patient is exposed.

## Treatment.

When atheroma of the aorta is associated with general arterio-sclerosis and high arterial tension, as is most commonly the case, treatment must be directed to lowering the latter, so that a minimum amount of strain may be thrown on the great vessels and heart.

Alcohol, tobacco, stimulants of all kinds, should be forbidden. Strict moderation in diet should be enjoined, and meat, game, and soups should be eschewed as far as possible. In some cases a strict milk diet may be advisable for a time. Undue exertion and excitement should, as far as possible, be avoided, but gentle walking exercise may be taken. Mild mercurial purgatives should be given once or twice a week, and these may be supplemented, if necessary, by a morning draught of a sulphated mineral water such as Hunyadi, Janos, Apenta, Friedrichshall, and the like.

Vaso-dilators, trinitrin, or erythrol tetranitrate should

be administered if the blood pressure is high, as they tend to lower the arterial tension by diminishing the peripheral resistance. Iodide of potassium may be given in addition, often with marked benefit.

When there is reason to believe that the degenerative change in the aorta is the result of syphilis, iodide of potassium should be freely administered for a long period, either alone or in combination with mercury.

# CHAPTER XXX.

## ANEURYSM OF THE ARCH OF THE AORTA.

MORBID ANATOMY — ETIOLOGY — PATHOGENY — RELATIONS OF THE ARCH OF THE AORTA—PHYSICAL SIGNS AND SYMPTOMS—ANEURYSM (1) OF THE INTRA-PERICARDIAL PORTION OF AORTA; (2) OF ASCENDING AORTA; (3) OF TRANSVERSE PART OF ARCH; (4) OF DESCENDING AORTA —DIAGNOSIS—PROGNOSIS—TREATMENT.

AN aneurysm is a pulsating tumour in connection with the interior of an artery. It is caused by the bulging or giving way, under the blood pressure of a portion of the wall of an artery weakened by injury or disease. It may be saccular, fusiform, or cylindrical in shape, according to the extent and area of the arterial wall which gives way in the first instance.

### MORBID ANATOMY.

A *cylindrical* or fusiform aneurysm is merely a general dilatation of the vessel in some part of its course.

A saccular aneurysm is caused by the giving way of a circumscribed portion of the vessel wall as the result of some morbid process affecting the deeper layers of the media. This weak spot gradually bulges and yields more and more under the blood pressure. The dilated portion is termed the sac, and the orifice by which it communicates with the interior of the vessel is termed the mouth of the sac.

The intima can usually be traced for a varying distance on to the interior of the sac.

The media is greatly thinned; the muscular fibres are atrophied and compressed, and have, to a great extent, disappeared; the elastic fibres are stretched and have lost their elasticity, and may be ruptured in places. The adventitia is thickened from formation of new fibrous tissue, so that the wall of the sac consists mainly of the thickened adventitia, with which may be incorporated adjacent structures to which it becomes adherent.

As the aneurysm increases in size and the mouth of the sac becomes relatively small in comparison with its interior, the circulation of blood in the sac becomes sluggish, and layers of laminated clot are deposited on the diseased walls.

The so-called dissecting aneurysm is not, strictly speaking, a true aneurysm. In this condition there is a rupture of the intima and of a portion of the media, through which the blood penetrates the media and tears its way downwards in its substance for a varying distance, sometimes finding its way back again into the interior of the vessel at a lower level.

## ETIOLOGY.

**Age.**—Aneurysm is a disease of middle and advanced life, but is met with also in young adults.

**Sex and Occupation.**—It is far more common in men than in women, which seems to point to hard work and laborious occupations as a factor in its production. It is frequently met with in soldiers and miners; the prolonged and severe exertion to which the former are subjected in campaigning and forced marches, together with the restraint on the free play of the chest wall by arms and accoutrements, the arduous nature of the work of the latter, and the constrained and cramped position in which they have to work, have been held to account for its common occurrence in men following these occupations.

Atheroma of the aorta, a comprehensive term, in ordinary parlance, for degenerative lesions of the aorta, of whatsoever origin, is one of the commonest causes of aneurysm. Its etiology has already been discussed in the last chapter, but as extensive and widespread atheroma of the aorta is of common occurrence without aneurysm, it is clear that certain factors must be more particularly concerned in the production of the latter. These are—

I. Affections which give rise to circumscribed or focal, rather than general, lesions of the aorta.

II. Conditions of varying and high blood pressure within the aorta.

Among the former are—

(*a*) **Syphilis.**—This is unquestionably one of the most important factors in the production of aneurysm, and about this opinion is almost unanimous. Welsh found a history of syphilis in 50 per cent., Fränkel in 47 per cent., and Huchard in 43 per cent. of cases of aneurysm of the aorta. Drummond of Newcastle considered that in a large proportion of cases of aneurysm in miners, attributed to strain, syphilis was mainly responsible, and this may be so, in soldiers, in whom, also, syphilis is very common.

It seems probable that syphilis may produce focal lesions of the aorta in two ways—

(1) In the secondary stage by a toxic action on the vessel wall similar to that of acute bacterial infections.

(2) In the later stages, by setting up endarteritis obliterans of the vasa vasorum of the aorta, at one or more points, and thus depriving its wall of the necessary nutriment, with resulting slow necrosis and degenerative change in the deeper layers of the media in corresponding circumscribed areas.

(*b*) **Acute Bacterial Infections.**—These I would suggest

as causes next in importance to syphilis. I am aware that they are not generally recognized etiological factors, but the experimental results of Boinet and Romary, detailed in Chapter XXVIII., afford strong support to this view, which has also certain pathological evidence in its favour. As already explained, it is probable that the toxins evolved by the micro-organisms reaching the aorta through the vasa vasorum give rise to areas of focal necrosis in the deeper layers of the media. Efficient repair does not take place, and a weak spot in the vessel wall results, which in later life, possibly some years after the primary lesion, when other factors have given rise to high arterial tension and increased blood pressure in the aorta, may become the site of an aneurysm.

Huchard * holds that whereas gout, atheroma, syphilis, alcoholism, and malaria, which may set up focal degeneration in the media, are predisposing causes, the supervention of some acute bacterial infection is commonly the immediate cause of aneurysm. In support of this, he instances the development of an aneurysm in syphilitic and gouty subjects, which he has observed subsequent to a severe attack of influenza.

(*c*) **Toxins other than Bacterial.**—Lead poisoning, which is a common cause of general arterio-sclerosis, can seldom be traced as a factor in aneurysm. We have little direct evidence as to the part played in the production of aneurysm by alcohol, or organic poisons such as may result from imperfect metabolism in gouty and plethoric subjects. Fischer † of Bonn has, however, recently published an account of experiments in which he was able to produce aneurysms in rabbits by repeated injections of adrenalin or digalen, and in the light of these it is possible that a variety of toxins may be etiological factors in aneurysm.

* "Mal. du Cœur," vol. ii. pp. 872, 873.

† *Deut. Med. Woch.*, October 26, 1905, pp. 1713 *et seq.*

These experiments will be referred to in more detail later on.

GROUP II. **Varying Conditions of High Blood Pressure in the Aorta.**—The strain to which the walls of the arch of the aorta are subjected by the varying conditions of the blood pressure within is greater than in any other vessel.

The blood, as it is forcibly expelled from the ventricle at each systole, rapidly expands the aorta, and impinges on the dome of the arch by which it is deflected. The respiratory variations of the blood pressure are also very considerable. The pressure is raised in inspiration, and in occupations which involve severe effort in cramped positions, frequently with the glottis closed, the strain imposed on the walls of the arch must be greatly increased. Strain on the vessel wall, more especially intermittent strain due to fluctuations in the blood pressure, which occur in these arduous occupations, such as those of the miner, collier, soldier, is unquestionably an important etiological factor in aneurysm.

I have seen two cases of spontaneous rupture of the intrapericardial portion of the aorta in which there was no patch of atheroma or indication of previous disease. The aorta was greatly dilated and stretched in both instances, and its walls were about the thickness of ordinary brown paper. One was in a man aged 42, who was brought in dead to St. Mary's Hospital; the other was in a boy aged 20, with pneumothorax on the left side. The rupture in this case occurred when the boy was apparently convalescent, three months after the onset of the pneumothorax.

## PATHOGENY.

The interesting paper of Fischer of Bonn already referred to throws much light on the pathogeny of aneurysm. He describes how he has been able to produce aneurysm of the aorta in rabbits experimentally by repeated injections of adrenalin.

Josué had previously produced arterio-sclerosis and atheroma in rabbits by injections of adrenalin, and his results have been confirmed by other investigators, including Fischer, who describes his results with adrenalin as follows :—

"The first alterations are circumscribed areas of necrosis of the smooth muscle fibres of the media. Dilatation of the aorta with straightening out of the elastic fibres, which normally have a wavy outline, is the next change. The thick elastic lamellæ are approximated, and the more delicate elastic fibres between them disappear. In most cases calcification of the necrotic area sets in early, so that a compact lamina of lime salts is found in the media, and the elastic fibres in the neighbourhood are torn and destroyed. I have thus demonstrated that this process differs materially from human arterio-sclerosis, and that a primary necrosis of the muscular fibres and the elastic lamellæ of the media is the cause of it. I have therefore given to this condition the name 'arterio-necrosis.'"

Fischer has also shown that various toxic substances besides adrenalin can produce this condition of arterio-necrosis in rabbits, but not aneurysm, which apparently requires, in addition, the increased blood pressure induced by the administration of adrenalin. He has produced a typical aneurysm of the aorta in a rabbit by twenty-one intravenous injections of adrenalin (1 in 1000), in doses of 0·3 to 0·5 ccm., and in one instance, a dissecting aneurysm of the aorta after twenty-three similar injections of adrenalin. He has also succeeded in producing aneurysm by repeated injections of digalen, a preparation of digitalis which would have similar effect to adrenalin in raising the blood pressure. He found that the arch of the aorta was most commonly affected first, and next in sequence, the thoracic aorta.

This experimental evidence would seem to point to a focal lesion of the deeper layers of the middle coat of the aorta as the primary lesion or predisposing cause, and to undue increase of the blood pressure within its walls as the exciting cause of aneurysm.

It is remarkable that in chronic interstitial nephritis, in which the blood pressure is higher, perhaps, than in any other affection, aneurysm is comparatively rare. The explanation of this would seem to be (1) that, as the rise in blood pressure is gradual, the vascular system has time to adapt itself to the increased strain by hypertrophy of its muscular coat, and is, moreover, maintained in a condition of hypertonus; (2) that the disease does not tend to produce a focal lesion in the aorta. MacWilliam* has demonstrated that in contracted arteries, the range of pulsatile expansion is much less than in relaxed vessels, and that there is a greater tendency to elongation and tortuosity, and consequently to dilatation of relaxed vessels subjected to strain. The maintenance of a condition of hypertonus is therefore protective against aneurysm.

In the arduous occupations which have been referred to above as predisposing to aneurysm, there is no protective hypertonus of the vessels; the strain is intermittent, and not constant, and may take place when the aorta is relaxed and more or less defenceless, so that the conditions are more favourable to aneurysm. It is, however, doubtful if this can result from strain alone, in the absence of a previous focal lesion of the vessel wall. The importance of a focal lesion as a factor in aneurysm is clearly demonstrated in syphilitic lesions of the aorta, in which no rise of blood pressure above the normal appears to be necessary to dilate the weakened area and give rise to aneurysm.

* Properties of Arterial and Venous Walls, *Proc. Roy. Soc.*, vol. lxx. p. 151.

## Anatomical Relations of the Arch of the Aorta.

Before discussing the physical signs of aneurysm, we must call to mind the *position and chief relations* of the arch of the aorta, as many of the symptoms and physical signs of aneurysm are directly dependent on pressure effects of the dilated portion of the vessel on the adjacent structures.

The aorta, as it emerges from the left ventricle behind the pulmonary artery, and overlapped by the appendix of the right auricle, takes an oblique course upwards, to the right and forwards, to the level of the upper border of the second right costal cartilage; this, anatomically, is termed the ascending aorta, but in discussing aneurysm it will be more convenient, clinically, to include under this head, the portion of the aorta from the pericardium to the origin of the innominate. The most important relations of the ascending portion of the arch with reference to the symptoms to which aneurysm of this part may give rise, are, the vena cava superior on the right or outer side, and the root of the right lung posteriorly; but, as there is free and extensive movement of this portion of the aorta at each cardiac systole, and provision is made for this, the surrounding structures are not in very close relation to the vessel: hence pressure symptoms will not arise till the aneurysm has attained a considerable size. It must not be forgotten that part of the aorta lies free in the pericardial cavity for a short distance from its origin; aneurysms of this intra-pericardial portion, more especially of one of the sinuses of Valsalva, are liable to rupture and cause sudden death before any physical signs or symptoms arise which would lead one to suspect their presence.

The second or transverse part of the arch of the aorta has a direction backward and to the left, and comprises the portion of the vessel between, and including the orifices of the innominate and left sub-clavian arteries. This portion has little freedom of movement, and lies in close relation to several important structures, pressure on which may early

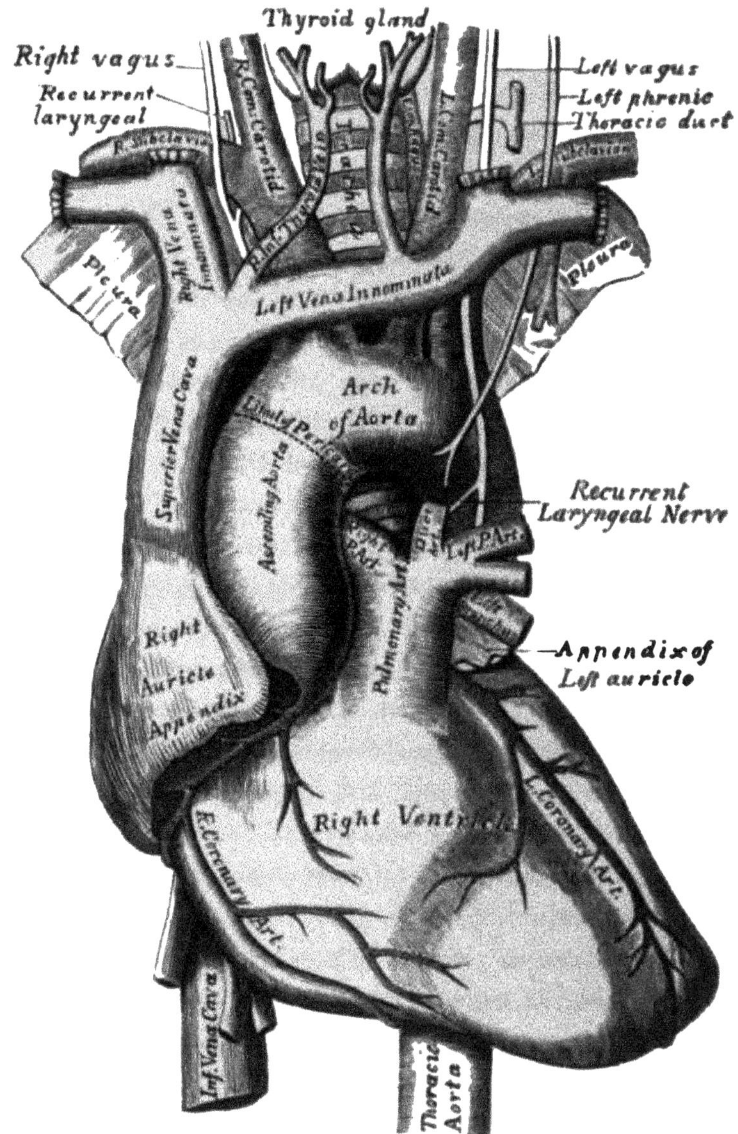


FIG. 28.—RELATIONS OF ARCH OF AORTA. From Gray's *Anatomy*.

give rise to characteristic symptoms. Behind it lie the trachea, œsophagus and thoracic duct: interposed between it and the trachea just above the bifurcation is the deep cardiac plexus; the left recurrent laryngeal nerve also curves round it and ascends towards the trachea on its posterior surface. In front the left vagus and left phrenic nerves and the two superficial cardiac nerves from the sympathetic and pneumogastric respectively, cross its anterior surface which, from its oblique course, looks to the left as well as forwards. Above is the left innominate vein; from its upper aspect are given off the innominate and left carotid and sub-clavian trunks. Below is the bifurcation of the pulmonary artery, the left bronchus, and the left recurrent laryngeal nerve as it winds round the aorta.

The third or descending part of the arch completes the curve downward and backward. It descends behind the root of the left lung to lie to the left of the body of the fourth dorsal vertebra.

As has been shown in the brief sketch of the course and relations of the arch of the aorta, the ascending portion is near the surface of the chest and accessible to physical examination, has no attachments to surrounding structures, and enjoys considerable freedom of movement. Aneurysm here often attains to considerable size before it begins to give rise to any symptoms from pressure on surrounding organs, so that the first indication of its presence may be a pulsating tumour visible on the chest wall to the right of the manubrium.

The transverse portion of the arch, on the contrary, is deeply placed, is more or less firmly fixed in position, and is in such close relation to various important structures, that a projection from its surface cannot elude or be eluded by the surrounding parts. Hence aneurysm of this portion of the aorta before it attains any great size, usually gives rise to symptoms from pressure on adjacent structures, of which a brassy cough and cracked voice, or tracheal breathing and difficulty of deglutition, may be the indications.

I have consequently been led to divide thoracic aneurysms into two classes, namely *Aneurysms of Physical Signs* and *Aneurysms of Symptoms*, from the predominance of physical signs and symptoms respectively, the former term applying to aneurysms of the ascending aorta and first part of the arch, the latter to aneurysms of the transverse and descending portions of the arch.

## Physical Signs of Aneurysm in general.

The most important and conclusive physical sign is *pulsation* at some part of the chest wall where it is not normally present. We must of course make sure that it is not due to the heart or great vessels being simply uncovered or displaced, as for example by the mediastinum being dragged to the right in consequence of retraction of the right lung, or by deformity of the chest wall bringing the heart or aorta into contact with the chest wall in some unusual situation. The pulsation may or may not be visible; when obscure it may sometimes be made more perceptible by pressing firmly on the part and watching the hand which is making the pressure; sometimes it can be seen by standing behind the patient and looking over his shoulders; it may be recognizable only during expiration; in doubtful cases the pulsation may sometimes be rendered evident by placing the small end of a wooden stethoscope on the spot, one half resting on a rib, the other pressed into the interspace, when the stethoscope will be tilted.

Pulsation when visible may be a localized protrusion or a general heave. Generally speaking it is best felt by placing the palm of the hand flat on the pulsating area, but it may be necessary to press the fingers well into the intercostal spaces. In estimating the significance of pulsation, whether in a tumour within the cavity of the thorax, or in a tumour which has made its way through the chest walls, there must be taken into account, not only the degree of its force or violence, and the extent of the area over which it is felt, but also its character, that is, whether it is distinctly expansile in some or all directions, or is simply firm and thrusting without marked expansion. In the former case the pulsating tumour will feel soft, and there will be no laminated fibrin lining supporting its wall; in the latter case this will probably be present. These conditions have an important bearing on the probable progress of the aneurysm, and consequently on the question of prognosis.

A characteristic vibratory thrill may be present, and is best felt by the palm of the hand pressed lightly on the tumour. Another point to be ascertained in the process of palpation is the presence or absence of a *diastolic shock*. This is a sharp vibration or shock, felt at the end of the true pulsation, synchronous with and due to the same cause as the second sound of the heart, viz. the recoil of the elastic walls of the aorta from the distension caused by the systolic injection of blood. This diastolic shock is the most absolutely pathognomonic of the signs of aneurysm; pulsation may be communicated to a tumour, or a malignant growth may itself be pulsatile, but there is no diastolic shock under such conditions.

The fingers may have to be pressed into intercostal spaces to recognize pulsation when an aneurysm of the ascending aorta is just projecting from under the right edge of the sternum; usually it is best felt at the end of expiration, when the border of the lung is withdrawn from over the vessel. It must be borne in mind that pulsation can often be made out in two or three spaces close to the right of the sternum, when the aorta is dilated from protracted high tension, or from incompetence of the aortic valves: it is when it is felt in one space only, and for a certain distance beyond the edge of the sternum, that it may be accepted as significant of aneurysm. More rarely can pulsation to the left of the manubrium be detected in this way in cases of aneurysm of the transverse portion of the arch.

The *tracheal tug* should be sought for while carrying out the examination by palpation. To detect this, the trachea is put gently on the stretch, by the fingers, which are placed just beneath the cricoid cartilage: if present a distinct short tug on the trachea is felt with each cardiac systole, superimposed on the slower up and down movements in respiration. It is a very important sign, but not absolutely conclusive, and in particular it does not help to distinguish between a sacculated projection from the aorta, and a general dilatation of the arch. A slight shock or communicated pulsation may sometimes be felt even in cases where there is no disease of heart or aorta.

**Percussion.**—When pulsation is distinct the evidence to be obtained by percussion is of secondary importance. Dulness around the pulsating area will merely serve to indicate the extent of the aneurysm. When pulsation is obscure, or absent, deep dulness on percussion over a certain area may corroborate and reinforce other indications of aneurysm, and be of great diagnostic value; such may be especially the case when the aneurysm is in the transverse or descending part of the arch, and is comparatively small: very slight physical signs may be then of great importance in the interpretation of the symptoms present; the area of dulness in such a case would probably be situated to the left of the manubrium and over the left half of the manubrium itself.

**Auscultation.**—Of the auscultatory indications, by far the most important is a low-pitched, musical second sound, which, when well marked, is loud and ringing. It is coincident with the diastolic shock, and when a rigid stethoscope is employed in auscultation the shock and sound will be felt and heard together. The significance of this ringing, low-pitched second sound is greater, the more remote its point of maximum intensity from the aortic valves—when, for example, it is heard far out in the right chest, and especially when it appears to the left of the manubrium: a reinforcement and change in character of the second sound in the course of the aorta can scarcely be due to any other cause than a dilatation or aneurysm.

This *aneurysmal second sound* is not simply an accentuation or intensification of the normal aortic second sound; the pitch is lower from the fact that the wall of the sac constitutes a larger area of resonating membrane than the tube of the aorta. The second sound is not produced by a click of the semi-lunar valves or by their sudden tension, but by the sudden tension of the walls of the aorta and valves together, as a vibrating membrane. When the aortic valves are incompetent, the aneurysmal second sound is impaired, but rarely extinguished.

The difference in the character and mode of production of the aortic and the aneurysmal second sound may be illustrated by suddenly putting on the stretch a small length of linen (say three inches of the border of a pocket-handkerchief) and comparing the sound thus produced with that which is generated when a portion double the length is similarly put on the stretch. In the latter instance the sound is lower pitched, of greater volume, less sharp in character than in the former, and corresponds to the aneurysmal second sound.

A *murmur* may or may not be heard in aneurysm. When present over a pulsating area, it adds nothing to the value of other physical signs, since a tumour pressing upon the aorta, or one of its branches, may give rise to a murmur, and its absence does not detract from their significance. Sometimes when no murmur is heard over the aneurysm itself, one may be heard on the distal side of the sac, caused by pressure on the aorta beyond it or on some of its branches. A murmur may be a sign of great value when, being absent over the aortic area, it is developed in the course of the arch and becomes audible over, or to the left of, the manubrium.

The auscultatory signs resulting from pressure on the root of one or other lung, will not be discussed here, but mention must be made of tracheal breath sounds conducted to the manubrium by means of an aneurysm in contact with the trachea; these may be heard over this bone loudly and distinctly before serious pressure is produced by the aneurysm on the trachea.

**The Pulse.**—An aneurysm may give rise to characteristic modification of, or difference between the two radial pulses.

The sac of an aneurysm is readily distended, and has little contractile power or elastic recoil, and its interposition in the course of the aorta will impair and delay the pressure or pulse-wave which is transmitted with great rapidity at each systole of the heart throughout the arterial system.

The combined effect on the pulse-wave will be, firstly to delay it, secondly to diminish its height, thirdly to cause its duration to be longer, and its subsidence more gradual and slower than normal.

As a further consequence, the artery will also be constantly full between the beats, as the sac acts like a blacksmith's bellows—being, in fact, a reservoir of blood.

These points are well illustrated by the sphygmographic tracings appended (Figs. 29 and 30).

It is obvious that if the aneurysm is situated in the ascending aorta, it will affect both pulses alike, and as there will then be no standard of comparison, such modification of the pulse, if it exist, will be of no great help in diagnosis. Moreover, the modification of the pulse is not, as a rule, so striking as to attract attention.

Difference between the two radial pulses is, however, frequently one of the most important physical signs in diagnosis of aneurysm, and may be present in the earlier stages, before pulsation is visible.

Difference between the pulses may arise: (1) From partial blocking of the mouth of one of the main branches of the aorta given off from an aneurysmal sac by projection into it of a portion of fibrin from the organized deposit on the walls of the sac. (2) From pressure on the innominate, or one of the sub-clavian arteries by an aneurysm; one of these

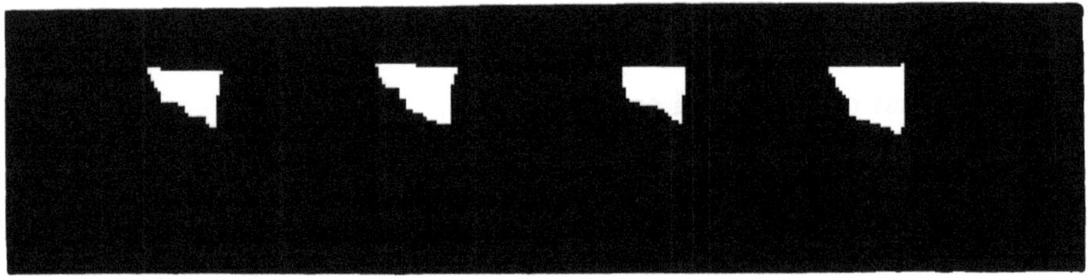

Walter Broadbent, *fecit.*

FIG. 29.—LEFT RADIAL PULSE IN ANEURYSM OF ASCENDING AORTA INVOLVING ORIFICE OF INNOMINATE ARTERY.

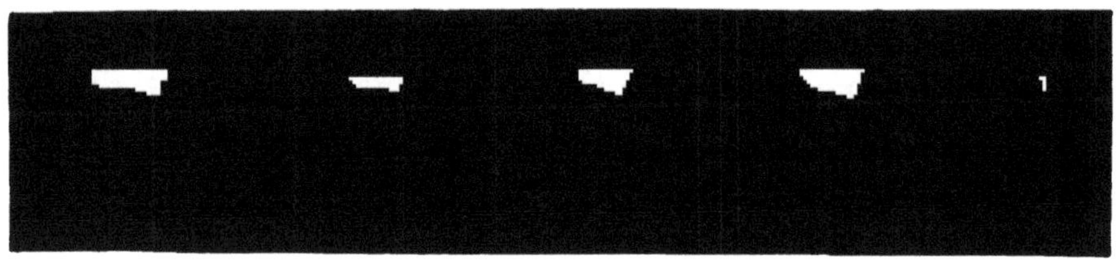

FIG. 30.—RIGHT RADIAL PULSE IN SAME CASE.

vessels may even be involved in the sac and run in its walls, so that its lumen becomes partially or totally obliterated. For instance, the right radial artery may be smaller than the left, and the pulsation in it weakened or altered in character, or entirely absent, from pressure of an aneurysm on the innominate artery, or from obstruction of its orifice. More frequently it is the left pulse which is affected, either by the interposition of an aneurysm between the origin of the innominate and the left sub-clavian artery, or by the

seemed to be no escape from a diagnosis of aneurysm of the transverse part of the arch involving the orifice of the left sub-clavian (*vide* tracings Figs. 33 and 34). The patient was fifty-eight years of age, and was admitted for shortness of breath and severe pain in the præcordial region. The heart was hypertrophied, and there was a double aortic murmur. There was no pulsation visible over the aortic or pulmonic area, and no dulness on percussion. There was, in fact, no other physical sign of aneurysm, except the

FIG. 33.—LEFT RADIAL PULSE, IN CASE WHERE ORIFICE OF LEFT SUB-CLAVIAN WAS OBSTRUCTED BY ATHEROMA.

FIG. 34.—RIGHT RADIAL PULSE.

marked difference in the pulses, though the severe pain in the chest and paroxysms of dyspnœa were symptoms consistent with, and in favour of aneurysm. At the post-mortem no aneurysm was found, but the orifice of the left sub-clavian artery was about one-half occluded by a thick calcareous plate projecting across it. The aorta was also dilated and atheromatous, and the aortic valves were incompetent.

*Delay of Pulse.*—One of the most characteristic differences between the two radial pulses which may be present in aneurysm is the apparent delay in one, when they are both felt at the same time. If one is affected by the interposition of the aneurysmal sac, the rise in pressure is more gradual, and reaches its maximum later; and as this is what is felt as the pulse, it will be delayed as compared with that of the other side.

**The Carotid Arteries.**—It must be borne in mind also that an aneurysm may affect pulsation in the carotids in the same way as in the radials. For, the orifice of the left carotid may be involved in the sac, or may be partially occluded by a plug of fibrin, and it is obvious that whatever affects the innominate artery will similarly affect the right sub-clavian and right carotid. The blocking of one carotid, partial or complete, or a difference between the pulsation in the carotids on either side, corresponding to that already noted in the radials, will be important confirmatory evidence of aneurysm.

**The Heart.**—It has been asserted by some authorities that aneurysm gives rise to hypertrophy of the heart. That this is *not* the case has been conclusively shown by Dr. James Calvert,* in a paper based on an analysis of 124 cases of aneurysm collected by Dr. Oswald Browne. In 68 of these cases aneurysm existed without giving rise to any hypertrophy of the heart. It is, however, true that cardiac hypertrophy is not infrequently found in association with aneurysm, but it may almost invariably be explained by causes other than aneurysm, such as arterio-sclerosis or prolonged high arterial tension due to kidney disease or other causes.

The heart may be displaced by aneurysm of the ascending aorta, or of the transverse part of the arch, so that the apex beat may be found below and outside its normal position, but this should not be mistaken for hypertrophy. More frequently the apex beat is displaced upwards: its position, and the extent to which the heart is displaced, will vary according to the size, shape, and situation of the aneurysm.

The physical signs that have been discussed thus far are mainly those directly dependent on the aneurysm itself, produced in and by it, and not on indirect or *pressure effects* of the aneurysm on adjacent structures, which will now be considered.

* *Trans. Med. Chir. Soc.*, 1899.

## Pressure Effects of Aneurysm on Adjacent Structures.

1. **The Great Veins.**—An aneurysm may compress and cause obstruction to the flow of blood through one of the large venous trunks, the vena cava superior, or the right or left innominate veins.

A sudden and complete block of the vena cava superior from thrombosis, or from compression by sudden extension of the aneurysm, may give rise to œdema of the head and neck and upper extremities, with a cyanotic appearance, the face being enormously swollen and disfigured, while severe dyspnœa is produced by œdema of the fauces and larynx. This, however, is an extremely rare event, only one example having come under my observation. Usually, the pressure takes effect gradually, and collateral venous channels are developed which carry the blood from the tributaries of the superior vena cava to the inferior, and obviate the effect described. Some of these are external, in the form of large tortuous veins crossing the clavicles, descending the surface of the chest, sometimes continued down the abdomen. A remarkable instance of this is shown in the photograph (Fig. 35) taken from a case of aneurysm of the first part of the arch, which was under observation for upwards of six years. The mass of dilated veins, some of which were of the size of the finger, on the surface of and below the tumour, was a striking feature. Below the mamma many of these veins disappeared, presumably anastomosing with the intercostal veins, but three large tortuous veins continued downward to anastomose apparently with the right epigastric veins. The direction of the current of blood, which should always be carefully ascertained, was found to be downwards. Other channels of communication, in which the azygos veins take part, are deep seated and not open to observation. The proportion of superficial and deep collateral venous circulation varies greatly in different cases.

The jugulars are distended, and an important point is that they are not emptied even partially by a deep inspiration, as is the case, more or less, when the veins of the neck are full from back pressure in the systemic venous system in mitral disease, or in emphysema and bronchitis.

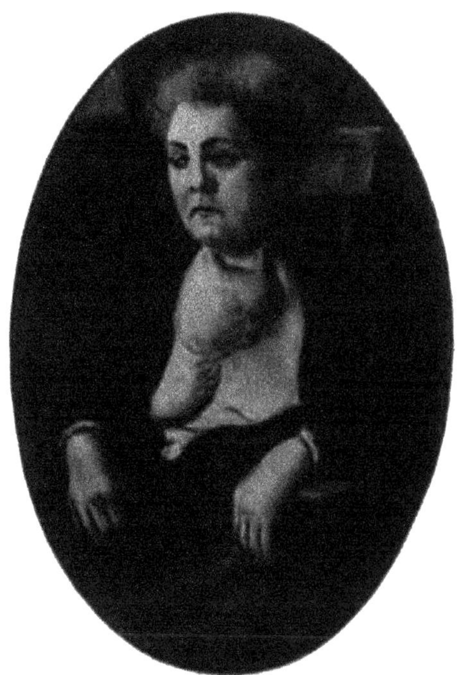

FIG. 35.—TORTUOUS DILATED VEINS ON SURFACE OF LARGE ANEURYSM OF ASCENDING AORTA.

Again, there is no true jugular pulsation such as is present in venous reflux from the tricuspid incompetence which supervenes as a result of dilatation of the right ventricle in mitral disease or emphysema. There may, however, be apparent pulsation in the veins caused by the subjacent carotid.

There may be pressure on the azygos vein which passes up behind the root of the right lung to open into the superior vena cava just before it enters the pericardium. This does not appear to give rise to any characteristic physical signs or symptoms, probably because of the free anastomosis with the lumbar veins, which enables the blood to return without difficulty viâ the iliac veins and inferior vena cava.

Even more interesting than obstruction of the vena cava is obstruction of one or other of the innominate veins. The discovery of a one-sided distension of the external and anterior jugulars, not disappearing in deep inspiration, especially if associated with dilatation of the veins of the upper extremity, is not unfrequently the first step towards the diagnosis of an aneurysm which might otherwise have eluded detection for some time. In such a case the collateral enlargement of veins is also one-sided.

2. **Pressure on the Root of the Lung.**—Pressure on the right or left bronchus will cause diminished entry of air to the corresponding lung, with characteristic alteration of the breath sounds. When the bronchus is obstructed without pressure on the pulmonary veins, the resonance will not be impaired, or will be only slightly modified. Resonance on percussion in association with silence on auscultation (pneumothorax, of course, being excluded) are highly characteristic of obstruction of a bronchus. The collapse of lung which eventually ensues will give rise to some falling in of the intercostal spaces, and impairment of resonance.

Pressure on the pulmonary veins may occur, giving rise to congestion of the lung tissue. As a rule, however, they escape compression in spite of their unresisting structure, probably because they are protected by the bronchi which usually suffer first. One case, nevertheless, has come under my notice in which the lung was found at the autopsy to be in a semi-gangrenous condition from this cause. The aneurysm was a large one, about the size of two fists, affecting the ascending aorta and extending backwards, and compressing the root of the right lung as well as presenting on the chest wall as a pulsating tumour.

3. Pressure on the cilio-spinal branches of the sympathetic may cause dilatation or contraction of the pupil on the corresponding side according as the dilator fibres are irritated or destroyed by compression.

4. Pressure on the left recurrent laryngeal nerve will cause paralysis of the left vocal cord.

The right recurrent laryngeal nerve is seldom affected by aneurysm of the aorta, since it winds round the right sub-clavian artery; occasionally it may be subjected to pressure by the sac of an aneurysm of the transverse part of the arch involving the orifice of the innominate, or by extension upwards of an aneurysm of the ascending part of the arch.

5. Pressure on the trachea, œsophagus, and thoracic duct may be caused by an aneurysm of the transverse or descending part of the arch.

There remains for discussion one symptom, namely pain, which is usually, at some period in the history of an aneurysm, a conspicuous feature.

Pain is very rarely absent, though it differs greatly in character and intensity in different cases. A feature common to aneurysmal pain of all kinds and in any situation, is the aggravation of it by exertion.

Pain may be the sole symptom, and may be of itself, without corroboration by physical signs, sufficient for a diagnosis of aneurysm.

Aneurysm at the very root of the aorta within the cavity of the pericardial sac, or aneurysm of the sinuses of Valsalva, may give rise to pain of anginoid character. It may indeed cause true angina by extension of disease from the sinuses of Valsalva along the coronary arteries, or by obstructing the openings of these vessels and consequently giving rise to degeneration of the walls of the heart. It is not always possible to distinguish between anginoid pain due to aneurysm in this situation and true angina; the sense of impending death is not as a rule so marked a feature of the attacks, and the pain often radiates down both arms instead of along the left only; occasionally it shoots down the right arm only. In angina, there may be no physical signs of disease in the great vessels; in aneurysm there will be the ringing second sound, and frequently a diastolic murmur, but rarely, dulness on percussion or recognizable pulsation.

In aneurysm of the ascending aorta, there is usually deep-seated pain of a vague kind which may be very severe while the aneurysm is extending, and may become quiescent when it has ceased to enlarge. It is usually aggravated by certain positions, relieved by others, so as to constrain the patient to a particular decubitus, different in different cases without obvious reasons. Pain in the right shoulder or scapular region may indicate backward extension of an aneurysm of the ascending aorta which is not revealed by physical signs.

Pain again attends the process of penetration of the chest wall, though it need not be severe. When the barrier of the ribs is overcome and the aneurysm projects on the surface of the chest, there is often relief, not only from the pain attending the pressure forward on the thoracic parietes, but from deep-seated pain.

A remarkable pain sometimes attends aneurysm in this situation, located in the tip of the right shoulder, and at the occipital insertion of the trapezius. When very severe, I have found the trapezius muscle in a state of spasm, and the head slightly rotated; but pain may be present when the muscular spasm is slight. Apparently the cause is reflex irritation of the spinal accessory nerve.

There is nothing specially remarkable about the pain

attending aneurysm of the transverse part of the arch, though it is often severe. It is when the descending part of the arch, or the thoracic aorta is the seat of aneurysm, that pain may be the sole symptom. The vessel is firmly held down to the vertebral column by the intercostal arteries; erosion of the bodies of the vertebræ takes place, and the intercostal nerves may be reached. Lancinating pain is then experienced of an extremely severe and persistent character before the aneurysm has reached a size which permits of its recognition by physical signs.

Thus far we have enumerated the general physical signs and symptoms to which aneurysm of the arch of the aorta may give rise. We shall now proceed to group these together around the various clinical types of aneurysm of which they are severally characteristic.

## Classification of Aneurysms of the Arch of the Aorta.

For clinical purposes we may divide aneurysms of the aorta into four groups, according to their anatomical situation—

(1) Aneurysm of the intra-pericardial portion of the aorta;

(2) Of the ascending aorta as far as the origin of the innominate;

(3) Of the transverse part of the arch;

(4) Of the descending part of the arch.

## (1) Aneurysm of the Intra-pericardial Portion of the Aorta.

The favourite site of an intra-pericardial aneurysm is one of the sinuses of Valsalva. As there are no adjacent structures to support the sac and contribute to its wall, it usually ruptures into the pericardium before it attains any considerable size. Should the aneurysm, however, extend towards the pulmonary artery or superior vena cava, its sac may become adherent to their wall, so that rupture is deferred for a time, eventually taking place, as a rule, into one of these vessels.

**Physical Signs and Symptoms.**—Angina pectoris may be present if the aneurysm involves the orifice of one of the coronary arteries, but frequently no physical signs or symptoms are present, and sudden death occurs from rupture of the aneurysm into the pericardium before any suspicion as to its presence has been aroused.

It may so happen that the sac of the aneurysm compresses the superior vena cava and obstructs the return of blood to the heart through this vessel, thus giving rise to characteristic symptoms.

An interesting instance of the latter condition occurred in a case under my care at St. Mary's Hospital in 1893. The patient, a man aged 30, was admitted suffering from shortness of breath and pain of an anginoid character. On examination, the heart was found to be hypertrophied, and there was evidence of aortic and mitral incompetence. The veins of the neck were distended and full, and it was noted that they did not empty on deep inspiration. This seemed to indicate that some tumour pressing on the superior vena cava, possibly aneurysm, was the cause of the obstruction to the return of blood to the heart. The liver was not enlarged, and there was no œdema of the extremities, so that it was clear there was no obstruction to the return of blood by the inferior vena cava. There was, however, no other definite evidence of aneurysm at the time of his admission, but on February 19th, a month later, he had an attack of severe pain in the region of the heart, and became very pale and almost pulseless; he rallied from this state of collapse, and in the evening vomited a little blood. Signs of pericardial effusion were present, and it was thought that a small rupture of the aneurysm into the pericardium had taken place.

He died four days later, becoming suddenly very pale and falling back dead in bed. At the autopsy the pericardium was found to be full of blood and recent clot, and there was also pale firm clot of older date due to the hæmorrhage four days before death.

There was a small aneurysm on the outer aspect of the aorta about one and a quarter inch above the valves, bulging into and partially embedded in the superior vena cava just below the point where it entered the pericardium. This had ruptured, and caused the sudden death.

## Rupture of an Aneurysm into the Pulmonary Artery.

A considerable number of cases of this incident have been recorded. In 1840 * Thurnam recorded five cases; in 1897 † Lamplough published a case which came under his observation, and gave a brief summary of fifteen cases which he had been able to collect, six of which had been published in the *Transactions of the Pathological Society*. In 1899 Sir William Gairdner published a case in the *Glasgow Hospital Reports*, and in 1900 ‡ Michell Clarke recorded a case. We have, therefore, although the condition is rare, a sufficient number of cases recorded for diagnostic data.

**Physical Signs and Symptoms.**—The immediate symptoms of rupture are, sudden pain in the chest with severe dyspnœa, followed by cough, sometimes with expectoration of blood-stained mucus. The attack does not, as a rule, prove rapidly fatal, but the patient may survive some weeks or several months, when definite physical signs and symptoms will usually develop. The earliest fatal termination in Lamplough's cases was in two weeks. The longest survival one year.

The most characteristic physical sign is a continuous roaring murmur, audible over the second and third left intercostal spaces. The murmur is loud and vibratory, its maximum intensity being systolic in time.

A vibratory thrill may sometimes be felt on palpation over the pulmonic area, and was present in 6 per cent. of Lamplough's cases. Pulsation is not present.

* *Trans. Med. Chi. Soc.*, vol. xxiii. p. 323.
† *B. M. J.*, 1897, vol. ii. p. 392.
‡ *B. M. J.*, 1900, vol. ii. p. 1701.

Subsequently, symptoms of dilatation of the right ventricle develop, and as this gives way, enlargement of the liver, tricuspid incompetence, and dropsy supervene, with engorgement of the lungs, and the patient dies with all the symptoms of right ventricle failure.

In a case recently under the care of Dr. Lees at St. Mary's Hospital, the patient was a man aged 49, who, ten months before admission, was suddenly seized with pain in the chest and severe dyspnœa. Three months after this attack, ascites and œdema of the legs set in. He was tapped for ascites seven times. On admission to St. Mary's Hospital, ten months after the onset of symptoms pointing to rupture of the aneurysm into the pulmonary artery, there was dyspnœa, slight cyanosis, dropsy, and ascites. Over the second and third intercostal spaces to the left of the sternum there was a well-marked vibratory thrill, but no actual pulsation. Over this area was a ceaseless, loud, roaring murmur, varying in intensity and most marked over the third left space. There was some hypertrophy of the left ventricle and great dilatation of the right. He died five weeks after admission. Post-mortem there was found to be a perforation in the aorta about half an inch in diameter, which opened into the pulmonary artery, obliterating one of the cusps of the pulmonic valve.

## Rupture of an Aneurysm into the Superior Vena Cava.

An interesting series of twenty-five cases, which they have collected from various sources, is recorded by Pepper and Griffiths.* Death frequently occurs in a few hours' time, but the patient may survive some months. The shortest period in which death occurred was six hours; the longest survival, seven months. One case is said to have recovered.

**Physical Signs and Symptoms.**—The immediate symptoms are sudden onset of severe dyspnœa, cyanosis, turgescence of the veins of the neck, rapidly followed by tense œdema of the neck and face. There is usually little or no actual pain. The dyspnœa, cyanosis, and œdema of the neck and face persist; distended veins make their appearance

* *American Journal of Medical Sciences*, 1890, vol. 100, p. 329.

on the front of the chest from collateral circulation established between the internal mammary and the intercostal and superficial epigastric veins. In course of time (from two to five weeks) a murmur develops, audible over the aortic area. The murmur may be systolic in time, or continuous, or a double murmur, systolic and diastolic, may be present. Pulsation over this area may make its appearance at a considerably later date, and is present in about 50 per cent. of cases. A thrill is felt in the majority of cases, but not in all.

The following case, which was under the care of Dr. Cheadle, at St. Mary's Hospital, in 1903, is of exceptional interest in that it was under observation from the onset of symptoms till death, some four months later, and a correct diagnosis was made on the day of admission.

Thomas M., aged 59, admitted to St. Mary's Hospital, March 28th, 1903.

*History.*—Was well till the evening before admission, when he suddenly, while in bed, became very short of breath and cyanosed. This was rapidly followed by swelling of the neck and face. There was no history of any previous symptoms pointing to aneurysm or affection of the heart.

*On admission* next morning he was very cyanosed and short of breath. The neck was swollen, brawny, and tense, somewhat resembling the condition of angina Ludovici, and did not pit on pressure. The face was also swollen, more especially the right side. The veins in the neck were full and distended. There was no pulsation visible, and no murmur was audible over the pulmonic area.

In the course of a week distended tortuous veins made their appearance on the front of the chest, and later all over the back above the scapulæ. The current of blood was downwards.

After three weeks a soft, blowing systolic murmur became audible over the aortic area, which gradually increased in intensity and became more prolonged. It remained soft and blowing and never became continuous, though the diastolic interval was very short.

A month after admission the œdema of the face and neck had, to a great extent, subsided, but the cyanosis persisted: the veins over the chest and back were very prominent, forming a diffuse network over the whole of the upper part of the front of the chest. The right internal jugular vein was thrombosed and filled with firm clot. The dyspnœa was less severe, and he was so much better that he insisted on going home.

He was readmitted three weeks later with severe dyspnœa, cyanosis, and œdema of the right arm and right side of the chest.

The murmur over the aortic area was louder and more prolonged. He became noisy and delirious at night, and his mental faculties were much impaired. Slight pulsation became evident over a localized area in the second right intercostal space. He died on May 10th, four and a half months after the onset of symptoms.

At the autopsy an aneurysm was found springing from the ascending aorta about one inch from its origin. The sac of the aneurysm was about three inches in diameter, and the pericardium was stretched over its upper aspect. There was a communication between the aneurysm and the superior vena cava about half an inch in diameter. The sac of the aneurysm was firmly united to the vena cava by adhesions, and there was no leakage into the pericardial cavity. The superior vena cava was greatly dilated, being nearly an inch in diameter, and its walls were greatly thickened. The right internal jugular vein was thrombosed, and occupied by firm adherent white clot. The left innominate vein was stretched over the front of the sac of the aneurysm, and its lumen was entirely obliterated. The right innominate and sub-clavian veins and the left sub-clavian and internal jugular veins were patent and free from clot. The azygos vein was greatly enlarged. The aorta was atheromatous.

## Rupture of an Aneurysm into the Auricles.

Cases are on record in which an aneurysm has ruptured into one of the auricles. In one case of rupture into the left auricle, described by King,* sudden dyspnœa, cough, and cyanosis supervened, and death took place in fifteen minutes. In another case, described by Ewart,† no symptoms were traceable to the perforation.

A case of rupture of an aneurysm into the right auricle is also recorded by Ewart,‡ and another by Norman Moore,§ in neither of which were any characteristic symptoms present.

## (2) Aneurysm of the Ascending Aorta beyond the Pericardium, or Aneurysm of Physical Signs.

Under this head are comprised aneurysms which involve the ascending aorta between the pericardium and the orifice

* *Transactions of the Pathological Society*, vol. 26, p. 37.
† *Ibid.*, vol. 31, p. 96.
‡ *Ibid.*, vol. 31, p. 95.
§ *Ibid.*, vol. 31, p. 82

of the innominate artery. As has already been stated, the name, "aneurysm of physical signs," has been given to aneurysms affecting this part of the aorta, since, from the nature of its anatomical relations, pressure symptoms do not readily arise, and frequently the first definite indication of the existence of an aneurysm is the appearance of an area of pulsation on the chest wall, usually in the second left

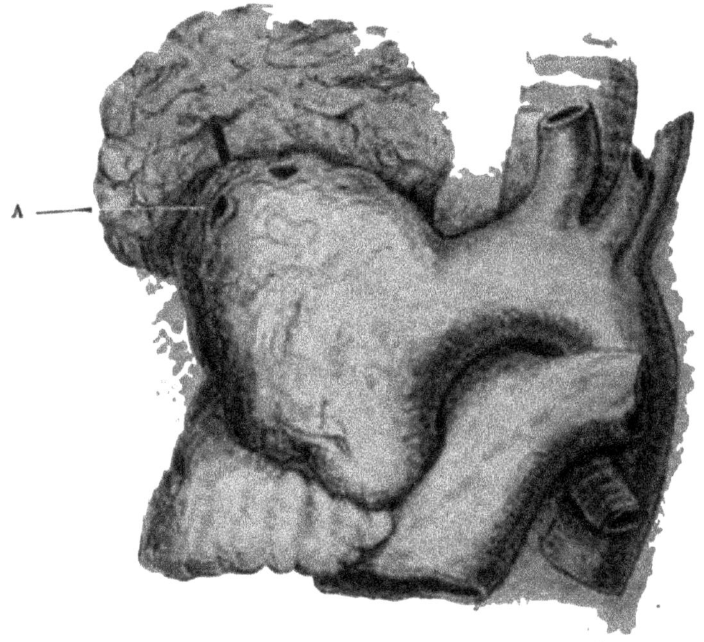


FIG. 36.—ANEURYSM OF ASCENDING AORTA WHICH RUPTURED INTO RIGHT PLEURAL CAVITY AT A.

intercostal space. Dulness or impaired resonance on percussion may be present before pulsation is visible, but dulness alone is not sufficient evidence of aneurysm, and pulsation may sometimes be recognizable in the second and third left intercostal spaces close to the sternum, when the aorta is dilated as in aortic incompetence. When pulsation is present, a diastolic shock may sometimes be felt on palpation over the tumour, and on auscultation the second sound is usually ringing in character and low pitched.

If the sac extends outwards, there will be evidence of

pressure on the superior vena cava, shown by distension and fulness of the veins on both sides of the neck; if it extends backwards, there may be symptoms of pressure on the root of the right lung.

Pain in the neighbourhood of the aneurysm is usually present in varying degree, being most severe, as a rule, when the tumour is being pressed up against the chest wall and is beginning to erode the ribs.

An aneurysm in this situation may attain very great size, sometimes being as large as a child's head. Usually it enlarges in the direction of the blood current, that is, towards the wall of the thorax, on reaching which it may erode the overlying ribs, and gradually force its way through them as they undergo atrophy from the pressure. It may rupture at any stage, sometimes into the right pleural cavity (vide Fig. 36).

It may also rupture into the lung, giving rise to hæmoptysis, which may be profuse and terminate fatally. If the perforation is small or at the base of a sacculus, it may become occluded by clot and the hæmorrhage be arrested, but attacks of hæmoptysis are liable to recur from time to time as the clot is dislodged. Sometimes the perforation is permanently closed by the development of adhesions. Frequently the lung tissue is compressed and adherent to the sac of the aneurysm, so that when a perforation occurs there may be little leakage at first. In one case, from which I put up a specimen for the St. Mary's Hospital Museum, there were no less than three separate perforations, and there was a history of recurrent attacks of hæmoptysis at intervals for over two years.

The patient was a man aged 59. The first attack of hæmoptysis occurred in December, 1900, the next in April, 1902, a third in September, a fourth in October, the patient dying in November, 1902. In the third attack 10 ozs., and in the fourth 20 ozs. of blood were coughed up. At the autopsy there was a large aneurysm involving the whole of the arch of the aorta, spreading out in a fan-like shape. There were two perforations on the outer aspect of the ascending part of the arch into the right lung, which were occluded by layers of laminated clot. The adjacent lung tissue was compressed, and adherent to the sac of the aneurysm over the bases of the perforations, which it helped to seal up. The perforations were about one-third of an inch in diameter. On the outer aspect of the descending portion of the arch was a third perforation into the left lung, which was engorged with blood, and it appeared that the recent attacks of hæmoptysis were due to leakage from this source.

Aneurysm of the ascending aorta is, however, compatible with life for a considerable number of years, as the cases appended will show.

Case 1.—Harriet H., aged 46, was admitted to St. Mary's Hospital in May, 1887, with the history that three years before she had noticed a small lump in the upper part of the right side of the chest. For a year previous to this she had felt pain in the chest of varying severity.

On admission, there was a small pulsating tumour about the size of a hen's egg just below the inner end of the clavicle immediately to the right of the manubrium.

The aneurysm had already made its way through the chest wall by erosion of the upper right costal cartilages, and was partially outside the thoracic cavity. There were some enlarged veins on the front of the chest wall, but the jugular veins were not markedly distended. There was no evidence of pressure on the air passages, or the recurrent laryngeal nerve. The second sound was accentuated and somewhat low pitched, but was not ringing in character or typical of aneurysm. After some weeks, she left the hospital, and was readmitted again in 1891, when the aneurysm had increased considerably in size, but she did not remain long in hospital. In September, 1892, she was again admitted. The aneurysm had then attained an enormous size, reaching upwards above the clavicle, and merging below the right mamma into a mass of dilated veins. The tumour was now firm and resistant, and the pulsation was scarcely perceptible, showing that a large amount of laminated clot had been deposited within the sac: there was no diastolic shock. The radial pulse on both sides was greatly modified, and the right was smaller than the left.

The jugulars on both sides were much distended, and did not empty on deep inspiration. The current of blood in the dilated veins was downwards, and they apparently anastomosed with the superficial epigastric and intercostal veins, showing that the vena cava superior was obstructed by pressure of the aneurysm, and that some of the blood normally returned by the superior vena cava was finding its way back to the heart by a devious route through the vena cava inferior. A photograph of this patient is given (Fig. 35).

The tumour measured 7 inches across, 9 inches long, and was about 19 inches in circumference.

She remained in hospital six months, and died at home eighteen months later. Unfortunately, an autopsy was not obtainable, but it was ascertained that she had not died suddenly; that is, from rupture of the aneurysm, but from some intercurrent pulmonary complication. She had thus survived nine or ten years from the first appearance of the aneurysm.

Case 2.—Lydia W., aged 40, first came under observation at St. Mary's Hospital about fifteen years ago. When first admitted, the aneurysm was so small that the diagnosis was difficult, more especially as she was also suffering from aortic incompetence in slight degree. Pulsation on the surface of the chest wall was not visible, but could be made out on firm palpation in the second and third right intercostal spaces. The aortic second sound was, however, low pitched and booming in character, and typical of aneurysm. While she was in hospital, the aneurysm steadily advanced, and pulsation soon became obvious. She suffered from pain and respiratory distress, and from attacks of palpitation and epistaxis. Treatment by pressure and iodide of potassium failed to arrest the progress of the aneurysm at this stage, and it was found necessary to keep her in hospital for eighteen months on account of the severity of the symptoms.

The aneurysm had greatly increased in size, and at the end of this period pulsation was visible in the second and third spaces as far out as the anterior axillary line with a corresponding increase of dulness on percussion. The administration of iodide of potassium, which had been discontinued, was now resumed in large doses, and consolidation rapidly took place. The tumour from being expansile became firm, showing evidence of the deposition of laminated clot on its inner surface. All her symptoms had greatly ameliorated, and she left comparatively well.

The reasons for this improvement, in spite of increase in the size of the aneurysm, seemed to be the following: When she came in, there was a small sac with a relatively large orifice communicating with the aorta, so that the current of blood swept through it, distending it more and more, and not allowing of the deposition of clot within the sac. When she left, conditions had changed; there was now a large sac with a relatively small mouth, so that the main current of blood rushed past the orifice instead of through the sac, and allowed of the formation of layers of laminated clot upon its walls.

She has come up to the hospital from time to time since, and when last seen, in 1905, she said she did not feel any special inconvenience from the aneurysm. There was then a pulsating tumour about the size of a hen's egg in the second and third right intercostal spaces, not projecting very much above the surface of the chest wall. A general heave was communicated to the chest wall around this area, and pulsation could be felt by deep palpation in the second and third spaces as far as the anterior axillary line, over which area there was dulness on percussion.

On palpation over the aneurysm, a well-marked diastolic shock was felt. The aortic second sound was low pitched and ringing, and a diastolic murmur was also audible.

There was no evidence of pressure on the superior vena cava, no difference in the pulses, no affection of the vocal cords. The pulse wave was forcible and sudden in character, but was sustained instead of collapsing, and presented the characters of the pulse of aortic incompetence scarcely modified by the aneurysm.

This is practically a case of cured aneurysm. The walls of the sac have become thick and strong from deposit of laminated clot within and chronic inflammatory changes without, and there is little chance of rupture. She has now survived fifteen years from the onset of the aneurysm, and seldom has any symptoms to remind her of its existence.

## (3) Aneurysm of the Transverse Part of the Arch. Aneurysm of Symptoms.

The name, aneurysm of symptoms, has been given to aneurysms affecting the transverse part of the arch because, as a rule, characteristic and important symptoms early arise which engender a suspicion of aneurysm some time before the physical signs are at all demonstrative of its existence.

Most of the symptoms which may arise have already been enumerated under the head of "Pressure Symptoms;" but, for the sake of clearness, it will be necessary to briefly discuss them here.

The symptoms will vary, and one or other of them will present themselves according as the aneurysm is situated in the convexity or concavity of the arch, or upon its anterior or posterior surface.

1. **Pressure on the Left Recurrent Laryngeal Nerve.**—

As this nerve winds round the aorta, an aneurysm on any aspect of the aortic arch may press upon it or stretch it, giving rise to characteristic symptoms.

One of these is the "cracked" voice, which is so peculiar as to be almost diagnostic.

Not infrequently the patient will come up to the throat department, or consult a throat specialist, complaining of hoarseness and alteration of voice; or, if he happens to have a cough, he may have also noticed that the sound made when he coughs has an altered, brassy character. There is not, as a rule, dyspnœa unless there is in addition pressure by the aneurysm on the trachea or one of the bronchi. On examination of the larynx, it will be found that these symptoms are due to paralysis of the left vocal cord.

The paralysis that results from pressure on the recurrent laryngeal nerve is that of the abductors of the larynx, so that the left vocal cord will be seen fixed and motionless in the median line in the position of phonation. This may be the first, and the only suspicious symptom of aneurysm, but it is very significant when present, as nothing except a tumour pressing on the recurrent nerve in some part of its course can give rise to one-sided laryngeal palsy, and of such tumours, by far the commonest is aneurysm. The right recurrent laryngeal nerve may be compressed by the sac of an aneurysm involving the innominate artery, as is illustrated in the second case described later on.

2. **Pressure on the Trachea, Œsophagus, and Thoracic Duct.**—Symptoms arising from pressure on these structures may be the earliest indications of an aneurysm on the posterior surface of the arch, or of a saccular aneurysm extending posteriorly.

Pressure on the trachea may give rise to slight dyspnœa, but this, as a rule, is only marked when there is in addition paralysis of one of the vocal cords. Auscultation of the lungs will show the modification of the breath sounds known as tracheal breathing. Rupture of the aneurysm into the trachea may occur as illustrated in Fig. 37, and give rise to profuse and fatal hæmoptysis.

The tracheal tug, already described, will as a rule be recognizable before the pressure gives rise to dyspnœa.

Pressure on the œsophagus will cause difficulty in swallowing, and it has happened ere now that adventurous persons seeking to ascertain the cause of some obscure œsophageal obstruction by passing a bougie, have unexpectedly done so by passing it through the sac of an aortic aneurysm. Many cases are on record of spontaneous rupture into the œsophagus with resulting profuse and fatal hæmatemesis.

Pressure on the thoracic duct gives rise to no very definite symptoms, but causes impairment of nutrition by obstructing the flow into the general circulation of lymph and products of digestion absorbed from the lacteals.

Pressure on the ciliospinal branch of the sympathetic may cause dilatation or contraction of the left pupil according as its fibres are irritated or destroyed.

3. **Pressure on the Root of the Left Lung.**—If the aneurysm is on the concavity of the arch, or the sac extends downwards, it may give rise to symptoms arising from pressure on the root of the left lung, already described above. The most marked of these will be diminished entry of air on the affected side.

**Difference between the Radial Pulses.**—Difference between the pulses is especially liable to occur in aneurysms involving this portion of the aortic arch, since the innominate or left sub-clavian may be given off from the sac or be compressed by it, or the sac may be interposed between the two vessels.

**Physical Signs. Pulsation.**—Usually some of the symptoms above described precede the appearance of pulsation on the chest wall. If the aneurysm is situated on the posterior aspect of the arch, visible pulsation may be absent throughout the course of the disease. More commonly, if the aneurysm attains any considerable size, it gives rise to an obscure general heave of the manubrium best appreciated by laying the palm of the hand on the part. When it

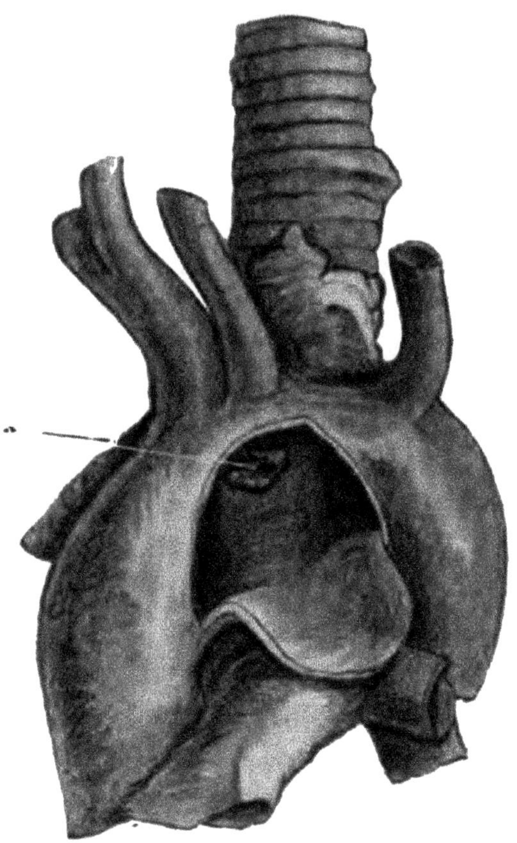

FIG. 37.—ANEURYSM OF THE TRANSVERSE PART OF THE ARCH WHICH RUPTURED INTO THE TRACHEA AT X. (FRONT VIEW.)

springs from the anterior aspect of the arch, the sac may present as a pulsating tumour in the second or third left intercostal space close to the margin of the sternum. Sometimes pulsation in the sac may be felt by pressing the finger down behind the sternal notch, before it is evident on the chest walls, but care must be taken not to mistake a dilated aorta for an aneurysm.

Dulness on percussion over the manubrium sterni, and immediately to the left of it, may often be made out before pulsation is visible, and when occurring in conjunction with some of the characteristic symptoms, is a valuable sign, though the possibility of its being due to enlarged glands or other mediastinal tumour, must be borne in mind.

On auscultation, tracheal breathing may sometimes be heard over the manubrium, conducted by an aneurysm in contact posteriorly with the trachea and anteriorly with the chest wall.

The aortic second sound may be reinforced, that is, may be louder and more distinct to the left of the manubrium than in the normal situation, and occasionally may be audible in the left supra-scapular space.

A systolic murmur is sometimes heard over the course of the aortic arch to the left of the manubrium, though no murmur is audible in the aortic area.

Course of the Disease.—An aneurysm in this situation on account of the important structures in immediate relation with it usually gives rise at an early stage to one or other of the symptoms enumerated above. It is only when it is situated on the upper and anterior aspect of the arch, and attains a considerable size, that physical signs such as dulness over the manubrium sterni, and to the left of it, or pulsation in the second left intercostal space may precede the appearance of symptoms. It never attains the great size sometimes seen in aneurysms of the ascending aorta, and usually proves fatal at a much earlier period.

If it is situated posteriorly and extends backwards, it may ulcerate through the trachea, and rupture into it when quite small, as seen in Figs. 37 and 38.

In this case the aneurysm was situated on the posterior aspect of the arch, and was only about the size of a plover's egg when it ruptured into the trachea.

It may ulcerate through and rupture into the left

bronchus or the œsophagus, or it may rupture into the left pleural cavity, left lung, or posterior mediastinum.

Death may occur from pulmonary complications caused by pressure on the trachea or root of left lung.

The two following cases illustrate the predominance of

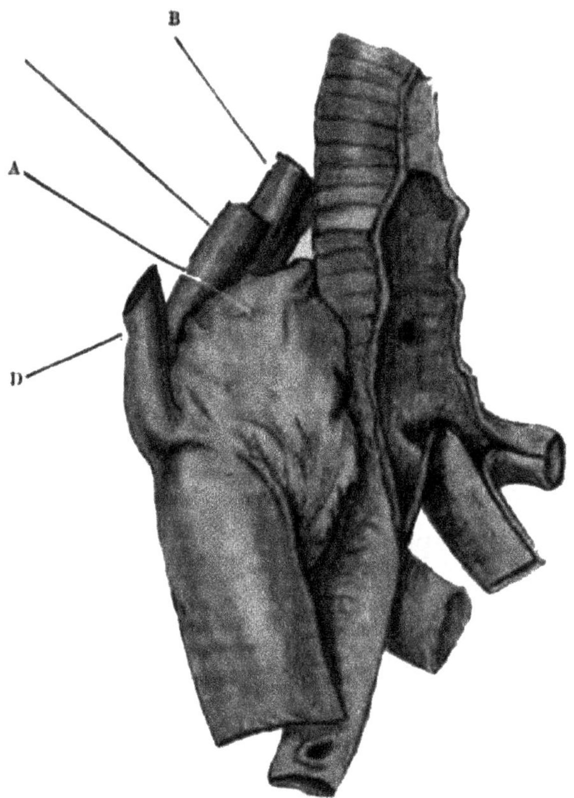


A. Sac of aneurysm; B. Innominate artery; C. Left carotid; D. Left sub-clavian.

FIG. 38.—ANEURYSM OF TRANSVERSE PART OF THE ARCH WHICH RUPTURED INTO THE TRACHEA. (SIDE VIEW, SHOWING SAC.)

symptoms over physical signs in the early stages of the disease, and the rapidity with which it may progress and cause death from pressure on the respiratory passages and other important structures. They are also especially interesting, clinically, from the number and variety of symptoms and physical signs which developed during the course of the disease. In the second of these two cases the right vocal cord was paralyzed, as the right sub-clavian artery was embedded in the sac of the aneurysm which had involved the orifice of the innominate artery.

Case 1.—The patient, a strong-looking, well-nourished man, aged 54, was admitted to St. Mary's Hospital in November, 1894, complaining of cough and shortness of breath; his lips were rather blue, and his face was congested. His chest was somewhat barrel-shaped, and the cardiac dulness was masked by emphysema: rhonchi were audible over both lungs. At first sight the case looked like one of simple emphysema and bronchitis. On careful observation it was noticed that the left external jugular vein was much more distended than the right, and did not empty on deep inspiration; the veins in the left arm were full and distended, and a large tortuous vein was also visible running across the front of the left shoulder, from the external jugular to the cephalic vein, in which the current of blood was downwards.

The carotid artery on the left side was difficult to see, and pulsation in it could scarcely be detected; in the right carotid pulsation could be seen and felt without difficulty.

The pupils were unequal in size, the left being larger than the right.

The left side of the chest was noticed not to move so well in respiration as the right, and on auscultation the entry of air was not so good. The percussion note was good on both sides. Tracheal breathing could be heard over the manubrium, and for a short distance on either side of it.

These indications seemed to point to a tumour which pressed on the trachea and left bronchus, compressed the left innominate vein hindering the return of blood through it to the heart, interfered with the flow of blood through the left carotid, and also stimulated a branch of the sympathetic, causing dilatation of the left pupil.

A tumour which would do this could scarcely be anything else than an aneurysm of the aorta. In support of this, it was found that there was marked tracheal tugging. There was, however, no difference in the radial pulses, no affection of the vocal cords, and there was no area of pulsation to be detected on the chest wall. At the end of five weeks, slight pulsation could be made out in the second left intercostal space at the end of expiration, and there was a small area of dulness to the left of the manubrium.

While the patient was under observation, the left pupil was seen to alter frequently in size, being sometimes smaller, sometimes larger than the right.

Rest and treatment failed to improve his condition, and on January 17th, seven weeks after admission, he had a severe attack of dyspnœa, sweating profusely, and becoming cyanosed. He was bled ten ounces from the arm, which relieved him considerably for a time.

Six days later he had another similar but more severe attack of dyspnœa, and this time inspiration was harsh and crowing, as if there was some laryngeal spasm, so that tracheotomy was contemplated, but was not deemed advisable. Venesection gave no relief, but inhalation of chloroform stopped the laryngeal stridor. He had several attacks of dyspnœa during the day, and became much exhausted. He died suddenly in the evening.

At the autopsy, an aneurysm about the size of a small cocoa-nut was found at the upper and posterior aspect of the transverse part of the arch where it crossed the trachea. The trachea at its bifurcation, and the left bronchus were compressed by the tumour, and the œsophagus was displaced to the left.

The left innominate vein was stretched over the sac, and its lumen was almost obliterated. A portion of the aneurysmal sac extended up behind the left common carotid artery, which was flattened and compressed by it.

The left sub-clavian artery was not involved in the aneurysm.

CASE 2.—Aneurysm affecting the anterior portion of the transverse part of the arch close to the origin of the innominate artery.

Samuel B——, age 27. This patient came to the Throat Department of St. Mary's Hospital complaining of hoarseness and attacks of difficulty in breathing. On examination of the larynx, it was found that the right vocal cord was paralyzed: aneurysm being suspected, he was sent up to the wards. On admission, his dyspnœa was very severe, his face was flushed and swollen, and when he was able to speak, his voice was noticed to be cracked and hoarse, and his inspiration was wheezing. He stated that he had been quite well till about six weeks previously, when he had a sudden attack of difficulty in breathing, which was considered to be croup and was treated as such. He also complained of a troublesome cough and difficulty in swallowing.

On inspection of the chest, on both sides large veins were seen over the front, in which the current of blood was downwards, carrying blood from the veins of the neck to the intercostal veins. The external jugulars on both sides were full and distended; and it was evident that the vena cava superior was occluded by pressure.

The pulse was absent in the right wrist, and in the right sub-clavian and carotid.

Examination of the chest showed dulness on percussion over the manubrium, and to the right and left of it for a short distance.

There was diffuse but faint pulsation over this region, best felt in expiration, and a loud ringing second sound was audible.

Over the front of the right lung there was absence of respiratory murmur and of vocal resonance, with normal resonance on percussion, a condition which was clearly due to pressure on the root of the lung. Posteriorly in the suprascapular region tubular breathing could be heard on both sides; over the bases the entry of air was good.

The pupils were unequal, the right being smaller than the left.

This was his condition on admission. He got gradually worse, in spite of rest in bed and treatment. Iodide of potash, ergot, and opium were administered; venesection was practised for the relief of pain, and was effectual at the time, but the relief only lasted two or three days. He died suddenly two months after admission.

At the autopsy an aneurysm the size of a large fist was found springing from the anterior wall of the arch, close to the origin of the innominate. The communication between the aneurysmal sac and the aorta was about the size of a shilling. The origin of the innominate artery was involved in the sac, and was not recognizable; the right sub-clavian was patent but small, it ran up the posterior wall of the sac, arising from it by a valvular opening. The right carotid contained a plug of coagulated fibrin, but there was a small passage by the side of the clot. The left carotid and sub-clavian came off beyond the sac and were not interfered with.

The vena cava superior was flattened out on the front of the sac, and was discoverable with difficulty, but it was not completely obliterated: the right innominate vein was quite destroyed; the left was flattened out, but the lumen was not entirely obliterated.

The trachea was compressed by the tumour, as were also the bronchi leading to the upper lobes of both lungs, more especially on the right side. The mucous membrane of the trachea was ulcerated. The oesophagus was also indirectly pressed upon, the trachea intervening between it and the sac. The right recurrent laryngeal nerve was compressed, and also the right vagus, which was involved in the adhesions round the aneurysmal sac.

Here the symptoms caused by the pressure effects of the aneurysm on the important structures surrounding it, occupied a more prominent position in the history of the case than the presence of abnormal pulsation on the chest wall, which was at no time well marked. The first symptoms were laryngeal, caused by pressure of the aneurysm on the right recurrent laryngeal nerve. The presence of the abnormal veins on the chest wall, and the absence of pulsation in the right carotid and radial vessels were striking features. The full jugulars, the distended veins on the front of the chest in which the current of blood was found to be downwards, pointed to some obstruction of the superior vena cava, and these phenomena, together with the paralysis of the right vocal cord, and disturbance of circulation in the right carotid and radial, would have been sufficient, even in the absence of pulsation on the chest wall, to enable one to come to a diagnosis of aneurysm.

## (4) Aneurysms of the Third or Descending Part of the Arch.

The descending aorta is deeply seated, lying to the left side of the bodies of the fourth and fifth dorsal vertebræ. The only important structures in immediate relation are the œsophagus and thoracic duct, which lie to the right of the aorta. Pressure symptoms are consequently not, as a rule, characteristic, and as the aneurysm rarely comes to the surface, physical signs are usually ill-marked. There may, however, be dysphagia from pressure on the œsophagus, and a not uncommon termination is rupture of the aneurysm into the œsophagus. Frequently the only symptom complained of is pain in the back, a pain radiating down the left arm or round the left side of the chest: there may be no other physical signs or symptoms present. The pain is due either to irritation of a spinal nerve, when it may radiate round the left side of the chest, or to erosion of the vertebræ, when smartly tapping the affected vertebra sometimes increases the pain. Diagnosis is in most cases a matter of considerable difficulty.

The aneurysmal sac may, however, enlarge in such a direction as to press on the root of the left lung and the recurrent laryngeal nerve. In one case, where the patient had been sent to the hospital for chronic laryngitis and attacks of paroxysmal dyspnœa, the left vocal cord was found to be paralyzed, and there were signs of pressure on the left bronchus, which seemed to point to aneurysm of the transverse part of the arch. At the autopsy, however, an aneurysm was found involving the aorta to the left of the bodies of the fourth and fifth dorsal vertebræ and adherent to them, and to the lower part of the body of the third dorsal vertebra.

In the accompanying illustration (Fig. 39), a large aneurysm of the descending aorta is shown, which compresses the œsophagus, and is adherent to the dorsal vertebræ from the fourth to the eighth.

## Diagnosis.

Little need be said here under this head, as the symptoms and physical signs characteristic of aneurysm have been fully discussed. It must, however, be borne in mind that a solid tumour in the mediastinum, such as a malignant growth, or enlarged mediastinal glands, may give rise to many of the pressure symptoms produced by aneurysm. Any mediastinal tumour may compress the great veins, the trachea, œsophagus, thoracic duct, the root of the lung, or may even involve the recurrent laryngeal nerve or sympathetic. In conjunction with symptoms produced by pressure on one or other of these structures, there may be an area of dulness over, and to one or both sides of the manubrium sterni. Pulsation will, as a rule, be absent, and there will not be the modification of the aortic second sound which is common in aneurysm. Cases may nevertheless occur in which pulsation is communicated from the arch of the aorta to a tumour intervening between it and the chest wall, and there is a diffuse general heave of the upper part of the thorax. If, on palpation, a diastolic shock is felt, all uncertainty will be at an end, as this could only be present in aneurysm.

On pressing the fingers down into the intercostal spaces a sense of resistance will be imparted by a solid tumour, and no true expansile pulsation will be felt. An aneurysm will sooner or later tend to present as a pulsatile swelling in one of the intercostal spaces, while the growth of a solid tumour will be indicated only by extension of dulness on percussion, without extension or localization of pulsation.

The history of the onset of the disease will be of service,

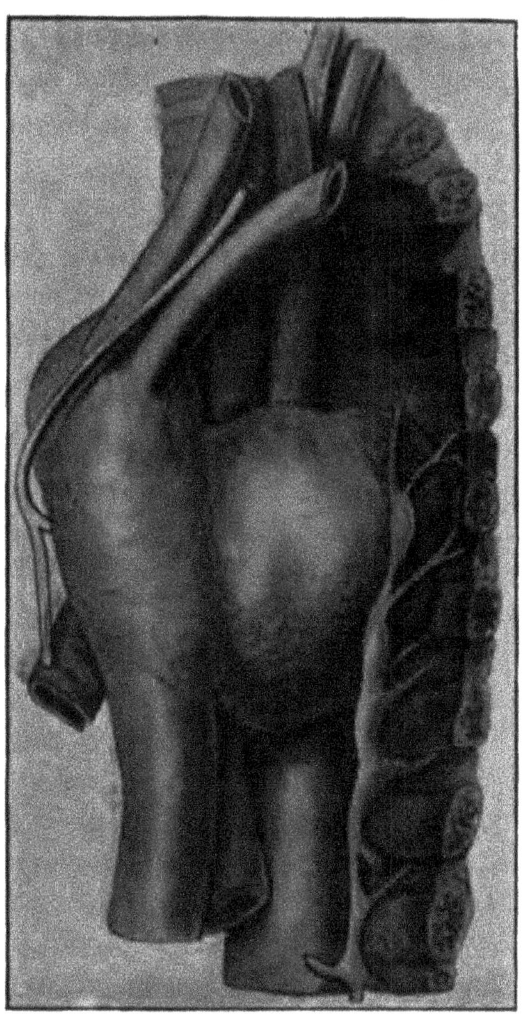

FIG. 39.—ANEURYSM OF DESCENDING AORTA.

and usually careful observation of the progress of the case will soon clear up all doubt.

It will be seen that a tumour in the mediastinum is most likely to be confused with aneurysm of the transverse part of the arch.

Aneurysm of the descending aorta may closely simulate spinal caries, when it compresses the spinal nerves and begins to erode the bodies of the vertebræ, and, as has already been stated, pain may be the only symptom to which it gives rise. The absence of rigidity of the spine will usually serve to exclude spinal caries, but the cause of the pain may be difficult to ascertain. If dysphagia is present in addition, this will be a help to diagnosis, but it may be impossible to diagnose with any certainty the existence of an aneurysm of the descending aorta, or that of an intra-pericardial aneurysm.

In doubtful cases an X-ray screen or photograph may be of great service.

## Prognosis.

The prognosis varies according to the situation of the aneurysm and the direction in which it extends, according to its shape, whether fusiform or sacculated, according as it increases rapidly or slowly in size.

When situated in the intra-pericardial portion of the aorta, it usually proves fatal by sudden rupture before it attains any considerable size. The vessel at this part lying free in the pericardial sac, there are no surrounding structures which the aneurysm can appropriate for its support, and there is also considerable up-and-down movement of the rest of the aorta. These conditions favour rapid extension and rupture of the aneurysm.

As the physical signs and symptoms are so indefinite, it is difficult to make an early or certain diagnosis, but where evidence points to the presence of an aneurysm in this situation, the condition of the patient is one of imminent danger, and little can be done to arrest the progress of the aneurysm.

When situated in the ascending portion of the arch above the pericardium, the aneurysm may attain an enormous size, and the patient live for some years without experiencing much inconvenience from it, especially if the aneurysm extends forwards, and makes its way through the chest wall. While the aneurysm is eroding the chest wall and making its way through, there may be considerable pain which will disappear later, but, the resistance offered by the chest wall in front being overcome, the pressure on deep-seated parts will be diminished.

If the aneurysm extends backwards, the prognosis is less favourable, as serious complications may arise from pressure on the root of the lung or the vena cava, or perhaps on the pneumogastric nerve.

When it involves the transverse portion of the arch, to the danger of the aneurysm *per se* must be added the danger of pressure effects on the important structures in its neighbourhood. Death may occur suddenly from rupture into the trachea or elsewhere, or, more slowly, from asphyxia and pulmonary collapse due to pressure on the trachea or on the root of one or other lung. If, however, the aneurysm extends forwards instead of backwards, and comes to the surface of the chest wall, the prognosis is less unfavourable.

With regard to the shape of the aneurysm, if it is of the sacculated variety, it may extend rapidly at first, and perhaps prove fatal by rupture at an early period; as it continues to enlarge, however, the mouth of the sac will become relatively small compared with the size of the tumour: thus less blood enters the sac, and the circulation in it is slowed. These conditions favour the deposition of fibrin, so that the progress of the aneurysm may be checked, or a spontaneous cure result. In fusiform aneurysm the progress of the aneurysm is usually slow; but little can be done to arrest it, as the blood sweeping through the whole of the sac gives little chance for the deposition of fibrin on its walls, and washes it away when deposited.

## TREATMENT.

In the treatment of aortic aneurysm the object to be attained is to keep down the blood pressure, to render the circulation as slow and equable as possible, to diminish the volume of blood, and to increase its coagulability. We shall thus reduce the strain on the walls of the aneurysm to a minimum, and favour the coagulation of blood in the sac. For this purpose the most important measure is *rest;* the patient should be kept in bed for six weeks or two months. It may be necessary to allow him to use a commode when the bowels act, as the straining attending the use of the bed pan may give rise to more effort than sitting up, but he should not get out of bed for any other purpose. Excitement of any kind must be avoided. Next in importance to rest is *feeding*. The amount of liquid taken with meals should be reduced to a minimum, 40 or, if practicable, 30 ounces only being taken in the 24 hours. Soups, game, salt fish, rich sauces, beer, and tea should be forbidden, and meat should be used in moderation, as extractives, rich foods, and excess of nitrogenous matter may lead to the retention of toxic materials in the blood, which give rise to increase in the peripheral resistance by their vaso-constrictor action. The food should not be bulky, that is, should not include too much farinaceous matter, such as potatoes, rice, etc.; the amount of food taken at each meal should be about the same, and should not be excessive, so as to avoid the extremes of repletion or depletion, and the varying rapidity of the circulation which would result were some meals copious and others small. The reduction of the volume of blood favours the repair of aneurysm in two ways—it lessens the distension of the entire vascular system, d therefore the internal pressure in the sac, and the rate flow of blood is diminished; further, the blood being ssated, fibrin is more readily deposited.

There is one drug which undoubtedly has a favourable influence on aneurysm, namely, iodide of potassium. This should be given in gradually increasing doses, till 20, 30, or 40 grains are taken three times a day. Its precise mode of action has been much discussed; chemically it has a solvent influence on fibrin, and cannot therefore be supposed to favour its precipitation on the wall of the sac; neither can the good effects of this drug in aneurysm be ascribed to its action on the aneurysm as a remote effect of syphilis. It is probable that it co-operates with the rest and diet, firstly, by its depressing influence on the action of the heart; secondly, by promoting diuresis, and thus helping to drain off water and inspissate the blood.

Aperients may have to be taken to obviate constipation, which would have a very injurious influence, and it may be necessary to counteract restlessness and assist sleep by bromides or opiates. Morphia may also be required for the relief of pain.

Sibson gave ergot in large doses in cases of aneurysm, and it could be easily demonstrated that the pulsation diminished in an aneurysm which had perforated the chest wall, and that its volume was lessened. This he attributed to the contraction of muscular fibres in the wall of the sac, but such fibres are non-existent. The cause was undoubtedly diminished output of blood by the left ventricle, due to limitation of its diastole by the ergot.

Venesection may be of the greatest service when there is severe pain. It usually affords immediate relief by lowering the tension within the aneurysm, and it may also so lessen the amount of blood in circulation as to afford a chance of fibrin being deposited. Surgery does not find much opportunity in the treatment of thoracic aneurysm, but ligature of the right sub-clavian and carotid arteries when the innominate is involved, or of the corresponding vessels on the left side when the origins of the left carotid and sub-clavian were implicated, has, in some instances, led to consolidation of the sac, by reducing the flow of blood through it. Other expedients have been tried, such as the introduction of coils of fine wire into the sac, passed in through a trocar, or the action of galvanic currents, with the object of the formation of a coagulum in the sac, but the results have not been encouraging. A risk sufficient in itself to prevent resource to either of these proceedings, except in an absolutely desperate case, is the possibility of a clot formed around the pole of a galvanic battery, or on the coils of wire, being carried into the carotid or vertebral arteries, and giving rise to a cerebral embolism.

Injections of a solution of gelatine into the buttock, with a view to increasing the coagulability of the blood and the tendency to clotting in the sac, have been practised, but the good results claimed in some cases are open to suspicion, and fatal cases of tetanus from imperfect sterilization of the gelatine employed have been recorded, so that this method of treatment is not to be recommended. Increase in coagulability of the blood can be more safely and efficiently effected by limitation of the amount of fluids, and by the administration of chloride or lactate of calcium in doses of from 10 to 15 grains two or three times a day. A milk diet may, to a certain extent, contribute to this object, as milk contains a considerable proportion of lime salts. It is also beneficial in that it contains no extractives or toxic materials, is non-stimulating, throws least work on the kidneys, and is slightly diuretic.

Satisfactory results from treatment can only be hoped r if the aneurysm is saccular, with a relatively small to the sac, so that the circulation in the sac is sluggand a chance is afforded for the deposition of fibrin s walls. The deposit of layers of laminated clot will support to the walls of the aneurysm, and help to nt its further extension, and will also tend gradually lude the blood from it by occluding the sac.

# INDEX.

## P



## R



## S



## T

THE END.

Lightning Source UK Ltd.
Milton Keynes UK
UKHW021900121118
332198UK00006B/146/P